65 Years On from Aflatoxin Discovery—a Themed Issue in Honor of Professor John D. Groopman

65 Years On from Aflatoxin Discovery—a Themed Issue in Honor of Professor John D. Groopman

Guest Editors

David L. Eaton
Thomas W. Kensler

MDPI

Basel • Beijing • Wuhan • Barcelona • Belgrade • Novi Sad • Cluj • Manchester

Guest Editors
David L. Eaton
Environmental &
Occupational Health Sciences
University of Washington
Seattle, WA
USA

Thomas W. Kensler
Departmental of
Environmental
Health Sciences
Johns Hopkins Bloomberg
School of Public Health
Baltimore, MD
USA

Editorial Office
MDPI AG
Grosspeteranlage 5
4052 Basel, Switzerland

This is a reprint of the Special Issue, published open access by the journal *Toxins* (ISSN 2072-6651), freely accessible at: https://www.mdpi.com/journal/toxins/special_issues/K456I1RH39.

For citation purposes, cite each article independently as indicated on the article page online and as indicated below:

Lastname, A.A.; Lastname, B.B. Article Title. *Journal Name* **Year**, *Volume Number*, Page Range.

ISBN 978-3-7258-7202-2 (Hbk)
ISBN 978-3-7258-7203-9 (PDF)
https://doi.org/10.3390/books978-3-7258-7203-9

Cover image courtesy of John D. Groopman

Contents

About the Editors

David L. Eaton

David L. Eaton received his PhD in Pharmacology and Toxicology from the Department of Pharmacology, Toxicology and Experimental Therapeutics at the University of Kansas Medical Center (KUMC) in 1978. He then joined the University of Washington (UW) faculty in 1979 as Assistant Professor in the Department of Environmental Health (School of Public Health). He spent his academic career of 40 years at the UW, in a variety of teaching, research and administrative positions.

Dr. Eaton has published ~130 peer-reviewed research papers, largely in toxicology-focused journals, and ~80 review articles, book chapters focused largely on toxicology education, and edited 5 books. His research focus was on the molecular processes that underlie how certain chemicals in the diet and environment, particularly aflatoxin B1, can cause cancer.

He served in numerous leadership roles, including the Society of Toxicology (Secretary, 1997–1998; President, 2001–2002); Chair of the Board of Scientific Councilors, National Toxicology Program (2019–2022), and ~two dozen National Academy of Sciences, Engineering and Medicine Committees. He has been Board Certified in General Toxicology by the American Board of Toxicology since 1981 and currently serves as the President of the Academy of Toxicological Sciences.

He was honored, awarded and recognized in toxicology numerous times, and his accomplishments include the Achievement Award, Society of Toxicology, 1993; Elected Fellow, American Association for the Advancement of Science (AAAS; 1995); elected Fellow, Academy of Toxicological Sciences (2000), Elected Member, National Academy of Medicine, (2011); the David Rall Medal for Outstanding Service to the National Academy of Medicine (2020); and the Merit Award (Lifetime Achievement Award) from the Society of Toxicology (2024).

Thomas W. Kensler

Thomas W. Kensler received his PhD in Toxicology from the Massachusetts Institute of Technology under the direction of Dr. Gerald Wogan in 1976. He completed a post-doctoral fellowship at the McArdle Cancer Research Institute in 1978. In 1980 he joined the faculty in the Department of Environmental Health Sciences at Johns Hopkins University. He remained at the Hopkins-Bloomberg School of Public Health in various faculty and administrative roles until 2010, when he moved to the University of Pittsburgh (while also maintaining an active collaborative role with colleagues at Johns Hopkins University). He moved to the Fred Hutchinson Cancer Research Center in 2017, where he remained active in research until his retirement in 2024.

Dr. Kensler was a prolific scientist, contributing nearly 400 peer-reviewed original research articles to the scientific literature, as well as 75+ book chapters and reviews. The primary focus of his research was on elucidation of the carcinogenic properties and public health impacts of aflatoxins, and on discovering new approaches to cancer chemoprevention through diet. He made many important contributions to our understanding of the role that diet plays in modifying oxidative stress via the 'antioxidant response pathway'.

His contributions to toxicology and cancer research have been broadly recognized through many awards and recognitions, including Honorary Professor, Qidong Liver Cancer Institute, Qidong, China; AACR-American Cancer Society Award for Research Excellence in Cancer Epidemiology and Prevention (2007); Society of Toxicology Translational Impact Award (2009); National Friendship Award, Beijing, People's Republic of China (2011); and NCI Outstanding Investigator Award (R35) (2015–2022).

Preface

This Reprint was developed in honor of the career contributions of Dr. John D. Groopman, for his lifelong contributions to our understanding of the carcinogenic properties of aflatoxin B1 (AFB), and the global public health consequences of dietary contamination of AFB. It features 8 reviews/original research articles related to the public health consequences of dietary AFB contamination, and emerging approaches to reducing the global impacts of AFB contamination of food and feed. It also includes an editorial overview of the reprint, and an obituary for Dr. Thomas W. Kensler, one of the editors of this reprint.

(Dr. Kensler died in a hiking accident in July 2024. Although he is not with us now to see the final results of this Special Edition, he made many contributions to this work. See the obituary for Dr. Kensler in this Special Issue).

David L. Eaton and Thomas W. Kensler
Guest Editors

toxins

MDPI

Editorial

Editorial: Introduction to the *Toxins* Special Edition Honoring Dr. John D. Groopman for His Contributions to the Field of Aflatoxin Carcinogenesis Research

David L. Eaton

Department of Environmental Occupational Health Sciences, School of Public Health, University of Washington, Seattle, WA 98195, USA; deaton@uw.edu

It is with both excitement and sorrow that I now write this brief introduction and overview to this Special Edition of Toxins. Excitement in honoring the tremendous, life-long contributions that my friend and colleague, Professor John D. Groopman, has made to our understanding of the important global public health impacts of the common dietary contaminant, aflatoxin B_1 (AFB_1)—one of the most potent human carcinogens ever identified. Sorrow, in that my co-editor and long-time friend and colleague, Dr. Thomas W. Kensler, is no longer with us to share the release of this momentous special edition of *Toxins* (please see the memorial article in this Special Issue titled: *Thomas W. Kensler (1948–2025): A Legend in Antioxidant Response Pathways and Aflatoxin Carcinogenesis Research)*.

When I was first asked if I would serve as editor of this Special Edition in honor of Dr. Groopman, I was both honored and enthusiastic to do so, but with one condition: that Dr. Kensler must also be invited as a co-editor so that he can share in the honor and effort needed to bring this to fruition. Tom enthusiastically agreed, and our journey began. Dr. Kensler was a career-long collaborator and friend of Dr. Groopman and contributed greatly to the field of aflatoxin research in his own right. Thus, this Special Issue also honors the lifelong contributions of Dr. Kensler to aflatoxin carcinogenesis research. The papers in this Special Issue have been published over the course of nearly two years of effort on the part of the multiple invited authors. The eight specific articles are divided into two main categories of aflatoxin research: the implications of aflatoxin contamination on public health and the evaluation of current and future approaches to mitigate the effects of aflatoxin contamination globally.

Part A: Public Health Significance of Aflatoxins: Recent Advances in the Toxicology and Epidemiology of Aflatoxins:

This volume begins with an introduction to the field of aflatoxin research, featuring a brief overview of the incredible contributions Dr. Groopman has made. Both Drs. Groopman and Kensler (and many other notable aflatoxin researchers) received their doctoral training in the laboratory of Dr. Gerald Wogan at MIT in the 1970s. Dr. Wogan basically 'founded' the field of aflatoxin toxicology, and his legacy lives on through the voluminous, productive research of Drs. Groopman, Kensler, and numerous other Wogan trainees, as well as their many successful students and post-docs, some of whom are co-authors on several of the papers in this Special Issue of Toxins. To put the field—and this Special Issue—in perspective, an introductory article, titled "65 Years on—Aflatoxin Biomarkers Blossoming: Whither Next", was written by the two co-editors (T.W. Kensler and D.L. Eaton) [1]. This article provides a brief overview of the remarkable scientific gains that have been made over the ~65 years since the initial reports of the fungal mycotoxins dubbed 'aflatoxins' (the name is derived from the fungal source (*Aspergillus flavus* toxins) and their fluorescing color under UV light (AFB1—blue, AFG1—green)), with an emphasis on the contributions of Dr. Groopman to our understanding of the global public health implications of dietary contaminations with AFB_1.

(1) Species differences in biotransformation of AFB_1.

There are widespread species differences in the hepatotoxic and carcinogenic effects of AFB1. The molecular basis for the toxicity differences between these species of AFB1 is discussed in detail in an article in this Special Issue [2]. Such differences are determined by genetic differences in hepatic cytochrome P450 (CYP)-mediated activation of AFB_1 to the AFB_1-8,9-*exo*-eoxide (AFBO) and especially genetic differences in the relative rate of detoxification of AFBO via hepatic glutathione S-transferase enzymes. For example, mice express a form of glutathione S-transferase (mGstA3-3) that has remarkably high affinity for AFBO and is expressed constitutively in the liver, making mice largely resistant to AFB_1-induced hepatocarcinogenesis, whereas human alpha class GSTs have no measurable detoxifying ability [3–7]. Rats have an orthologous alpha class form to mice with relatively high detoxifying activity toward AFBO, but it is not constitutively expressed in the liver, and thus rats are quite sensitive to the hepatotoxic and carcinogenic effects of AFB_1. Avians have a wide range of relative sensitivity to AFB1. Domestic turkeys are quite sensitive to the hepatic effects of AFB. Indeed, the initial discovery of aflatoxins was from an outbreak of liver disease in a turkey facility and dubbed 'Turkey X Disease' [1,8,9]. Hepatic CYP enzymes effectively activate AFB to AFBO, but an alpha-class GST with significant AFBO activity is not constitutively expressed in the liver of turkeys, similar to rats [10]. Fish, especially salmonids, are remarkably sensitive to the carcinogenic effects of AFB_1. A single 1 h exposure of rainbow trout embryos to 0.5 ppm AFB_1 produced liver tumors in 60% of exposed embryos 1 year later [11]. One reason for the extraordinary susceptibility of trout to AFB_1 is the absence of any GST with significant detoxifying activity toward AFBO and reduced DNA repair capacity [12].

(2) Epidemiology of Aflatoxin carcinogenesis in populations across the globe

The risk of AFB_1-induced hepatocellular carcinoma has been recognized for decades, especially in populations with endemic hepatitis B virus. Drs. Groopman, Kensler, and co-workers were among the first to establish highly sensitive and specific effects-related biomarkers of aflatoxin exposure, such as AFB-albumin adducts in the plasma and AFB-N7guanine adducts in urine [13]. Many of the early population-based epidemiologic studies of AFB_1 carcinogenesis occurred in Qidong Province [14]. It was within this highly exposed population that the potent interaction between HBV and AFB_1 was first demonstrated and where AFB_1-specific molecular biomarkers were developed by Groopman and Kensler [15–17]. Although public health interventions and altered agricultural practices have greatly reduced the AFB_1-associated cancer burden in China [18], AFB remains a significant public health concern in many other parts of the world. In this Special Issue, Dr. Katherine McGlynn and colleagues at the National Cancer Institute, along with Dr. Groopman, provide an overview of the global estimated exposures to dietary AFB using biomarker data [19]. Of substantial importance is the relatively recent identification of substantial exposures from maize (corn) products in Mexico and Central America, described in detail in this article.

(3) Unique and distinct mutational spectrum of aflatoxin B1 and sterigmatocystin

It has been known since the early days of aflatoxin research that the carcinogenic and hepatotoxic effects of AFB1 are the result of DNA damage and subsequent mutagenesis. Sterigmatocystin (ST), a structural analog of AFB_1 and a naturally occurring mycotoxin

 https://doi.org/10.3390/toxins18020097

produced by certain strains of *Aspergillus*, is significantly less extensively studied than AFB1. Although both molecules share the difuran moiety with a double bond, where metabolic activation occurs, they differ in the cyclopentanone ring structure area of AFB1 (ST contains a phenolic ring structure in place of cyclopentanone). In this Special Issue, the mutational spectra of metabolically activated AFB_1 and ST are compared using ultra-high-resolution DNA sequencing techniques [20]. Although the two molecules are both genotoxic, the mutational spectra of the two were quite different. AFB1 mutations were largely focused on G-->T transversions that escaped DNA repair, whereas ST generated fewer G-->T transversions. However, the mutational spectrum generated by activated ST was reflective of more extensive oxidative damage to DNA compared to AFB1. The authors speculate that the detailed mutational spectra for each compound might provide *"unique genomic fingerprints that could be future biomarkers aiding the fields of risk assessment and cancer prevention"*.

(4) Challenges with assessing the potential impact of dietary aflatoxin exposure on childhood development in under-resourced areas of the world

Although the primary public health focus on dietary aflatoxin exposures has focused on liver cancer and, in rare instances, liver toxicity, there are numerous suggestive studies of other adverse effects of aflatoxins, particularly in early life growth and development [21–24]. It is possible that subtle AFB_1-induced toxic effects on the liver, especially in malnourished children, could enhance the consequences of malnourishment, leading to decreased growth (stunting). In this Special Issue, this topic is reviewed in detail [24]. Although not a systematic review, the authors evaluated the study design and outcomes of 5 cross-sectional studies, 9 longitudinal studies, and two intervention trials focused on aflatoxin exposure and early childhood growth (stunting). All the studies used AFB_1-albumin adduct biomarkers to evaluate AFB_1 exposure. Although many of the studies found associations between AFB_1-albumin biomarkers and a common measure of stunting (low body height for age), the article discusses the many challenges to comparing such studies. The authors note that many previous reviews often find mixed associations but often lack a critical assessment of study design and little data on patterns of aflatoxin exposure. The paper provides an interesting discussion of the diverse patterns of aflatoxin exposure over time and how such patterns influence study design to address public health consequences of childhood aflatoxin exposure in under-resourced parts of the world.

Part B: Recent Approaches to Mitigation of Dietary Contamination of Aflatoxins:

The identification of aflatoxins as a significant public health concern in many parts of the world has led to the development of strategies to mitigate the potential adverse health impacts of aflatoxin contamination in food staples such as corn (maize) and peanuts. This requires an understanding of both the molecular biology of how aflatoxins are formed by *Aspergillus* spp. and a variety of host-specific factors that determine the extent of mold growth, both pre- and post-harvest.

Three articles in this Special Issue review the status of a wide variety of efforts to mitigate aflatoxin contamination.

(1) Review of approaches to reducing AFB_1 production, growth of *Aspergillus* on food crops, and modifying host resistance to aflatoxin contamination

In their comprehensive review, Guo et al. [25] examine the historical approaches that have been used to alter the growth of *Aspergillus* and/or aflatoxin production, genetic approaches to modifying host (crop) resistance to mold infection, and recent advances in genome editing for enhancing drought tolerance and increasing plant immune responses. The authors note in their conclusions, *"For decades, the research community has sought the*

https://doi.org/10.3390/toxins18020097

proverbial "Silver Bullet"—a single intervention that could reliably and consistently eliminate preharvest aflatoxin contamination. No individual solution is likely to succeed in isolation. Instead, durable progress will require coordinated, multi-component strategies that combine knowledge of host resistance and breeding, fungal biology, and environmental influences with modern tools such as CRISPR genome editing, biotechnology, nanotechnology, and improve forecasting and detection systems." [25].

(2) Approaches to decrease the bioavailability of aflatoxins in food and feed via administration of binding agents

In order to mitigate the risks to public health from dietary aflatoxin exposure, the Phillips laboratory and other investigators have been working for years to identify ways to reduce or eliminate aflatoxin absorption by binding to various clays, which, if effective, could be used *as* AFB_1 binders in feed and food. This could be beneficial for both public health prevention in areas where food contamination is unavoidable and for reducing the impacts of contaminated feed on livestock. In this Special Issue, the Phillips laboratory (Oladele et al. [26]) discusses recent results of studies on chlorophyll- and chlorophyllin-amended montmorillonite clays for the binding of AFB_1. Their data demonstrated that the green engineered clays significantly detoxified AFB_1 (86% to 100%) and provided complete protection at levels as low as 0.1%.

(3) New approaches to aflatoxin mitigation using artificial intelligence

Gamlath and Wu [27] look into the future and discuss how artificial intelligence, combined with the plethora of new genomics tools and biotechnologies, could be used to identify novel approaches to reducing the public health impacts of aflatoxin contamination. They include a discussion of how such new approaches need to be accommodated by regulatory frameworks throughout the world. Using a 'case study' of aflatoxin-contaminated corn, they propose a conceptual scenario to demonstrate how AI and biotechnology could be incorporated into the entire food supply chain to manage aflatoxin contamination.

Conflicts of Interest: The author declares no conflict of interest.

References

1. Kensler, T.W.; Eaton, D.L. 65 Years on-Aflatoxin Biomarkers Blossoming: Whither Next? *Toxins* **2024**, *16*, 496. [CrossRef]
2. Eaton, D.L.; Williams, D.E.; Coulombe, R.A. Species Differences in the Biotransformation of Aflatoxin B1: Primary Determinants of Relative Carcinogenic Potency in Different Species. *Toxins* **2025**, *17*, 30. [CrossRef]
3. Borroz, K.I.; Ramsdell, H.S.; Eaton, D.L. Mouse strain differences in glutathione S-transferase activity and aflatoxin B1 biotransformation. *Toxicol. Lett.* **1991**, *58*, 97–105. [CrossRef]
4. Eaton, D.L.; Bammler, T.K. Concise review of the glutathione S-transferases and their significance to toxicology. *Toxicol. Sci.* **1999**, *49*, 156–164. [CrossRef] [PubMed]
5. Hayes, J.D.; Judah, D.J.; Neal, G.E.; Nguyen, T. Molecular cloning and heterologous expression of a cDNA encoding a mouse glutathione S-transferase Yc subunit possessing high catalytic activity for aflatoxin B1-8,9-epoxide. *Biochem. J.* **1992**, *285*, 173–180. [CrossRef] [PubMed]
6. Ilic, Z.; Crawford, D.; Vakharia, D.; Egner, P.A.; Sell, S. Glutathione-S-transferase A3 knockout mice are sensitive to acute cytotoxic and genotoxic effects of aflatoxin B1. *Toxicol. Appl. Pharmacol.* **2010**, *242*, 241–246. [CrossRef]
7. Monroe, D.H.; Eaton, D.L. Effects of modulation of hepatic glutathione on biotransformation and covalent binding of aflatoxin B1 to DNA in the mouse. *Toxicol. Appl. Pharmacol.* **1988**, *94*, 118–127. [CrossRef] [PubMed]
8. Nesbitt, B.F.; O'Kelly, J.; Sargeant, K.; Sheridan, A.N.N. Aspergillus Flavus and Turkey X Disease. Toxic Metabolites of Aspergillus Flavus. *Nature* **1962**, *195*, 1062–1063. [CrossRef]
9. Van der Zijden, A.S.M.; Koelensmid, W.; Boldingh, J.; Barrett, C.B.; Ord, W.O.; Philip, J. Aspergillus Flavus and Turkey X Disease: Isolation in Crystalline Form of a Toxin Responsible for Turkey X-Disease. *Nature* **1962**, *195*, 1060–1062. [CrossRef]
10. Kim, J.E.; Bunderson, B.R.; Croasdell, A.; Reed, K.M.; Coulombe, R.A., Jr. Alpha-class glutathione S-transferases in wild turkeys (Meleagris gallopavo): Characterization and role in resistance to the carcinogenic mycotoxin aflatoxin B1. *PLoS ONE* **2013**, *8*, e60662. [CrossRef] [PubMed]

 https://doi.org/10.3390/toxins18020097

11. Croy, R.G.; Nixon, J.E.; Sinnhuber, R.O.; Wogan, G.N. Investigation of covalent aflatoxin B1-DNA adducts formed in vivo in rainbow trout (Salmo gairdneri) embryos and liver. *Carcinogenesis* **1980**, *1*, 903–909. [CrossRef]
12. Bailey, G.S.; Williams, D.E.; Hendricks, J.D. Fish models for environmental carcinogenesis: The rainbow trout. *Environ. Health Perspect.* **1996**, *104*, 5–21. [CrossRef]
13. Groopman, J.D.; DeMatos, P.; Egner, P.A.; Love-Hunt, A.; Kensler, T.W. Molecular dosimetry of urinary aflatoxin-N7-guanine and serum aflatoxin-albumin adducts predicts chemoprotection by 1,2-dithiole-3-thione in rats. *Carcinogenesis* **1992**, *13*, 101–106. [CrossRef] [PubMed]
14. Chen, J.G.; Zhu, Y.R.; Qian, G.S.; Wang, J.B.; Lu, J.H.; Kensler, T.W.; Jacobson, L.P.; Munoz, A.; Groopman, J.D. Fifty Years of Aflatoxin Research in Qidong, China: A Celebration of Team Science to Improve Public Health. *Toxins* **2025**, *17*, 79. [CrossRef] [PubMed]
15. Groopman, J.D.; Wild, C.P.; Hasler, J.; Junshi, C.; Wogan, G.N.; Kensler, T.W. Molecular epidemiology of aflatoxin exposures: Validation of aflatoxin-N7-guanine levels in urine as a biomarker in experimental rat models and humans. *Environ. Health Perspect.* **1993**, *99*, 107–113. [CrossRef]
16. Jackson, P.E.; Groopman, J.D. Aflatoxin and liver cancer. *Baillieres Best. Pract. Res. Clin. Gastroenterol.* **1999**, *13*, 545–555. [CrossRef] [PubMed]
17. Kensler, T.W.; Roebuck, B.D.; Wogan, G.N.; Groopman, J.D. Aflatoxin: A 50-year odyssey of mechanistic and translational toxicology. *Toxicol. Sci.* **2011**, *120*, S28–S48. [CrossRef]
18. Chen, J.G.; Kensler, T.W.; Zhu, J.; Zhu, Y.R.; Wang, J.B.; Lu, J.H.; Munoz, A.; Groopman, J.D. Profound primary prevention of liver cancer following a natural experiment in China: A 50-year perspective and public health implications. *Int. J. Cancer* **2024**, *156*, 756–763. [CrossRef] [PubMed]
19. Corleto, K.A.; Alvarez, C.S.; Ramirez-Zea, M.; Groopman, J.D.; McGlynn, K.A. Aflatoxin Exposure and Human Health with a Focus on Northern Latin America. *Toxins* **2026**, *18*, 58. [CrossRef] [PubMed]
20. Thongararm, P.; Chancharoen, M.; Suwanwong, N.; Ruchirawat, S.; Ruchirawat, M.; Fedeles, B.I.; Croy, R.G.; Essigmann, J.M. Structurally Similar Mycotoxins Aflatoxin B(1) and Sterigmatocystin Trigger Different and Distinctive High-Resolution Mutational Spectra in Mammalian Cells. *Toxins* **2025**, *17*, 112. [CrossRef]
21. Khlangwiset, P.; Shephard, G.S.; Wu, F. Aflatoxins and growth impairment: A review. *Crit. Rev. Toxicol.* **2011**, *41*, 740–755. [CrossRef] [PubMed]
22. Smith, L.E.; Prendergast, A.J.; Turner, P.C.; Mbuya, M.N.; Mutasa, K.; Kembo, G.; Stoltzfus, R.J.; Sanitation Hygiene Infant Nutrition Efficacy Trial Team. The Potential Role of Mycotoxins as a Contributor to Stunting in the SHINE Trial. *Clin. Infect. Dis.* **2015**, *61*, S733–S737. [CrossRef]
23. Phillips, E.; Ngure, F.; Smith, L.E.; Makule, E.; Turner, P.C.; Nelson, R.; Kimanya, M.; Stoltzfus, R.; Kassim, N. Protocol for the trial to establish a causal linkage between mycotoxin exposure and child stunting: A cluster randomized trial. *BMC Public Health* **2020**, *20*, 598. [CrossRef]
24. Turner, P.C.; Phillips, E. The Difficulties in Demonstrating That Aflatoxin Reduction Improves Stunting in Developing World Regions. *Toxins* **2026**, *18*, 32. [CrossRef]
25. Guo, B.; Foka, I.C.K.; Wu, D.; Clevenger, J.P.; Di, R.; Fountain, J.C. Fifty Years and Counting: Searching for the "Silver Bullet" or the "Silver Shotgun" to Mitigate Preharvest Aflatoxin Contamination. *Toxins* **2025**, *17*, 596. [CrossRef] [PubMed]
26. Oladele, J.O.; Xenophontos, X.; Elizondo, G.M., 3rd; Daasari, Y.; Wang, M.; Tamamis, P.; Johnson, N.M.; Phillips, T.D. Green-Engineered Montmorillonite Clays for the Adsorption, Detoxification, and Mitigation of Aflatoxin B1 Toxicity. *Toxins* **2025**, *17*, 131. [CrossRef]
27. Gamlath, C.J.; Wu, F. AI and Biotechnology to Combat Aflatoxins: Future Directions for Modern Technologies in Reducing Aflatoxin Risk. *Toxins* **2025**, *17*, 524. [CrossRef] [PubMed]

 https://doi.org/10.3390/toxins18020097

toxins

MDPI

Review

65 Years on—Aflatoxin Biomarkers Blossoming: Whither Next?

Thomas W. Kensler [1,*] and David L. Eaton [2,*]

1 Department of Environmental Health and Engineering, Johns Hopkins Bloomberg School of Public Health, Baltimore, MD 21205, USA
2 Department of Environmental and Occupational Health Sciences, School of Public Health, University of Washington, Seattle, WA 98195, USA
* Correspondence: tkensle1@jhu.edu (T.W.K.); deaton@uw.edu (D.L.E.)

Abstract: Aflatoxins are mycotoxins produced by *Aspergillus flavus* and several other related organisms and are common contaminants of numerous grains and nuts, especially maize (corn) and peanuts. Although, undoubtedly, aflatoxins have been present in the food of humans for millennia, their toxic effects were not discovered until 1960, first becoming evident as a non-infectious outbreak of poisoning of turkeys (Turkey X disease) arising from contaminated groundnut meal. The elucidation of specific chemical structures in 1963 led to the rapid characterization of aflatoxins as among the most potent chemical carcinogens of natural origin ever discovered. As a frontispiece to the Special Issue "65 Years on from Aflatoxin Discovery—A Themed Issue in Honor of Professor John D. Groopman", we highlight many of Professor Groopman's important contributions utilizing urinary (aflatoxin–N^7–guanine) and, especially, serum (aflatoxin–albumin adducts) biomarkers; this work focused on over 40+ years of the development of analytical methods to measure biomarkers of aflatoxin exposure and their application in experimental and clinical studies. Collectively, this work serves as a template for using chemical-specific biomarkers as key tools to probe 'exposure–disease relationships'—in this instance, dietary aflatoxins and liver cancer. New approaches to measuring carcinogen biomarkers will build upon this 'aflatoxin paradigm' to inform the public health implications of diverse exposures around the world.

Keywords: aflatoxin B_1; aflatoxin–N^7–guanine; aflatoxin–albumin adduct; biomarkers; validation; exposome; liver cancer

Key Contribution: This manuscript highlights the important role of analytically rigorous, well-validated biomarkers to establish 'exposure–disease relationships' in at-risk populations. The work of Professor John D. Groopman using aflatoxin–albumin adducts in populations at risk for exposures to dietary aflatoxins and the development of liver cancer serves as a prototypic paradigm for the development and implementation of such studies.

1. Introduction

Aflatoxins derive their name from their fungal origin: *Aspergillus flavus* toxin. Although these mycotoxins have undoubtedly been around for millennia, they were not discovered until ~1960, when an outbreak of hepatotoxicity killed over 100,000 turkeys in England, dubbed 'Turkey X disease [1–3]. The origin of the poisonings was traced to Brazilian groundnut meal ("Rosetta meal"), and, from there, the *Aspergillus flavus* mold was identified as the likely culprit. Soon after, the toxic effects of the Brazilian groundnut meal were confirmed in numerous other species, including ducklings, chicken, young pheasants, cattle, rats, and pigs. Necropsies of some of the animals identified the liver as the primary organ of toxicity, including evidence of liver cancer development (see [2,4] for excellent reviews of the history of aflatoxin discovery).

The characterization of the toxic entity produced by *A. flavus* was described in 1962. The initial extract had a blue fluorescence—thus, the moniker "Aflatoxin B". A second material separated by thin-layer chromatography had a green fluorescence—thus, the moniker for aflatoxin G [5]. Subsequent work identified the structures of both aflatoxin B and aflatoxin G in 1963 [6,7].

The outbreak of poisonings among turkeys was characteristic of the acute or sub-acute toxicity of aflatoxin, with typical histopathological findings that include enlarged and mottled livers with periportal necrosis, hemorrhaging, and the accumulation of fat [8]. The acute/sub-acute toxicity of aflatoxins is relatively high (<20 mg/kg) in most vertebrate species tested but can vary substantially among species. Ducks, trout, and rabbits tend to be the most sensitive, with LD_{50} values less than 1 mg/kg, whereas the chicken and Porton rat exhibit the highest LD_{50} of ~18 mg/kg [4]. Acute toxicity, however, is not a good predictor of relative species sensitivity to the carcinogenic effects of aflatoxin, as discussed in more detail in the papers in this Special Issue.

Although the evident toxic effects of *A. flavus*-contaminated diets were largely associated with acute and sub-acute hepatotoxicity, the discovery of the potent carcinogenic effects of aflatoxin B_1 [AFB_1] followed quickly. The first reports of the evidence of the carcinogenicity of the toxic components of groundnut meal was reported in 1961 [9]. In 1958–1959, liver tumors were identified in guinea pigs given a 'routine', standardized Medical Research Council (MRC) diet containing 15% groundnut meal. However, the etiologic factor(s) in the diet that caused the liver tumors was unknown. In 1960–1961, 'Turkey X disease' stimulated numerous studies to identify the causal agents within the groundnut meal. The association between the groundnut meal that caused Turkey X disease and the fact that groundnut meal was a constituent in the guinea pig diet led Schoental [9] to deduce that fungal contaminants in the groundnut meal were carcinogenic. Several subsequent experimental studies demonstrated the potent hepatocarcinogenic effects of the major isolate, AFB_1 [10–12]. Barnes and Butler [11] carried out what was perhaps the first 'controlled study' in rats of aflatoxin carcinogenesis. The availability of reasonably pure AFB_1 was limiting for such studies. A summary of the study illustrates well the challenges of conducting such studies: "*Thus 3/3 rats receiving a diet containing 1·75 p.p.m. aflatoxin for 89 days ultimately developed liver cancer after a further 300 or more days on a diet that produces no liver changes in control rats. The rats ate on average 16 g of the food containing aflatoxin each day, so that it is possible to calculate that the carcinogenic dose of aflatoxin for rats is certainly not greater than 2·5 mg per rat*". Although the sample size was small and the duration of exposure was limited, this study clearly illustrated the strong hepatocarcinogenic potential of AFB_1. Another study with ducks reported in 1965 [13] also demonstrated the potent hepatotoxic and hepatoxic carcinogenic effects of AFB_1 in groundnut meal.

In 1967, Gerald Wogan and Paul Newberne at MIT conducted the first controlled, dose–response study of AFB_1 administered in the diet for up to 80 weeks in rats [14]. Although previous studies had demonstrated the potential toxicity and hepatocarcinogenic effects of extracts of *A. flavus*-contaminated groundnut meal [12,15,16], this was the first study that directly utilized purified AFB_1 with relatively long-term exposures of 60–80 weeks. Multiple different studies and design protocols were used, with several to assess acute as well as chronic toxicity. Perhaps the most informative study involved the administration of 15, 300, or 1000 ppb AFB_1 daily for 60 weeks or longer. The study demonstrated the remarkable potency of AFB_1 following prolonged feeding to both male and female Fischer rats. Even at the lowest dose of 15 ppb in the diet, 100% of both male (12/12 at 68 weeks) and female (13/13 at 80 weeks) rats had developed hepatocellular carcinomas.

Based on the remarkable potency of AFB_1 from this initial study, Wogan et al. [17], in 1974, conducted a lifetime carcinogenicity study using male Fischer rats fed with five different doses incorporated into the diet, ranging from 1 to 100 ppm, plus a control group. The results are shown in Figure 1.

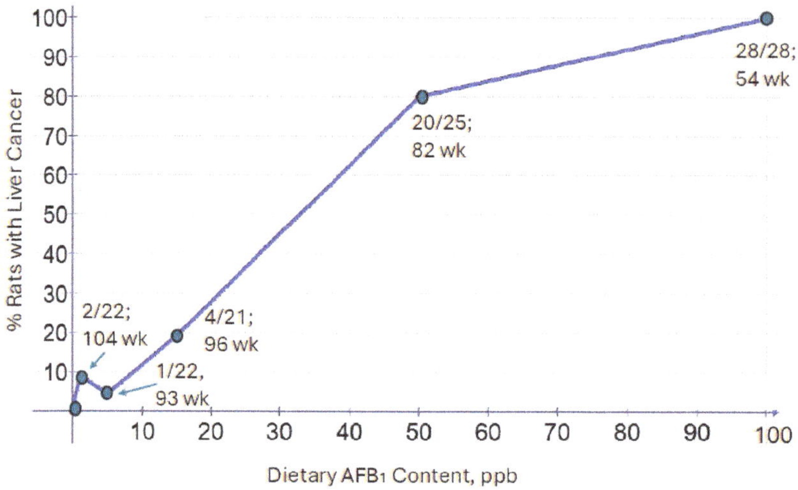

Figure 1. Dose–response relationship between AFB_1 dose and malignant liver tumors in male rats. The numbers of animals with tumors out of the total number of animals is shown for each dose point. Also shown are the first 'time to tumor' data for each dose point. See Wogan et al., 1974 for details [17].

As with the initial study, there were some suggestions that a dose as low as 1 ppb in the diet was sufficient to induce hepatocellular carcinomas (HCCs) when given over the lifetime of the animals. All 28 rats given 100 ppb developed HCCs, with the first carcinoma-related fatality occurring at 54 weeks at that dose. At a concentration of only 15 ppb, which is below the current FDA action limit (20 ppb) for aflatoxin (the sum of the B- and G-series) in food in the U.S., nearly 20% of the animals developed liver cancer by the end of the two-year study. Based on these results, and numerous other studies in other species, aflatoxin appears to be the most potent genotoxic carcinogen of natural origin ever identified. The molecule referred to commonly as 'dioxin' (2,3,7,8-tetrachlorodibenzo-p-dioxin; TCDD) has a TD50 (see the Lhasa Carcinogen Potency Database, that also includes TD50 data from the Ames and Gold Carcinogen Database: https://lcdb.lhasacloud.org/study-information/44411599 accessed on 11 November 2024)) (estimated dose where 50% of exposed animals would develop cancer) about 15-times lower (more potent) than that for AFB_1 (0.00014 μg/kg-d for TCDD, versus 0.0020 μg/kg-d for AFB_1, using the Ames and Gold Carcinogen Potency Database). The mode of action for the hepatocarcinogenic effects of TCDD is via a receptor-mediated enhancement of a signaling pathway (Aryl hydrocarbon Receptor, or AhR) that promotes tumorigenesis, rather than genotoxic events that initiate carcinogenesis. A more appropriate comparison of carcinogenic potency would be with the nitrosamine, N-nitroso-dimethylamine (NDMA). Like AFB_1, NDMA is a potent genotoxic hepatocarcinogen. The TD50 for NDMA in rats is 0.09 μg/kg-d, or about 45-times less potent than AFB_1. The FDA acceptable intake for pharmaceuticals contaminated with NDMA is 96 ng. Using the TD50 values for a relative potency comparison, that would equate to an acceptable daily intake of AFB_1 of about 2 ng. If a commodity (say, corn or peanuts) is contaminated with AFB_1 at 15 ppb (15 μg/kg), which is below the FDA action level of 20 ppb, a one ounce (28 g) serving would contain 420 ng of AFB_1, which is more than 200-times the potential carcinogenic dose of a pharmaceutical containing the FDA allowable limit of NDMA. Of course, this exercise assumes that the potency for both NDMA and AFB_1 determined in rats is similar in humans. As discussed in detail by Eaton et al. in this series, there are important differences among species in how AFB_1 is metabolized that largely determine the relative carcinogenic potency across species. There are also important species differences in the carcinogenicity of NDMA between humans and rats [18]. The point here is that it was known in the 1960s that AFB_1 was a very potent carcinogen in several species and, thus, human studies were of paramount importance to determining the public health significance of dietary contamination with AFB_1. One of the biggest challenges in designing such epidemiology studies is assessing the extent of exposure, or dose. The use of biological markers (biomarkers) has thus played a critical role in the design and conducting of many epidemiology studies over the past 4+ decades that have established AFB_1 as a potent human liver carcinogen. The contributions of Professor John Groopman in the development of biomarkers of AFB_1 exposure were essential for these studies.

2. Identification and Development of Aflatoxin Biomarkers of Internal Dose and Effective Dose

Urinary Aflatoxin Metabolites: As discussed in a review elsewhere in this Special Issue (Eaton et al.), the metabolism of AFB_1 has been well-characterized in multiple species including humans. Figure 2 summarizes the oxidative, conjugation, and adduct products of AFB_1 metabolism that have been used as biomarkers of the internal dose and, sometimes, early biological effect. In some instances, they can be quantitatively linked to estimates of dietary exposure.

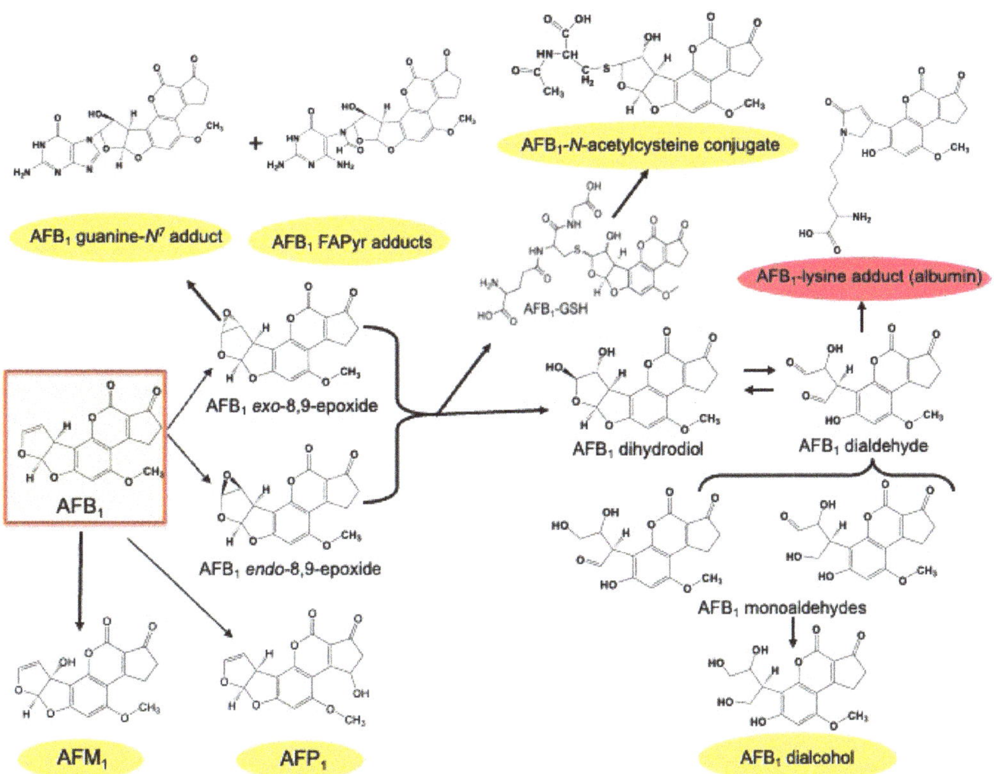

Figure 2. AFB_1 metabolites used as biomarkers from biofluids. Various cytochromes, P450, form oxidative metabolites, of varying toxicity. AFB-8,9-oxide is highly toxic and responsible for most, if not all, of the toxic and carcinogenic effects of AFB_1. However, it can be detoxified by conjugation with glutathione, via specific glutathione S-transferases. Formation of DNA and protein adducts provide stable urinary and serum biomarkers of exposure with biological half-lives of ~8 h and ~30 days, respectively. Yellow: urine; red: serum or plasma.

Several metabolites, notably, aflatoxin M_1 (AFM_1) along with aflatoxin-8,9-epoxide-derived adducts with DNA, RNA, and protein, were used for the initial monitoring of human exposures. These studies used urine as the biospecimen source due its role as a major portal for excretion, the ease of collection, and the simplicity of processing for analyses. However, the short whole-body half-lives of these metabolites, coupled with typically heterogenous exposures, renders evaluations of the associations of individual levels with the risk of disease challenging. Studies of aflatoxin biomarkers in human populations began in the Philippines, where investigators first demonstrated that an oxidative metabolite of AFB_1, AFM_1, could be measured in urine as an internal dose marker for people consuming aflatoxin-contaminated peanut butter [19]. Studies in two areas with a high incidence of liver cancer, the People's Republic of China and The Gambia, West Africa, reported that urinary levels of oxidative aflatoxin metabolites followed a dose-dependent relationship with aflatoxin ingestion for AFM_1 but not for aflatoxin P_1 (AFP_1), another oxidative metabolite [20]. From initial measures using thin-layer chromatography and fluorescence detection to the use of immunoaffinity antibodies for sample enrichment coupled with high-performance liquid chromatography with spectrometric or fluorescence detectors to mass spectrometry, the methods for quantitating urinary biomarkers have improved vastly the sensitivity and specificity of such measures. Professor John Groopman contributed greatly to these advancements [20–26] (Figure 3, panels B, C, E, and F).

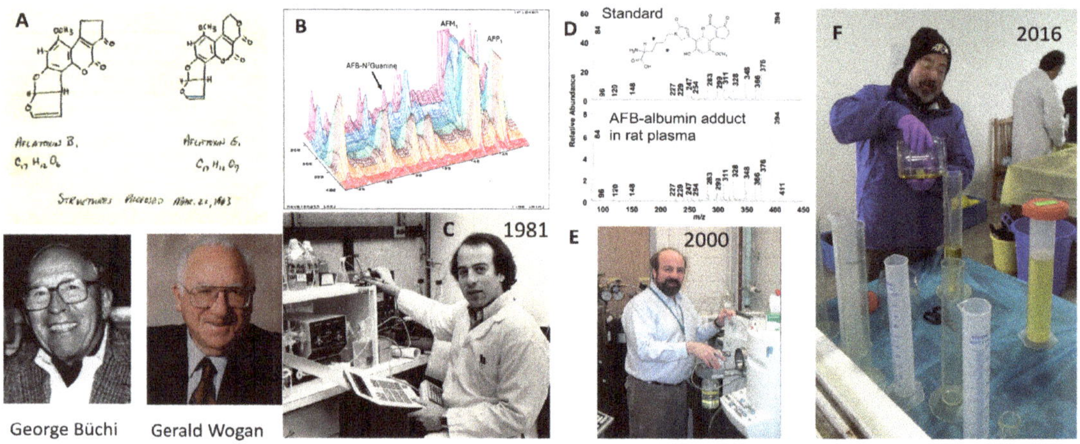

Figure 3. Pioneers of AFB_1 discovery and biomarker development. (**A**) Proposed structures of AFB_1 and AFG_1 by George Büchi on 22 March 1963 and reported later that year by Büchi, Wogan and colleagues [6]. Professor Gerald Wogan was the doctoral mentor for Prof. Groopman. Courtesy of Prof John Essigmann, MIT. (**B**) Initial chromatography of aflatoxin–N^7–guanine by HPLC and photodiode array detection in human urine in 1987 by Groopman. (**C**) Dr Groopman with his first HPLC (1981). Courtesy of Prof. John Groopman. (**D**) Mass spectrometry of aflatoxin–lysine adduct standard and in rat serum. * Indicates position of stable isotope labels for internal standard. (**E**) John Groopman with his first mass spectrometer for biomarker quantification, a Thermo LCQ (2000). Photo courtesy of Thomas Kensler. (**F**) John Groopman measuring volumes of urine in samples collected during molecular epidemiology studies and chemoprevention clinical trials in Qidong, China, an endemic area for aflatoxin exposure, with a high incidence of liver cancer (2016). Photo courtesy of Thomas Kensler.

While oxidative metabolites reflect the internal dose, aflatoxin–DNA adducts excreted in urine following either spontaneous depurination or excision repair offer direct insights into the ultimately carcinogenic dose, given the potent genotoxicity of aflatoxin–DNA damage products that are critical to the carcinogenic properties of AFB_1. The ultimate carcinogenic form of AFB_1, the 8,9-epoxide (originally termed the 2,3-oxide), was described in the mid-1970s [27] and determined to mediate the formation of the principal AFB_1–DNA adduct formed in vivo in rat liver [28–30] and later found to be excreted in rat urine as well [31]. Validation studies in rats reported a linear relationship between AFB_1 dose and the excretion of the aflatoxin–N^7–guanine adduct in urine over the initial 24 h period [32]. Subsequent biomonitoring studies in The Gambia and The Peoples' Republic of China demonstrated the feasibility of measuring this DNA damage biomarker in urine from humans exposed to aflatoxins and further characterized its kinetic features [33,34]. While the classic dose–response is a critical element for biomarker performance, the modulation of internal dose, in addition to the external or administered dose, is a valuable tool for validation. Chemopreventive interventions that reduce the absorption of AFB_1 from the gastrointestinal tract (e.g., chlorophyllin) or alter hepatic metabolism to block epoxide formation or enhance its detoxication through conjugation with glutathione (e.g., ethoxyquin, oltipraz, and 2-cyano-3,12-dioxooleana-1,9(11)-dien-28-imidazolide [CDDO-Im]) confirm this element of biomarker modulability. In rats, the decreased formation of aflatoxin–N^7–guanine adducts in liver are associated with a reduction in tumor burden following chemopreventive interventions with the agents ethoxyquin, oltipraz, and CDDO-Im [35–37].

Chlorophyllin, a water-soluble derivative of chlorophyll, inhibits liver cancer development in aflatoxin-treated trout [38], wherein the primary mode of action is thought to be the sequestration of aflatoxin by chlorophyllin by forming a non-covalent complex in a 1:1 stacking ratio [39]. In 1997, a randomized, double-blind, placebo-controlled chemoprevention trial with chlorophyllin was conducted in Qidong, China. The ingestion of chlorophyllin tablets (100 mg) at each meal led to an overall 55% reduction in median urinary levels of aflatoxin–N^7–guanine adducts collected 3 months into the intervention compared with those subjects taking a placebo [40]. An earlier clinical trial in this aflatoxin-endemic area with oltipraz led to the diminished excretion of AFM_1 and increased excretion of aflatoxin–*N*–acetylcysteine in urine [41], suggesting a likely reduction of DNA damage in the individuals receiving the repurposed drug compared to a placebo.

Serum Aflatoxin–Albumin Adducts: Day-to-day aflatoxin exposure through the diet can be very heterogeneous, reflecting the varied contamination within dietary staples such as ground nuts, maize, and grains and across growing and storage seasons. Consequently, biomarkers with short whole-body half-lives (~8 h), such as AFM_1, aflatoxin–*N*–acetylcysteine, or aflatoxin–N^7–guanine excreted in urine reflect only the most recent of exposures. Longer half-life biomarkers offer a promise of more integrated exposure assessments, smoothing the day-to-day variability to better reflect a steady-state level of exposure. Towards that end, aflatoxin–albumin adducts measured in serum samples have been used widely in animal studies as well as human ecological surveys and interventional trials. Importantly, they have been used to understand dose–response relationships between exposures and health outcomes, both acute toxicities and chronic manifestations including liver cancer. The biological half-life of aflatoxin–albumin adducts in serum is estimated to be about 30 days; in rats, it is much shorter (2–3 days).

Albumin is now recognized as a reservoir for binding many xenobiotics and endobiotics, especially at the cysteine in position 34. However, several other amino acids serve as targets for adduct formation [42]. The major aflatoxin–albumin adduct forms at a lysine residue. Sabbioni and colleagues [43] initially described the properties of the major serum albumin adduct formed by AFB_1 in vivo in rats. Subsequently, they examined the relationships between dose (dietary exposure), yield, and steady-state levels in humans. A split bowl assessment of aflatoxin in foods eaten by study participants and the measurement of serum albumin adducts examined the dose relationship between ingestion and biomarker levels over a one-week period [44]. Regression analysis indicated a highly significant association between the amount of aflatoxin ingested and biomarker levels. An average aflatoxin–lysine adduct yield of 0.38 ng aflatoxin–lysine/μg AFB_1 from the diet was proposed. No differences by gender were observed. Similar values have been estimated from dosimetry experiments in rats [43]. Despite the differences in half-lives of the serum and urinary aflatoxin biomarkers, the levels of both aflatoxin–albumin adducts and/or aflatoxin–N^7–guanine adducts have been shown to correlate with aflatoxin exposure [33,34,45].

3. Validation of Aflatoxin Biomarkers: Are They Risk Markers Too?

The validation of aflatoxin metabolites and albumin adducts as exposure biomarkers has been accomplished successfully [46,47]. Beginning with the recognition of AFB_1 as a hepatocarcinogen in trout and rats, and, as a suspected human carcinogen, the development of rigorous methodologies for sensitive and selective measures of biomarkers in biofluids occurred in lockstep with general analytical advancements. The current levels of detection are more than suitable for biomonitoring in human populations. Animal studies determined the dose–response and temporal relationships to exposures. Cross-sectional studies of these biomarkers in human populations with high exposures to aflatoxins confirmed the major elements of the rodent studies. Longitudinal studies, albeit few, have noted that the tracking of repeated measures over months to years is low, unlike measures of blood pressure or blood cholesterol in individuals as examples. This outcome suggests that, while population-based monitoring may be robust, linking individual levels to health outcomes may be an overreach. The long-term stability of the aflatoxin analytes stored in frozen urine and serum have also been confirmed [48]. Confidence in the interpretation of aflatoxin biomarker levels, even at the population level, required additional steps of inquiry. Once more, animal models were critical in defining linkages between biomarkers and health outcomes, typically hepatocarcinogenesis. Most informative have been case–control, cohort, and interventional studies in humans.

Animal studies. Several studies in rats have directly examined the predictive value of aflatoxin biomarkers in the subsequent tumor burden (presumptive, preneoplastic lesions such as GGT+ or GSTP+ foci) or the lifetime incidence of hepatocarcinogenesis. These were two-armed studies examining the chemopreventive efficacy of agents now known to be inducers of the nuclear factor erythroid 2–related factor 2 (NRF2) cytoprotective, stress response network [49]. The earliest studies looked at the magnitude of reduced hepatic levels of aflatoxin–DNA adducts relative to a reduced tumor burden. The diminution of hepatic aflatoxin–DNA adduct levels consistently underestimated the chemopreventive efficacy [50], highlighting a quantitative disconnect between biologically effective dose markers and risk reduction. Lifetime bioassays evaluating interventions with oltipraz [37] or CDDO-Im [35] compared the initial effects on the urinary excretion of aflatoxin–N^7–guanine to cancer reduction. In both studies, the protection against cancers was 100%, whereas the urinary biomarker, while significantly diminished, was detectable in all samples. Clearly, the notion of a threshold for DNA damage within the context of cancer risk muddles the associations between the two outcomes [51].

Studies focused on serum aflatoxin–albumin adducts led to similar conclusions. In a dietary intervention with the oltipraz analog 1,2-dithiole-3-thione, the overall diminutions in the levels of hepatic DNA adducts, urinary aflatoxin–N^7–guanine, and serum aflatoxin–albumin adducts over a two-week exposure period were remarkably similar [32]. In a follow-up study, the rats were dosed with AFB_1 daily for 5 weeks after randomization into no intervention, delayed-transient intervention (weeks 2 and 3 relative to AFB_1), or persistent oltipraz intervention (weeks −1 to 5) groups [52]. Serial blood samples were collected from each animal at weekly intervals. The area under the curve (AUC) values for aflatoxin–albumin adducts decreased 20 and 39% in the delayed-transient and persistent oltipraz intervention groups, respectively, as compared to the value with no intervention. The total incidence of HCC dropped from 83 to 60% ($p = 0.03$) and 48% ($p < 0.01$) in these groups, highlighting a concordance between these two end points. Overall, a significant association was seen between biomarker AUC and the risk of HCC ($p < 0.01$). However, when the predictive value of aflatoxin–albumin adducts was assessed within treatment groups, there was no association between AUC and the risk of HCC ($p = 0.56$). Thus, aflatoxin–albumin adducts can be useful for monitoring population-based changes induced by interventions, such as in chemoprevention trials, but have limited utility in identifying individuals destined to develop HCC.

Human studies. The seminal study on aflatoxin biomarkers and cancer risk was conducted in Shanghai, China by an international team including Professor Groopman. A prospective study of more than 18,000 men during the 1980s and 1990s revealed a statistically significant increase in the risk of liver cancer (relative risk, 3.4) when aflatoxin biomarkers were detected. For persons seropositive for HBsAg (a biomarker of hepatitis B virus (HBV) infection), the relative risk was 7.3, but, for individuals positive for both aflatoxin and HBsAg, the relative risk was 59.4, thus demonstrating a synergistic effect of these joint risk factors [53,54]. These results contributed to the International Agency for Research on Cancer classifying aflatoxins as Group 1 human carcinogens [55]. Subsequent cohort studies in Taiwan have substantially confirmed the results from the Shanghai investigation [56,57]. Notably, as in the Shanghai cohort, the liver cancer risk associated with AFB_1 exposure was most striking among HBV carriers with detectable aflatoxin–N^7–guanine adducts in urine.

Using a population-based cancer registry established by the Qidong Liver Cancer Institute in 1972 and aflatoxin-specific biomarkers, Groopman and colleagues documented that the reduction in aflatoxin exposure from exceedingly high to nearly undetectable levels has likely contributed to a nearly 70% decline in age-standardized liver cancer incidence over the past 30 years despite an unchanging prevalence of HBV infection in cases [58]. A natural experiment of economic reform in the 1980s drove a rapid switch from the consumption of heavily contaminated maize to minimally, if any, contaminated rice and, subsequently, the expansion to dietary diversity. Serum levels of aflatoxin–albumin adducts in the Qidong population began declining after that switch and are now virtually undetectable [59]. The time to liver cancer diagnosis was extended as well: in 1990, the median age of diagnosis was 48 years, whilst increasing to 67 years by 2021. Perhaps aflatoxin exposures were also accelerating the time to tumors in the background of HBV-infected people. These findings have important translational public health implications, since >5 billion people in developing countries worldwide are at risk of the chronic exposure to aflatoxins through contaminated foods, especially in societies using maize as the staple food [60]. Using aflatoxin–albumin adduct biomarkers, and observations that aflatoxin exposure may affect child growth and susceptibility to infection [61], as well the liver cancer risk, served to further emphasize the public health need for the development and implementation of interventions in these populations.

A timeline of key milestones in the discovery, biomarker development and molecular epidemiology, and the regulation of aflatoxins is presented in Figure 4. The key contributions of Professor Groopman to these events are highlighted.

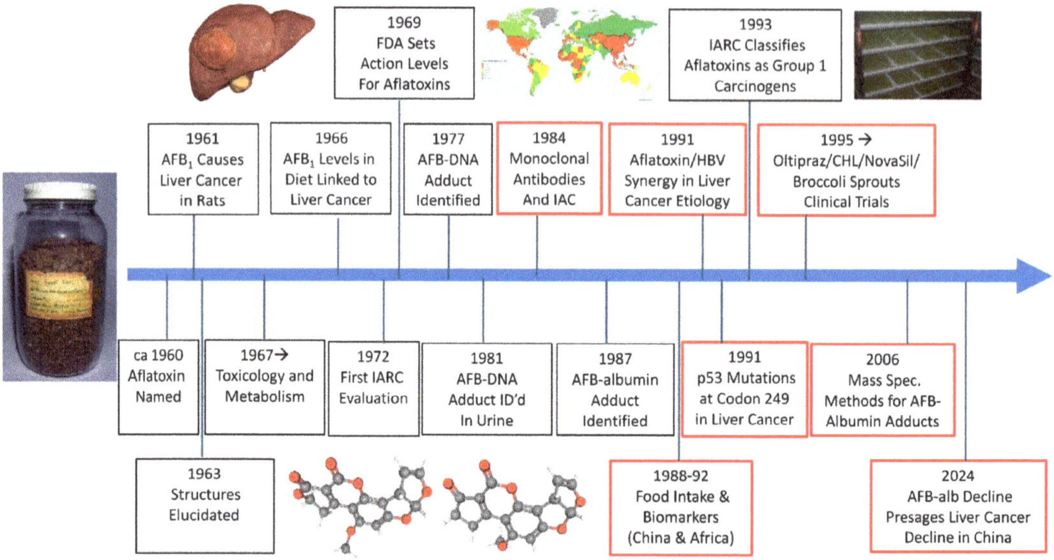

Figure 4. Timeline for key events in the discovery, biomarker development and molecular epidemiology, and regulation of aflatoxins. FDA, Food and Drug Administration; IARC, International Agency for Research on Cancer; IAC, immunoaffinity chromatography; CHL, chlorophyllin. Red boxes highlight seminal contributions of Professor John Groopman over the last 4 decades. Photo credits: original "Rosetta" groundnut meal used in initial characterization of aflatoxin toxicities, courtesy of John Groopman; and broccoli sprouts grown in the Qidong Liver Cancer Institute, China for the first clinical trials, courtesy of Thomas Kensler.

4. Analytic Approaches to Aflatoxin Biomarker Development

Many different analytical methods have been applied for the quantitation of chemical adducts in biological samples. Thin-layer chromatrography, HPLC coupled with UV or fluorescence detection, and isotope-dilution mass pectrometry with ever improving detection modalities have been used in population biomonitoring. Key in biomarker development and application has been the serial improvements in sensitivity and specificity as these methodologies came online. Each methodology has unique features of specificity and sensitivity. For example, to measure a single aflatoxin metabolite, a chromatographic method can resolve mixtures of aflatoxins into individual compounds, providing that the extraction procedure does not introduce large amounts of interfering chemicals. Antibody-based methods often are more sensitive than chromatography, but immunoassays are less selective because the antibody may cross-react with multiple metabolites. Current studies using isotope-dilution and tandem mass spectrometry with liquid chromatography separation and improved detection methods have demonstrated an increase in sensitivity of at least 1000-fold over technologies previously used for the detection of aflatoxin biomarkers. Exquisite technologies are not useful, however, if they are not amenable to the high throughput needed for population-based studies at a reasonable cost.

Biomarker measurements in biofluids have typically involved a normalization step to either urinary creatinine levels to account for variations in urine flow rates or serum albumin levels where the albumin content is measured. While the use of urinary creatinine is broadly accepted for many types of urinary biomarker measures, the use of albumin levels for normalization has been questioned recently. As discussed by Smith et al. [62], the normalization of human serum albumin adds complexity and error due to the quantitative biases of various albumin assays used across disparate studies, which are typically of much lower sensitivity than current measures of AFB_1-lys levels. Coupled with the added time, financial costs, and sample consumption required to perform albumin normalization, there is little compelling justification for their use.

An important advance lies in the use of both aflatoxin–DNA adduct in urine and aflatoxin-serum albumin adduct determinations to estimate daily dietary exposures. To date, the estimates using the aflatoxin–albumin adduct have been found to be of great utility for comparisons of the exposure across different populations at risk [63]. In a study in Fusui County, Guangxi, China, aflatoxin was measured in the corn porridge that was the staple food; it was calculated that 2.9% of the daily dietary exposure was converted to the aflatoxin–albumin adduct [44]. Assuming the steady-state accumulation of albumin adduct formation occurring over a 30-day time frame, the measured value by mass spectrometry of the albumin adduct level is divided by 30 to provide a daily exposure measure. A daily exposure over 1 month of 1 μg aflatoxin per day would result in a value of 17.5 pg AFB-lysine/mg albumin. The limit of detection for daily exposure by the mass spectrometry method is 14 ng AFB_1 per day.

5. Whither Next?

The concept of the 'exposome', as originally proposed by Professor Christopher Wild, is "composed of every exposure to which an individual is subjected from conception to death" [64]. Miller and Jones [65] have expanded this concept as "the cumulative measure of environmental influences and associated biological responses throughout the lifespan, including exposures from the environment, diet, behavior, and endogenous processes". Aflatoxin biomarkers ably assist in the former and fall short of the later. At their best, these markers accurately reflect individual exposures of the internal dose (oxidation and conjugation metabolites and albumin adducts) and the biologically effective dose (aflatoxin–N^7–guanine adducts). These are targeted or knowledge-based biomarkers in which the methods were optimized for each analyte. Such exposure biomarkers are powerful tools in epidemiologic studies to dampen the prevalence of exposure misclassification in case–control and cohort studies. However, their half-lives are relatively short and do not reflect the chronic, cumulative exposures throughout a lifespan, nor do they reflect the biological responses. However, because of their chemical stability in frozen biological fluids, now verified for decades, coupled with the analytical need for very minimal specimen volumes, longitudinal collections of urine or serum samples provide opportunities for retrospective reconstructions of past aflatoxin exposures and the linkage to disease outcomes at the population, if not at the individual, level.

Analytical methods and their associated costs are now amenable to large-scale assessments of exposures from the past, present, and future (prospectively) using aflatoxin–albumin adducts. Excellent correlation between three independent methodologies has been reported [66], as has a recognition that a simple normalization to serum volume rather than additional albumin measures is superior [62]. It is conceivable to design studies to consider whether the current regulatory standards for aflatoxin levels in human diets adequately protect public health. Enough is known about the relationships between contamination levels in foodstuffs, biomarker levels in humans, and some disease outcomes, notably, liver cancer, to consider such a fundamental question. Of course, it is not simple, as multiple confounders including infections with hepatitis B or C viruses exert additive to multiplicative perturbations to the calculus for cancer, as well as the long latency between the initial exposure and disease outcome. Further, do current levels of aflatoxin exposure contribute equally to liver cancer risk in economically developed versus less developed countries?

Biomonitoring can also address whether subpopulations exist within the U.S. or elsewhere who may experience elevated aflatoxin exposures through dietary habits involving the consumption of large amounts of food products especially prone to aflatoxin contamination. If so, does this exposure put them at a significantly elevated risk of adverse health outcomes? A cross-sectional study of aflatoxin–lysine adduct levels in samples from the National Health and Nutrition Examination Survey (NHANES) reported that about 1% of the U.S. population had detectable levels and that additional target surveillance may be warranted [67]. Such possibilities have been carried out or are being considered in Texas [68], Guatemala [69], China [70], South Asia [71,72], and Africa [62,73,74]. Can we use biomarkers to track the consequences of climate change on aflatoxin exposures and downstream health outcomes? Do regulatory changes or active interventions (dietary diversification, the introduction of stress-resistant crops or non-toxigenic forms of *Aspergillus* into farmlands, better storage practices for dietary staples, or targeted chemopreventive interventions) adequately and sustainably dampen the internal dose levels—and, presumptively, the effects on health? Aflatoxin biomarkers are essential tools for answering questions such as these.

Analytically, only a few forms of aflatoxins need to be monitored given the dominant toxicities of AFB_1 within the family of aflatoxins. Lysine is the primary, if not sole, amino acid for adduction in albumin. However, methods are being developed for multiplexing measures of environmental exposures within albumin. Many amino acid residues are known to be sites of covalent modifications by exogenous and endogenous electrophiles (principally Cys, but also His, Tyr, Ser, Met, and Arg in addition to Lys). Thus, albumin represents a stable macromolecular platform for discerning diverse exposures through the untargeted profiling of adducts. The Rappaport [75] and Groopman [42] labs, among others, have been leaders in the application of such proteomic technologies including data deconvolution in biomarker measures of complex exposures such as air pollution that include products of exogenous (SO_2, and benzene) and endogenous (oxidation, lipid peroxidation, glycation, and carbamylation) origin. The characterization of the exposome as envisioned by Professor Wild is becoming a reality. The inclusion of other -omic technologies, particularly metabolomics, will enable conjoined perspectives on the resultant biological responses.

The paradigm of discovery, validation, and utilization of aflatoxin biomarkers sits at the current high point of biomarker development and the application for environmental carcinogens. Perhaps the only other chemical-specific biomarkers to reach this perch are the targeted, tobacco-specific biomarkers which arise from a very complex exposure milieu in smokers. Their use has demonstrably contributed to regulatory changes in the prohibitions of smoking in public places, the extent and impact of secondary smoke exposures, and the nature and extent of possible health risks from newer nicotine-delivery products [76]. The continued development of biomarkers reflecting exogenous agents and the resultant endogenous processes coupled to rapid, inexpensive, multiplexing platforms is needed to fulfill the goals of lifelong exposome characterizations.

Author Contributions: Both authors contributed equally to the conceptualization, writing, review and editing, and project administration. All authors have read and agreed to the published version of the manuscript.

Funding: This review received no external funding.

Institutional Review Board Statement: Not applicable.

Informed Consent Statement: Not applicable.

Data Availability Statement: No new data were created or analyzed in this study. Data sharing is not applicable to this article.

Acknowledgments: The authors thank our mentors, Groopman, along with his and our students, fellows, and other collaborators for the aflatoxin journeys we have undertaken. We thank the National Institutes of Health (NCI and NIEHS) for the decades of support for our research on aflatoxin and related topics.

Conflicts of Interest: The authors declare no conflicts of interest.

References

1. Blount, W.P. Turkey "X" Disease. **1961**, *9*, 55–58. *J. Br. Turkey* **1961**, *9*, 55–58.
2. Pickova, D.; Ostry, V.; Toman, J.; Malir, F. Aflatoxins: History, Significant Milestones, Recent Data on Their Toxicity and Ways to Mitigation. *Toxins* **2021**, *13*, 399. [CrossRef] [PubMed]

3. Wannop, C.C. Groundnut Toxicity in Poultry: Turkey X Disease. *Br. Vet. J.* **1963**, *119*, 174–177. [CrossRef]
4. Cullen, J.M.; Newberne, P.M. Acute Hepatotoxicity of Aflatoxins. In *The Toxicology of Aflatoxins: Human Health, Veterinary and Agricultural Significance*; Eaton, D.L., Groopman, J.D., Eds.; Academic Press, Inc.: Boston, MA, USA, 1994; pp. 3–26.
5. Van der Zijden, A.S.M.; Koelensmid, W.; Boldingh, J.; Barrett, C.B.; Ord, W.O.; Philip, J. Aspergillus Flavus and Turkey X Disease: Isolation in Crystalline Form of a Toxin Responsible for Turkey X-Disease. *Nature* **1962**, *195*, 1060–1062. [CrossRef]
6. Asao, T.; Buechi, G.; Abdel-Kader, M.M.; Chang, S.B.; Wick, E.L.; Wogan, G.N. the Structures of Aflatoxins B and G. *J. Am. Chem. Soc.* **1965**, *87*, 882–886. [CrossRef]
7. Nesbitt, B.F.; O'Kelly, J.; Sargeant, K.; Sheridan, A.N.N. Aspergillus Flavus and Turkey X Disease. Toxic Metabolites of Aspergillus Flavus. *Nature* **1962**, *195*, 1062–1063. [CrossRef]
8. Hendrix, J.D. Carcinogenicity of Aflatoxins in Nonmammalian Organisms. In *The Toxicology of Aflatoxins: Human Health, Veterinary and Agricultural Significance*; Eaton, D.L., Groopman, J.D., Eds.; Academic Press, Inc.: Boston, MA, USA, 1994; pp. 103–136.
9. Schoental, R. Liver Changes and Primary Liver Tumours in Rats given Toxic Guinea Pig Diet (M.R.C. Diet 18). *Br. J. Cancer* **1961**, *15*, 812–815. [CrossRef]
10. Allcroft, R.; Carnaghan, R.B.A. Toxic Products in Groundnuts. Biological Effects. *Chem. Ind.* **1963**, *2*, 50–53.
11. Barnes, J.M.; Butler, W.H. Carcinogenic Activity of Aflatoxin to Rats. *Nature* **1964**, *202*, 1016. [CrossRef]
12. Butler, W.H.; Barnes, J.M. Toxic Effects of Groundnut Meal Containing Aflatoxin to Rats and Guinea-Pigs. *Br. J. Cancer* **1963**, *17*, 699–710. [CrossRef]
13. Carnaghan, R.B. Hepatic tumours in ducks fed a low level of toxic groundnut meal. *Nature* **1965**, *208*, 308. [CrossRef] [PubMed]
14. Wogan, G.N.; Newberne, P.M. Dose-response characteristics of aflatoxin B1 carcinogenesis in the rat. *Cancer Res.* **1967**, *27*, 2370–2376. [PubMed]
15. Lancaster, M.C.; Jenkins, F.P.; Philp, J.M. Toxicity Associated with Certain Samples of Groundnuts. *Nature* **1961**, *192*, 1095–1096. [CrossRef]
16. Newberne, P.M.; Harrington, D.H.; Wogan, G.N. Effects of cirrhosis and other liver insults on induction of liver tumors by aflatoxin in rats. *Lab. Investig.* **1966**, *15*, 962–969.
17. Wogan, G.N.; Paglialunga, S.; Newberne, P.M. Carcinogenic effects of low dietary levels of aflatoxin B1 in rats. *Food Cosmet. Toxicol.* **1974**, *12*, 681–685. [CrossRef]
18. Paustenbach, D.J.; Brown, S.E.; Heywood, J.J.; Donnell, M.T.; Eaton, D.L. Risk characterization of N-nitrosodimethylamine in pharmaceuticals. *Food Chem. Toxicol.* **2024**, *186*, 114498. [CrossRef]
19. Campbell, T.C.; Caedo, J.P., Jr.; Bulatao-Jayme, J.; Salamat, L.; Engel, R.W. Aflatoxin M1 in human urine. *Nature* **1970**, *227*, 403–404. [CrossRef]
20. Groopman, J.D.; Roebuck, B.D.; Kensler, T.W. Molecular dosimetry of aflatoxin DNA adducts in humans and experimental rat models. *Prog. Clin. Biol. Res.* **1992**, *374*, 139–155.
21. Groopman, J.D.; Donahue, P.R.; Zhu, J.Q.; Chen, J.S.; Wogan, G.N. Aflatoxin metabolism in humans: Detection of metabolites and nucleic acid adducts in urine by affinity chromatography. *Proc. Natl. Acad. Sci. USA* **1985**, *82*, 6492–6496. [CrossRef]
22. Sabbioni, G.; Ambs, S.; Wogan, G.N.; Groopman, J.D. The aflatoxin-lysine adduct quantified by high-performance liquid chromatography from human serum albumin samples. *Carcinogenesis* **1990**, *11*, 2063–2066. [CrossRef]
23. Scholl, P.F.; Musser, S.M.; Groopman, J.D. Synthesis and characterization of aflatoxin B1 mercapturic acids and their identification in rat urine. *Chem. Res. Toxicol.* **1997**, *10*, 1144–1151. [CrossRef]
24. Scholl, P.F.; Turner, P.C.; Sutcliffe, A.E.; Sylla, A.; Diallo, M.S.; Friesen, M.D.; Groopman, J.D.; Wild, C.P. Quantitative comparison of aflatoxin B1 serum albumin adducts in humans by isotope dilution mass spectrometry and ELISA. *Cancer Epidemiol. Biomarkers Prev.* **2006**, *15*, 823–826. [CrossRef]
25. Sheabar, F.Z.; Groopman, J.D.; Qian, G.S.; Wogan, G.N. Quantitative analysis of aflatoxin-albumin adducts. *Carcinogenesis* **1993**, *14*, 1203–1208. [CrossRef] [PubMed]
26. Walton, M.; Egner, P.; Scholl, P.F.; Walker, J.; Kensler, T.W.; Groopman, J.D. Liquid chromatography electrospray-mass spectrometry of urinary aflatoxin biomarkers: Characterization and application to dosimetry and chemoprevention in rats. *Chem. Res. Toxicol.* **2001**, *14*, 919–926. [CrossRef] [PubMed]
27. Swenson, D.H.; Miller, E.C.; Miller, J.A. Aflatoxin B1-2,3-oxide: Evidence for its formation in rat liver in vivo and by human liver microsomes in vitro. *Biochem. Biophys. Res. Commun.* **1974**, *60*, 1036–1043. [CrossRef] [PubMed]
28. Croy, R.G.; Essigmann, J.M.; Reinhold, V.N.; Wogan, G.N. Identification of the principal aflatoxin B1-DNA adduct formed in vivo in rat liver. *Proc. Natl. Acad. Sci. USA* **1978**, *75*, 1745–1749. [CrossRef]
29. Essigmann, J.M.; Croy, R.G.; Nadzan, A.M.; Busby, W.F., Jr.; Reinhold, V.N.; Buchi, G.; Wogan, G.N. Structural identification of the major DNA adduct formed by aflatoxin B1 in vitro. *Proc. Natl. Acad. Sci. USA* **1977**, *74*, 1870–1874. [CrossRef]
30. Swenson, D.H.; Lin, J.K.; Miller, E.C.; Miller, J.A. Aflatoxin B1-2,3-oxide as a probable intermediate in the covalent binding of aflatoxins B1 and B2 to rat liver DNA and ribosomal RNA in vivo. *Cancer Res.* **1977**, *37*, 172–181.
31. Bennett, R.A.; Essigmann, J.M.; Wogan, G.N. Excretion of an aflatoxin-guanine adduct in the urine of aflatoxin B1-treated rats. *Cancer Res.* **1981**, *41*, 650–654.
32. Groopman, J.D.; DeMatos, P.; Egner, P.A.; Love-Hunt, A.; Kensler, T.W. Molecular dosimetry of urinary aflatoxin-N7-guanine and serum aflatoxin-albumin adducts predicts chemoprotection by 1,2-dithiole-3-thione in rats. *Carcinogenesis* **1992**, *13*, 101–106. [CrossRef]

33. Groopman, J.D.; Hall, A.J.; Whittle, H.; Hudson, G.J.; Wogan, G.N.; Montesano, R.; Wild, C.P. Molecular dosimetry of aflatoxin-N7-guanine in human urine obtained in The Gambia, West Africa. *Cancer Epidemiol. Biomarkers Prev.* **1992**, *1*, 221–227. [PubMed]
34. Groopman, J.D.; Hasler, J.A.; Trudel, L.J.; Pikul, A.; Donahue, P.R.; Wogan, G.N. Molecular dosimetry in rat urine of aflatoxin-N7-guanine and other aflatoxin metabolites by multiple monoclonal antibody affinity chromatography and immunoaffinity/high performance liquid chromatography. *Cancer Res.* **1992**, *52*, 267–274. [PubMed]
35. Johnson, N.M.; Egner, P.A.; Baxter, V.K.; Sporn, M.B.; Wible, R.S.; Sutter, T.R.; Groopman, J.D.; Kensler, T.W.; Roebuck, B.D. Complete protection against aflatoxin B(1)-induced liver cancer with a triterpenoid: DNA adduct dosimetry, molecular signature, and genotoxicity threshold. *Cancer Prev. Res.* **2014**, *7*, 658–665. [CrossRef]
36. Kensler, T.W.; Egner, P.A.; Davidson, N.E.; Roebuck, B.D.; Pikul, A.; Groopman, J.D. Modulation of aflatoxin metabolism, aflatoxin-N7-guanine formation, and hepatic tumorigenesis in rats fed ethoxyquin: Role of induction of glutathione S-transferases. *Cancer Res.* **1986**, *46*, 3924–3931.
37. Roebuck, B.D.; Liu, Y.L.; Rogers, A.E.; Groopman, J.D.; Kensler, T.W. Protection against aflatoxin B1-induced hepatocarcinogenesis in F344 rats by 5-(2-pyrazinyl)-4-methyl-1,2-dithiole-3-thione (oltipraz): Predictive role for short-term molecular dosimetry. *Cancer Res.* **1991**, *51*, 5501–5506. [PubMed]
38. Breinholt, V.; Hendricks, J.; Pereira, C.; Arbogast, D.; Bailey, G. Dietary chlorophyllin is a potent inhibitor of aflatoxin B1 hepatocarcinogenesis in rainbow trout. *Cancer Res.* **1995**, *55*, 57–62. [PubMed]
39. Breinholt, V.; Schimerlik, M.; Dashwood, R.; Bailey, G. Mechanisms of chlorophyllin anticarcinogenesis against aflatoxin B1: Complex formation with the carcinogen. *Chem. Res. Toxicol.* **1995**, *8*, 506–514. [CrossRef]
40. Egner, P.A.; Wang, J.B.; Zhu, Y.R.; Zhang, B.C.; Wu, Y.; Zhang, Q.N.; Qian, G.S.; Kuang, S.Y.; Gange, S.J.; Jacobson, L.P.; et al. Chlorophyllin intervention reduces aflatoxin-DNA adducts in individuals at high risk for liver cancer. *Proc. Natl. Acad. Sci. USA* **2001**, *98*, 14601–14606. [CrossRef]
41. Wang, J.S.; Shen, X.; He, X.; Zhu, Y.R.; Zhang, B.C.; Wang, J.B.; Qian, G.S.; Kuang, S.Y.; Zarba, A.; Egner, P.A.; et al. Protective alterations in phase 1 and 2 metabolism of aflatoxin B1 by oltipraz in residents of Qidong, People's Republic of China. *J. Natl. Cancer Inst.* **1999**, *91*, 347–354. [CrossRef]
42. Smith, J.W.; O'Meally, R.N.; Burke, S.M.; Ng, D.K.; Chen, J.G.; Kensler, T.W.; Groopman, J.D.; Cole, R.N. Global Discovery and Temporal Changes of Human Albumin Modifications by Pan-Protein Adductomics: Initial Application to Air Pollution Exposure. *J. Am. Soc. Mass. Spectrom.* **2023**, *34*, 595–607. [CrossRef]
43. Sabbioni, G.; Skipper, P.L.; Buchi, G.; Tannenbaum, S.R. Isolation and characterization of the major serum albumin adduct formed by aflatoxin B1 in vivo in rats. *Carcinogenesis* **1987**, *8*, 819–824. [CrossRef] [PubMed]
44. Gan, L.S.; Skipper, P.L.; Peng, X.C.; Groopman, J.D.; Chen, J.S.; Wogan, G.N.; Tannenbaum, S.R. Serum albumin adducts in the molecular epidemiology of aflatoxin carcinogenesis: Correlation with aflatoxin B1 intake and urinary excretion of aflatoxin M1. *Carcinogenesis* **1988**, *9*, 1323–1325. [CrossRef]
45. Wild, C.P.; Hudson, G.J.; Sabbioni, G.; Chapot, B.; Hall, A.J.; Wogan, G.N.; Whittle, H.; Montesano, R.; Groopman, J.D. Dietary intake of aflatoxins and the level of albumin-bound aflatoxin in peripheral blood in The Gambia, West Africa. *Cancer Epidemiol. Biomarkers Prev.* **1992**, *1*, 229–234.
46. Groopman, J.D.; Kensler, T.W. The light at the end of the tunnel for chemical-specific biomarkers: Daylight or headlight? *Carcinogenesis* **1999**, *20*, 1–11. [CrossRef]
47. Kensler, T.W.; Roebuck, B.D.; Wogan, G.N.; Groopman, J.D. Aflatoxin: A 50-year odyssey of mechanistic and translational toxicology. *Toxicol. Sci.* **2011**, *120* (Suppl. S1), S28–S48. [CrossRef]
48. Scholl, P.F.; Groopman, J.D. Long-term stability of human aflatoxin B1 albumin adducts assessed by isotope dilution mass spectrometry and high-performance liquid chromatography-fluorescence. *Cancer Epidemiol. Biomarkers Prev.* **2008**, *17*, 1436–1439. [CrossRef] [PubMed]
49. Yamamoto, M.; Kensler, T.W.; Motohashi, H. The KEAP1-NRF2 System: A Thiol-Based Sensor-Effector Apparatus for Maintaining Redox Homeostasis. *Physiol. Rev.* **2018**, *98*, 1169–1203. [CrossRef] [PubMed]
50. Kensler, T.W.; Groopman, J.D.; Sutter, T.R.; Curphey, T.J.; Roebuck, B.D. Development of cancer chemopreventive agents: Oltipraz as a paradigm. *Chem. Res. Toxicol.* **1999**, *12*, 113–126. [CrossRef]
51. Eaton, D.L.; Schaupp, C.M. Of mice, rats, and men: Could Nrf2 activation protect against aflatoxin heptocarcinogenesis in humans? *Cancer Prev. Res.* **2014**, *7*, 653–657. [CrossRef]
52. Kensler, T.W.; Gange, S.J.; Egner, P.A.; Dolan, P.M.; Munoz, A.; Groopman, J.D.; Rogers, A.E.; Roebuck, B.D. Predictive value of molecular dosimetry: Individual versus group effects of oltipraz on aflatoxin-albumin adducts and risk of liver cancer. *Cancer Epidemiol. Biomarkers Prev.* **1997**, *6*, 603–610.
53. Qian, G.S.; Ross, R.K.; Yu, M.C.; Yuan, J.M.; Gao, Y.T.; Henderson, B.E.; Wogan, G.N.; Groopman, J.D. A follow-up study of urinary markers of aflatoxin exposure and liver cancer risk in Shanghai, People's Republic of China. *Cancer Epidemiol. Biomarkers Prev.* **1994**, *3*, 3–10. [PubMed]
54. Ross, R.K.; Yuan, J.M.; Yu, M.C.; Wogan, G.N.; Qian, G.S.; Tu, J.T.; Groopman, J.D.; Gao, Y.T.; Henderson, B.E. Urinary aflatoxin biomarkers and risk of hepatocellular carcinoma. *Lancet* **1992**, *339*, 943–946. [CrossRef] [PubMed]
55. IARC. *Some Naturally Occurring Substances: Food Items and Constituents, Heterocyclic Aromatic Amines and Mycotoxins*; IARC Press: Lyon, France, 1993; Volume 56.

56. Chen, C.J.; Wang, L.Y.; Lu, S.N.; Wu, M.H.; You, S.L.; Zhang, Y.J.; Wang, L.W.; Santella, R.M. Elevated aflatoxin exposure and increased risk of hepatocellular carcinoma. *Hepatology* **1996**, *24*, 38–42. [CrossRef]
57. Wang, L.Y.; Hatch, M.; Chen, C.J.; Levin, B.; You, S.L.; Lu, S.N.; Wu, M.H.; Wu, W.P.; Wang, L.W.; Wang, Q.; et al. Aflatoxin exposure and risk of hepatocellular carcinoma in Taiwan. *Int. J. Cancer* **1996**, *67*, 620–625. [CrossRef]
58. Chen, J.G.; Kensler, T.W.; Zhu, J.; Zhu, Y.R.; Wang, J.B.; Lu, J.H.; Munoz, A.; Groopman, J.D. Profound primary prevention of liver cancer following a natural experiment in China: A 50-year perspective and public health implications. *Int. J. Cancer* **2024**. [CrossRef] [PubMed]
59. Chen, J.G.; Egner, P.A.; Ng, D.; Jacobson, L.P.; Munoz, A.; Zhu, Y.R.; Qian, G.S.; Wu, F.; Yuan, J.M.; Groopman, J.D.; et al. Reduced aflatoxin exposure presages decline in liver cancer mortality in an endemic region of China. *Cancer Prev. Res.* **2013**, *6*, 1038–1045. [CrossRef]
60. Strosnider, H.; Azziz-Baumgartner, E.; Banziger, M.; Bhat, R.V.; Breiman, R.; Brune, M.N.; DeCock, K.; Dilley, A.; Groopman, J.; Hell, K.; et al. Workgroup report: Public health strategies for reducing aflatoxin exposure in developing countries. *Environ. Health Perspect.* **2006**, *114*, 1898–1903. [CrossRef]
61. Gong, Y.Y.; Cardwell, K.; Hounsa, A.; Egal, S.; Turner, P.C.; Hall, A.J.; Wild, C.P. Dietary aflatoxin exposure and impaired growth in young children from Benin and Togo: Cross sectional study. *BMJ* **2002**, *325*, 20–21. [CrossRef]
62. Smith, J.W.; Ng, D.K.; Alvarez, C.S.; Egner, P.A.; Burke, S.M.; Chen, J.G.; Kensler, T.W.; Koshiol, J.; Rivera-Andrade, A.; Kroker-Lobos, M.F.; et al. Assessing the Validity of Normalizing Aflatoxin B(1)-Lysine Albumin Adduct Biomarker Measurements to Total Serum Albumin Concentration across Multiple Human Population Studies. *Toxins* **2022**, *14*, 162. [CrossRef]
63. Groopman, J.D.; Egner, P.A.; Schulze, K.J.; Wu, L.S.; Merrill, R.; Mehra, S.; Shamim, A.A.; Ali, H.; Shaikh, S.; Gernand, A.; et al. Aflatoxin exposure during the first 1000 days of life in rural South Asia assessed by aflatoxin B(1)-lysine albumin biomarkers. *Food Chem Toxicol* **2014**, *74*, 184–189. [CrossRef]
64. Wild, C.P. The exposome: From concept to utility. *Int. J. Epidemiol.* **2012**, *41*, 24–32. [CrossRef] [PubMed]
65. Miller, G.W.; Jones, D.P. The nature of nurture: Refining the definition of the exposome. *Toxicol. Sci.* **2014**, *137*, 1–2. [CrossRef] [PubMed]
66. McCoy, L.F.; Scholl, P.F.; Sutcliffe, A.E.; Kieszak, S.M.; Powers, C.D.; Rogers, H.S.; Gong, Y.Y.; Groopman, J.D.; Wild, C.P.; Schleicher, R.L. Human aflatoxin albumin adducts quantitatively compared by ELISA, HPLC with fluorescence detection, and HPLC with isotope dilution mass spectrometry. *Cancer Epidemiol. Biomarkers Prev.* **2008**, *17*, 1653–1657. [CrossRef]
67. Schleicher, R.L.; McCoy, L.F.; Powers, C.D.; Sternberg, M.R.; Pfeiffer, C.M. Serum concentrations of an aflatoxin-albumin adduct in the National Health and Nutrition Examination Survey (NHANES) 1999–2000. *Clin. Chim. Acta* **2013**, *423*, 46–50. [CrossRef]
68. Xue, K.S.; Tang, L.; Shen, C.L.; Pollock, B.H.; Guerra, F.; Phillips, T.D.; Wang, J.S. Increase in aflatoxin exposure in two populations residing in East and West Texas, United States. *Int. J. Hyg. Environ. Health* **2021**, *231*, 113662. [CrossRef] [PubMed]
69. Kroker-Lobos, M.F.; Alvarez, C.S.; Rivera-Andrade, A.; Smith, J.W.; Egner, P.; Torres, O.; Lazo, M.; Freedman, N.D.; Guallar, E.; Graubard, B.I.; et al. Association between aflatoxin-albumin adduct levels and tortilla consumption in Guatemalan adults. *Toxicol. Rep.* **2019**, *6*, 465–471. [CrossRef]
70. Wang, S.; Pan, D.; Zhang, T.; Su, M.; Sun, G.; Wei, J.; Guo, Z.; Wang, K.; Song, G.; Yan, Q. Corn Flour Intake, Aflatoxin B(1) Exposure, and Risk of Esophageal Precancerous Lesions in a High-Risk Area of Huai'an, China: A Case-Control Study. *Toxins* **2020**, *12*, 299. [CrossRef]
71. Mahfuz, M.; Alam, M.A.; Fahim, S.M.; Gazi, M.A.; Raihan, M.J.; Hossain, M.; Egner, P.A.; Bessong, P.O.; Petri, W.A.; Groopman, J.D.; et al. Aflatoxin exposure in children living in Mirpur, Dhaka: Data from MAL-ED companion study. *J. Expo. Sci. Environ. Epidemiol.* **2019**, *29*, 655–662. [CrossRef]
72. Mahfuz, M.; Hasan, S.M.T.; Alam, M.A.; Das, S.; Fahim, S.M.; Islam, M.M.; Gazi, M.A.; Hossain, M.; Egner, P.A.; Groopman, J.D.; et al. Aflatoxin exposure was not associated with childhood stunting: Results from a birth cohort study in a resource-poor setting of Dhaka, Bangladesh. *Public. Health Nutr.* **2021**, *24*, 3361–3370. [CrossRef]
73. Azziz-Baumgartner, E.; Lindblade, K.; Gieseker, K.; Rogers, H.S.; Kieszak, S.; Njapau, H.; Schleicher, R.; McCoy, L.F.; Misore, A.; DeCock, K.; et al. Case-control study of an acute aflatoxicosis outbreak, Kenya, 2004. *Environ. Health Perspect.* **2005**, *113*, 1779–1783. [CrossRef]
74. Smith, J.W.; Matchado, A.J.; Wu, L.S.; Arnold, C.D.; Burke, S.M.; Maleta, K.M.; Ashorn, P.; Stewart, C.P.; Shaikh, S.; Ali, H.; et al. Longitudinal Assessment of Prenatal, Perinatal, and Early-Life Aflatoxin B(1) Exposure in 828 Mother-Child Dyads from Bangladesh and Malawi. *Curr. Dev. Nutr.* **2022**, *6*, nzab153. [CrossRef] [PubMed]
75. Carlsson, H.; Rappaport, S.M.; Tornqvist, M. Protein Adductomics: Methodologies for Untargeted Screening of Adducts to Serum Albumin and Hemoglobin in Human Blood Samples. *High. Throughput* **2019**, *8*, 6. [CrossRef] [PubMed]
76. Yuan, J.M.; Butler, L.M.; Stepanov, I.; Hecht, S.S. Urinary tobacco smoke-constituent biomarkers for assessing risk of lung cancer. *Cancer Res.* **2014**, *74*, 401–411. [CrossRef] [PubMed]

toxins

MDPI

Review

Species Differences in the Biotransformation of Aflatoxin B1: Primary Determinants of Relative Carcinogenic Potency in Different Animal Species

David L. Eaton [1,*], David E. Williams [2] and Roger A. Coulombe [3]

1 Department of Environmental and Occupational Health Sciences, School of Public Health, University of Washington, Seattle, WA 98195, USA
2 Environmental and Molecular Toxicology, College of Agricultural Sciences, Oregon State University, Corvalis, OR 97331, USA; david.williams@oregonstate.edu
3 Graduate Toxicology Program, Department of Veterinary Sciences, Utah State University, Logan, UT 84322, USA; roger@usu.edu
* Correspondence: deaton@uw.edu

Abstract: It has been known since the early days of the discovery of aflatoxin B1 (AFB1) that there were large species differences in susceptibility to AFB1. It was also evident early on that AFB1 itself was not toxic but required bioactivation to a reactive form. Over the past 60 years there have been thousands of studies to delineate the role of ~10 specific biotransformation pathways of AFB1, both phase I (oxidation, reduction) and phase II (hydrolysis, conjugation, secondary oxidations, and reductions of phase I metabolites). This review provides a historical context and substantive analysis of each of these pathways as contributors to species differences in AFB1 hepatoxicity and carcinogenicity. Since the discovery of AFB1 as the toxic contaminant in groundnut meal that led to Turkey X diseases in 1960, there have been over 15,000 publications related to aflatoxins, of which nearly 8000 have addressed the significance of biotransformation (metabolism, in the older literature) of AFB1. While it is impossible to give justice to all of these studies, this review provides a historical perspective on the major discoveries related to species differences in the biotransformation of AFB1 and sets the stage for discussion of other papers in this Special Issue of the important role that AFB1 metabolites have played as biomarkers of exposure and effect in thousands of human studies on the toxic effects of aflatoxins. Dr. John Groopman has played a leading role in every step of the way—from initial laboratory studies on specific AFB1 metabolites to the application of molecular biomarkers in epidemiological studies associating dietary AFB1 exposure with liver cancer, and the design and conduct of chemoprevention clinical trials to reduce cancer risk from unavoidable aflatoxin exposures by alteration of specific AFB1 biotransformation pathways. This article is written in honor of Dr. Groopman's many contributions in this area.

Keywords: aflatoxin; biotransformation; species differences; cytochrome P450; glutathione S-transferase; biomarkers

Key Contribution: Evolutionary differences in the function and expression of biotransformation enzymes have led to remarkable species differences in sensitivity to the potent liver toxin and carcinogen, aflatoxin B1. This paper reviews the extensive literature on this topic and identifies that subtle structural differences in numerous biotransformation enzymes confer most of the well-recognized difference in susceptibility to AFB1 toxicity and carcinogenicity across species.

1. Introduction

The initial discoveries of aflatoxin as a potent hepatotoxin among turkeys, ducks, and certain strains of trout in the early 1960s provided the first insights into the potential long-term risk of cancer in humans [1–4]. However, tumors were not evident in the turkeys, perhaps because the potent hepatotoxic effects caused mortality well before tumors had a chance to develop. However, at approximately the same time, a strain of rainbow trout was identified as susceptible to the toxicities of *A. flavus*-contaminated feed, including the occurrence of liver tumors. Even just 5 days of exposure to 20 ppb aflatoxin B1 (AFB1) in the diet of young rainbow trout resulted in a 12% incidence of liver tumors 12 months later [2]. Soon after, rainbow trout were identified as perhaps being the most sensitive animal to the carcinogenic effects of AFB1, wherein trout fed a diet containing only 8 parts per billion of AFB1 developed liver tumors at a 70% incidence 12 months later [1]. The potent hepatocarcinogenic effects of purified AFB1 in mammals was demonstrated in 1967 by Wogan and Newberne [3]. A few years later they completed a more in-depth dose–response lifetime assessment of the hepatocarcinogenicity of aflatoxin in male Fisher rats, further highlighting the potent, dose-related carcinogenic effects of AFB1 in mammals [4]. However, Wogan's group also found that a standard strain of laboratory mice (Swiss mice) seemed completely resistant to the carcinogenic effects of AFB1, with doses as high as 150,000 ppb producing no tumors [5].

Although there are likely numerous fundamental biochemical differences that contribute to such remarkable species differences in susceptibility to the carcinogenic effects of aflatoxin, it is now well recognized that such differences are predominantly related to specific biotransformation pathways. The biotransformation of AFB1 is somewhat complex, involving multiple steps of oxidation, reduction, conjugation, and macromolecular adduct formation. Although the metabolic pathways that AFB1 undergoes are qualitatively similar in most, if not all, vertebrate species, there are important quantitative differences in the expression and catalytic activity of the enzymes responsible for AFB1 biotransformation that impart large differences in the relative species sensitivity to the carcinogenic—as well as other toxic—effects of AFB1. While aflatoxin metabolism has been reviewed extensively over the past decade (see the following references as examples: [6–17]), this review provides a detailed historical context to the development of our current understanding of the important role that subtle differences in both the expression and catalytic activity of a variety of biotransformation enzymes play in determining relative species susceptibility to the carcinogenic effects of AFB1.

2. Phase I Biotransformation of AFB1: Oxidation Reactions

There are numerous different oxidative pathways for AFB1, nearly all of which are mediated via one or more cytochromes P450 (CYPs; Figure 1).

2.1. Step #1 Oxidation of AFB1 to Aflatoxin-8,9-Epoxide

There is little question that the initial oxidation of AFB1 to the unstable aflatoxin B1-8,9-epoxide (AFBO) represents the single most important step involved in most, if not all, toxic effects, including carcinogenesis. There are two stereoisomers of AFBO, designated 'exo-' and 'endo-' AFBO, where the epoxide structure is either above or below the plane of the rest of molecule. Only the exo- isomer reacts with DNA [18]. The importance of the double bond in the cyclopentanone ring is illustrated by the much lower toxicity and carcinogenicity of aflatoxin B2 (AFB2) [19], which is chemically identical to AFB1 except that this double bond is absent.

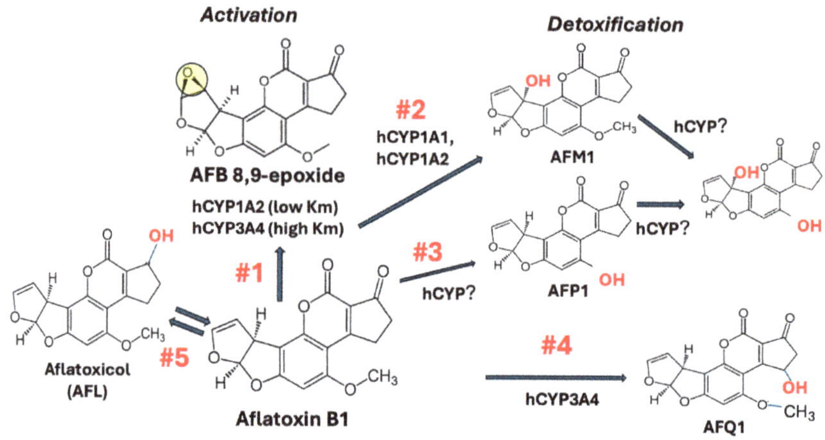

Figure 1. Basic steps in the oxidation of AFB1 to various metabolites. The human enzymes, where known, catalyzing these oxidations are listed. Each oxidation step shown in Figure 1 is discussed in detail below, with a focus on understanding important species differences in each oxidation step, as well as the specific enzyme isoforms that contribute to each reaction.

The oxidation of AFB1 to AFBO is mediated almost exclusively by the cytochrome P450 (CYPs) family of enzymes. There is a large body of in vitro and in vivo data on liver microsomal biotransformation of AFB1 in a variety of species. Ramsdell and Eaton [16] compared the initial rates of oxidation of AFB1 in human, rat, mouse, and Macaca liver microsomes under identical experimental conditions, using a high AFB1 concentration of 124 μM (Figure 2). Formation of AFBO, measured by trapping the epoxide with BHA-induced mouse liver cytosol, occurred in the rat at a rate of 0.6 nmol of product/mg of microsomal protein/min, which was about 3 times higher than human, but less than mouse and Macaca microsomes (Figure 2).

More recently, Gerdemann et al. [6] compared the disposition of AFB1 in primary cultures of isolated hepatocytes obtained from mouse, rat, and human liver, using LC-MS-MS to characterize individual biotransformation products (Figure 3).

An important advantage of using intact hepatocytes, versus microsomal or post-mitochondrial fractions of the liver, is that both cytosolic and microsomal enzymes are present and organized in a manner similar to what occurs in vivo. However, a disadvantage is that gene expression can change substantially during the isolation process and over the time course of experimentation. Thus, primary hepatocytes may not accurately reflect the quantitative distribution of specific biotransformation enzymes seen in vivo, including enzymes involved in the biotransformation of AFB1 [20,21]. It is evident from Figure 3 that there are large differences in metabolite distribution across the three species, and that the ratios of different metabolites vary substantially when comparing a low (1 μM) to relatively higher (10 μM) initial AFB1 concentration. Mouse hepatocytes demonstrated nearly complete (99%) biotransformation of the added AFB1 at 1 μM, whereas human hepatocytes metabolized only about 20% of the added AFB1. Rats eliminated 78% of the administered dose over the 4 h incubation. However, at 10 μM AFB1, the intrinsic clearance increased from 19% to 32% in human hepatocytes. Other important species differences in AFB1 metabolites found in this and other studies are discussed in the following sections.

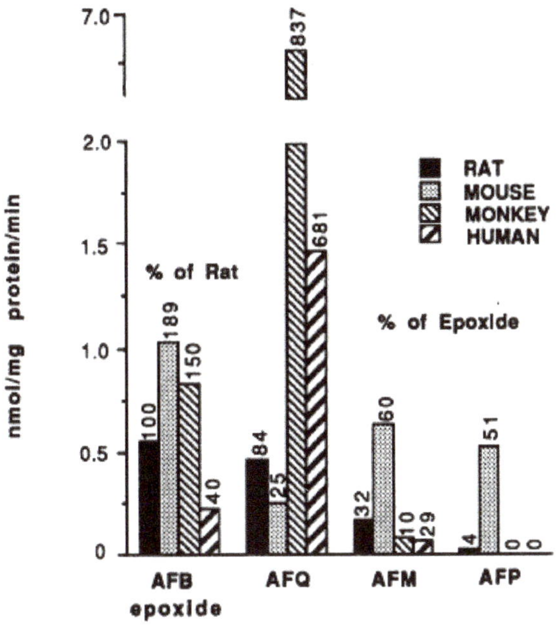

Figure 2. Hepatic microsomal oxidation of AFB1 to various oxidative metabolites in different species. The initial rates of formation (Vo) were determined in hepatic microsomes from rat, mouse, monkey, and human microsomes under identical experimental conditions. AFBO was determined by trapping as the GSH conjugate using BHA-induced mouse liver cytosol, which contains a high level of mGSTA3-3. Each metabolite was separated and quantitated by HPLC. Rates of AFBO formation as a percentage of that observed with rat liver microsomes are also shown. The rates of formation of AFQ1, AFM1, and AFP1 were calculated as a percentage of the rate of epoxidation observed for the respective species; these values are shown above each column. (From Ramsdell and Eaton [16]). Reprinted under AACR copyright permissions to authors.

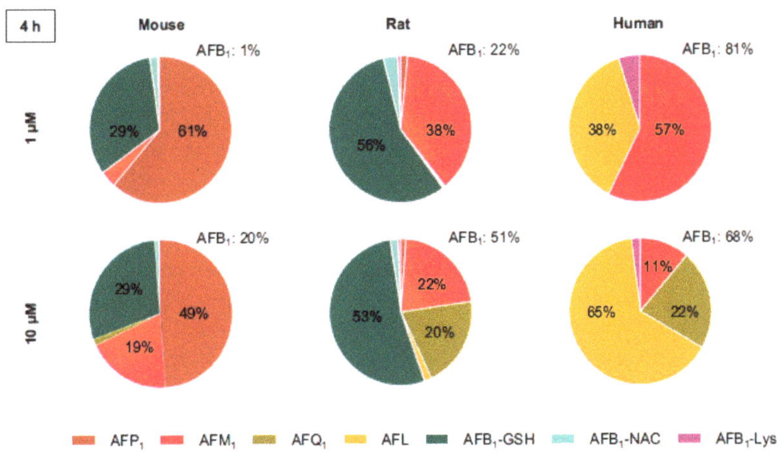

Figure 3. AFB1 metabolite distribution at 1 µM and 10 µM in mouse, rat, and human hepatocytes. Isolated hepatocytes from each species were incubated for 4 h in cell culture medium. Metabolites were identified by HPLC-MS/MS. (From: Gerdemann et al. [6]; figure is reprinted under Creative Commons Attribution 4.0 International License).

Role of Specific Isoforms of CYPs in Activating AFB1 to AFBO, by Species

a. Humans

The role of specific human CYPs in biotransformation of AFB1 is well established. Human hCYP1A2, hCYP3A4, hCYP3A5, hCYP3A7 and hCYP2A13 are all capable of activating AFB1 to AFB-8,9-epoxide [18,22–25], but the kinetic characteristics are distinct and important [23]. hCYP3A5 is variably expressed at relatively low levels in the human liver. CYP3A7 is primarily a fetal form that has been shown to activate AFB1 to the 8,9-epoxide [26,27] and, thus, could play an important role in AFB1 disposition if exposure occurs in utero [28]. Aflatoxin–albumin adducts have also been identified in cord blood of newborns whose mothers were exposed to aflatoxin in the diet in The Gambia [29].

In contrast to CYP3A4, which preferentially forms AFQ1, CYP3A5 metabolizes aflatoxin B1 mainly to the exo-8,9 epoxide but is ~100-fold less efficient compared to the formation of AFQ1 [30]. There is a large genetically determined variability in expression of hepatic CYP3A5 between individuals, with many individuals showing no expression. For example, ~40% of African Americans do not express this enzyme [31]. Therefore, differences in expression of CYP3A5 could influence susceptibility to aflatoxins.

hCYP2A13 is expressed in human lung tissue, but not liver. Thus, it is generally agreed that hCYPs 1A2 and 3A4 are the predominant CYP enzymes that can generate AFBO in human liver. hCYP1A2 forms roughly equal amounts of both endo- and exo-AFB-8,9-epoxide, whereas hCYP3A4 appears to form predominantly the exo form of epoxide [18] (and relatively greater amounts of AFQ1). This is important, because AFB1 exo-8,9-epoxide reacts with DNA to give adducts in high yield (>98%). This interaction is characterized by a K_d of ~1.4 μM, intercalation between base pairs, and rapid reaction to form AFB-N7-guanine adduct [32]. Although some studies suggested that hCYP3A4 is the predominant hCYP in forming AFBO in vitro [33], these and other studies have utilized relatively high concentrations (e.g., >50 μM) of AFB. However, Gallagher et al. [23] examined the reaction kinetics of AFB1 oxidation by hCYP1A2 and hCYP3A4 in both human liver microsomes (HLMs) and in human CYP3A4 and CYP1A2 cDNA-expressed lymphoblastoid microsomes using relatively low concentrations. AFBO formation by cDNA-expressed human CYP1A2 followed Michaelis–Menten kinetics, with a Km of 41 μM and a Vmax = 2.63 nmol/min/nmol P450. In contrast, hCYP3A4 formation of AFBO in cDNA-expressed hCYP3A4 microsomes was sigmoidal and exhibited the kinetic characteristics of "substrate activation". Application of a sigmoid Vmax model equivalent to the Hill equation produced excellent fits to the cDNA-expressed CYP3A4 data and to the data from HLMs pretreated with the specific hCYP1A2 inhibitor, furafylline, which selectively inhibits hCYP1A2 activity. The Hill model predicted that two substrate binding sites are involved in hCYP3A4-mediated AFB1 catalysis and that the average affinity of AFB1 for the two sites was 140–180 μM, about 4 times higher than the Km for hCYP1A2. However, the hCYP3A4 Vmax values for AFBO formation were substantially greater than that for hCYP1A2, reflective of the relative amounts of the two proteins in human liver microsomes [23].

Using the derived kinetic parameters for hCYP1A2 and h3A4 to model the in vitro rates of AFB1 activation at low substrate concentrations, Gallagher et al. [23] predicted that CYP1A2 contributes to over 95% of AFB1 activation in human liver microsomes at 0.1 μM AFB. However, at in vitro concentrations of AFB1 greater than about 10 μM, CYP3A4 appears to the dominant contributor to AFBO formation. Kamdem et al. [24] conducted a similar kinetic study with baculovirus-expressed hCYP1A2, 3A4, 3A5, and 3A7, as well as human liver microsomes, and concluded that CYP3A4 was the dominant human CYP that forms exo-AFBO. They disagreed with Gallagher et al., stating that "*However, the critically important hepatic expression levels of P450 1A2 and P450 3A4 were not considered in the calculation. The postulated dominant role of P450 1A2 in AFBO production was also not supported by the Vmax of AFBO production, which was highest in the liver with the highest P450 3A4 expression and not in the liver with the highest P450 1A2 expression, as would be expected (in Gallagher et al.* [23]*)".*

But Kamdem et al. [24] used only five concentrations of AFB1, ranging from 25 to 500 μM, to assess their kinetics, and at these relatively high concentrations were not able to observe the important Hill kinetics characteristics that occur when an enzyme has more than one substrate binding site, one of which serves as a "self-activator" of activity, as shown by Gallagher et al. for AFB1 [23]. Gallagher et al. used nine different substrate concentrations, ranging from 0.5 to 512 μM, which was sufficient to demonstrate non-linearity at low doses, consistent with Hill, but not Michaelis–Menten, kinetics. Numerous other studies have demonstrated non-linear Hill kinetics for hCYP3A4 with numerous substrates [34–38]. Hill kinetics dictate that, at low substrate concentrations (<1 μM for AFB1), the high apparent Km (low binding affinity) for AFB1 precludes any significant catalytic activity by hCYP3A4, even if there are relatively large amounts (high Vmax) of protein available. And Gallagher et al. did consider the relative amounts of CYP1A2 and 3A4, as they used human liver microsomes, which have substantially greater amounts of CYP3A4 protein compared to CYP1A2. Kamdem et al. [24] did not include any substrate concentrations below 25 μM in their kinetic assessment, and thus did not observe Hill kinetics, versus Michaelis–Menten, in their evaluation. This led them to conclude that CYP3A4 was far more important in exo-AFBO formation than CYP1A2, even at low substrate concentrations.

Most importantly the role of hCYP1A2 in the hepatic in vitro activation of AFB1 at low substrate concentrations (0.13 μM) was supported by DNA binding studies using human liver microsomes in the Gallagher et al. study. AFB1-DNA binding in control HLMs (reflecting the contributions of both CYP1A2 and CYP3A4) and furafylline-pretreated microsomes (reflecting the contribution of CYP3A4 only) catalyzed the binding of 1.71 and 0.085 pmol equivalents of AFB1 to DNA, respectively, demonstrating that hCYP1A2 was responsible for 95% of AFB1-DNA adduct formation, even though the amount of CYP3A4 protein was much higher than that of CYP1A2.

The results of Gerdemann et al. [6] from human hepatocytes also illustrate the important kinetic differences in AFBO formation between high and low concentrations of AFB1 and the relative contribution of hCYP1A2 and hCYP3A4 to oxidative metabolism of AFB1 (Figure 3, human). At 1 μM AFB1, AFM1 represents 57% of total metabolites, and AFQ1 is less than 1% of epoxide formation (sum of dihydrodiol, AFB-GSH, and AFB-Lys). However, at 10 μM, AFM1 drops to 11%, AFQ1 increases to 22%, and AFBO increases to 66%. This change in metabolite distribution, and the overall increase in the rate of total biotransformation, is consistent with Hill kinetics for CYP3A4 formation of AFBO and AFQ1. The 10 μM concentration of AFB1 in the hepatocytes was sufficient to induce substrate activation of CYP3A4. Thus, at a low AFB1 concentration of 1 μM, CYP1A2 dominates biotransformation, resulting in large amounts of both AFM1 and AFBO, whereas at a high substrate concentration (10 μM), CYP3A4 is allosterically activated and contributes substantially to overall clearance and increases the amount of both AFBO and AFQ1 formation.

Thus, the studies of Gallagher et al. [23,39,40] and Gerdemann et al. [6] demonstrate that CYP1A2 dominates the activation of AFB1 in human liver microsomes in vitro at sub-micromolar concentrations and support the hypothesis that hCYP1A2 is the predominant CYP responsible for AFBO activation (exo-AFBO) in human liver in vivo at the relatively low dietary concentrations encountered in the human diet, even in high-AFB1-exposure regions of the world.

Finally, it is worth noting that CYP1A2 is a hepatic-specific CYP, consistent with the relatively selective toxicity and carcinogenicity of AFB1 in the liver. However, inhalation exposure to aflatoxin can occur and could potentially cause lung toxicity or cancer if there were CYPs in the lung capable of activating AFB1 to AFBO. Indeed, several studies have demonstrated this potential. Putt et al. [41] demonstrated that rabbit and rat nasal mucosa microsomes were highly active in forming AFBO from AFB1, and demonstrated that cDNA-expressed rabbit CYP2A10 and 2A11, which are expressed in nasal mucosa, were effective at forming AFB-DNA adducts when incubated with AFB1. Several studies have found that human CYP2A6 does have AFBO formation activity, although this is less active than that of either CYP1A2 or 3A4 in cDNA expression assays for AFBO-generating activity [22,42]. hCYP3A4 is also expressed in the human lung, albeit at relatively low levels, and has been shown to activate AFB1 in human lung microsomes [43]. A recent review of occupational exposure studies on mycotoxins [44] found nine reports in the literature that have identified AFB1 in dusts in a variety of settings (animal husbandry (three studies), agriculture (four studies), and waste plants (two studies)). However, few studies have examined lung cancer risk among workers exposed to AFB1-contaminated dust. One small occupational epidemiology study of workers in a plant that extracted oil from linseed and peanuts during the period 1961–1968 assessed the potential for inhalation exposure to AFB1 to cause cancer, including lung cancer [45]. Aflatoxins were measured in the plant, and estimates of exposure were based on inhalation of dust particles containing trace amounts of AFB1. Although the study was small (N = 71), there were seven cases of lung cancer identified among the AFB1-exposed workers, with only three in a matched control group (N = 68). But information was not available on individual smoking histories, so no strong conclusions can be drawn from this small cohort study. No liver cancers were detected in the small cohort.

Since CYP3A4 is expressed in human intestinal tissue, including colon [46,47], and is capable of activating AFB1 to exo-AFBO, it is possible that relatively high concentrations of AFB1 in the diet could induce DNA damage and possibly cancer in the human intestinal tract. Harrison et al. [48] found AFB1-DNA adducts in human colon tissues, and hypothesized that AFB1 could contribute to colon cancer risk. However, to date there is little evidence demonstrating an association between dietary aflatoxin exposure and colon cancer.

b. Non-human primates

There is relatively little information on the role of specific CYPs in the biotransformation of AFB1 by non-human primates. One study [49] compared the microsomal oxidation of AFB1 to AFBO, AFM1, AFP1 and AFQ1 in human liver with two species of non-human primates (*Macaca* and Marmoset). The mean activation of AFB1 to AFBO in human, Macaque, and Marmoset liver microsomes (N = 3 for each) was 68.7, 55.2, and 25.3 pmol/min/mg microsomal protein, respectively, at an AFB1 concentration of 16 μM, with a 2.8-fold range of activity in the three human liver samples. However, an earlier study that compared AFB1 metabolism in hepatic microsomal fractions from human, rat, mouse, and non-human primates (*Macaca nemestrina*) found that, at a relatively high substrate concentration of 124 μM, Macaque liver microsomal activity of AFBO formation was about 3 times higher than that of human liver microsomes (Figure 2; [16]). Thus, it appears that the livers of these two species of non-human primates have a roughly similar AFB1 activation potential as human liver, although there are no studies evaluating which specific CYP enzymes are responsible, nor any studies assessing relative activities at lower substrate concentrations relevant to human exposures (e.g., <0.1 μM).

c. Rats

In 1991 Ch'ih et al. [50] conducted an experiment with isolated rat hepatocytes to evaluate the role of various biotransformation pathways in the overall disposition of AFB1 and determine whether AFB1 metabolites are excreted into the extracellular environment. Cells were incubated with 1500 pmol/10^8 cells for 60 min, and then the cells and the media were analyzed for the presence of various AFB1 metabolites (Table 1).

Table 1. Distribution of oxidative metabolites of AFB1 (1500 pmol/10^8 cells, or approximately 20 μM) following 1 h of incubation in isolated rat hepatocytes. (Data from Ch'ih et al [50]).

AFB1 Form	% of Total	% Extracellular
Unchanged AFB1	5%	6%
Bound to DNA + proteins	23%	BDL
AFB-GSH	60%	72.4%
Distribution of Oxidative Metabolites		
AFBO (Bound + AFB-GSH)	83%	-
AFM1 (15% conjugated)	3%	92%
AFP1 (93% conjugated)	13%	95%
AFQ1 (<31% conjugated)	1%	89%

BDL: Below limit of detection.

The key points here are as follows: (1) ~95% of the AFB1 was metabolized; (2) of that, 83% was biotransformed to AFBO (sum of "bound" and AFB-GSH), and (3) only 1% of the overall oxidative metabolism was attributed to hydroxylated forms (AFM1, AFP1, and AFQ1); (4) of those, AFP1 was the dominant form in rat liver hepatocytes; and (5) there was a remarkable capacity of liver cells to transport metabolites out of the cells and into the extracellular media.

The results of Gerdemann et al. (Figure 3; [6]) in primary cultures of isolated rat hepatocytes are consistent with this finding, showing AFBO formation of about 60% of total biotransformation products. These results also suggest that rat CYP3A2 may exhibit similar allosteric activation as human CYP3A4, since AFQ1 was less than 1% of overall metabolites at 1 μM but increased to 20% of overall metabolites at 10 μM.

Perhaps surprisingly, few studies have evaluated which specific rat CYPs are involved in AFBO formation. Although the specific rat CYPs involved in AFBO formation are not known for certain, there is some evidence suggesting that rCYP3A2 (orthologous to hCYP3A4) and rCYP2C11 are involved in metabolic activation of AFB1 in the rat [51,52]. In contrast to humans, rat CYP1A2 appears to play little role in hepatic activation of AFB1 [53], and it is likely that rCYP3A2 is the predominant CYP in rats that forms AFBO.

d. Mice

As illustrated in Figure 2, mouse liver microsomes have relatively high activity to form AFBO from AFB1, nearly twice that of rat and about 5 times greater than human liver microsomes. As noted previously, adult mice are highly resistant to the carcinogenic effects of AFB1, but apparently it is not because they cannot form the genotoxic AFBO. As with rats, there is relatively little information on which specific CYPs form AFBO in mouse liver, although mouse Cyp3a11 and 3a13 have been shown to possess AFBO-forming activity [54,55]. However, there is some evidence that mouse Cyp2a5 may also be involved in AFB1 activation [56]. The role of mouse Cyp1 enzymes in AFB1 is unclear. However, one study found that inhibitory antibodies to mouse Cyp1a2 had less inhibitory effect on AFB1 activation than did inhibitory antibodies to mCyp2b or mCyp3a, suggesting that mCyp1a2 may play only a minor role in AFB1 activation in mouse liver [57]. Thus, it remains uncertain exactly which mouse Cyp enzyme(s) is/are responsible for activation of AFB1 to AFBO, although the Cyp3 family is likely to contribute significantly.

e. Fish/salmonids

The sensitivity of rainbow trout to hepatocellular carcinoma induction by AFB1 is due in large part to trout CYP2K1, a constitutively expressed CYP in liver [58]. Trout CYP2K1 (previously designated as trout liver LM2) was purified from liver of BNF-treated trout [59,60]. CYP2K1, down-regulated by BNF treatment, could be distinguished from the BNF-induced CYP1A1 (previously designated as trout liver LM4b) by its *lambda* max of 450 nm in the CO-reduced versus CO spectra compared to LM4, and by immunochemical specificity with rabbit antibodies raised to either CYP [60,61]. The isozymes could also be distinguished by substrate specificity. CYP2K1 did not display any activity in vitro toward benzo[*a*]pyrene but exhibited high activity toward AFB1 [58,60]. Conversely, trout CYP1A1 had only 15% of the turnover with AFB1 compared to CYP2K1 and failed to produce any adducts with added calf thymus DNA.

Purified trout CYP2K1 was incubated with ^{14}C-AFB1 and metabolites separated by HPLC and quantified by scintillation counting of peaks (365 nm) corresponding to AFB1-8,9-diol (hydrolysis product of the epoxide), AFQ1, and AFM1 (Figure 1). CYP2K1 exhibited high regioselectivity (72% of metabolites produced) toward production of the 8,9-*exo*-epoxide (Table 2). In addition to AFB1, purified hepatic CYP2K1 and BV-CYP2K1 (expressed with baculovirus) exhibit regioselectivity toward omega-1 hydroxylation of lauric acid [62–64]. AFB1 is also epoxygenated to produce covalent DNA adducts in vivo in zebrafish [65]. Although zebrafish are only 4-fold less efficient than trout at AFB1-DNA adduction in vivo, they exhibit relative resistance to AFB1-induced HCC [66]. CYP2K6, expressed from zebrafish, has activity toward conversion of AFB1 to the exo-8,9-epoxide but, unlike trout CYP2K1, has no activity toward lauric acid [67].

Table 2. Metabolic profile [^{14}C]-AFB1 and DNA binding of [^{3}H]-AFB1 catalyzed by reconstituted rat CYP3A1 or CYP1A1 and trout CYP2K1 or CYP1A1.

Enzyme [a]	Water Fraction [b]	Peak 1 [c]	AFBO	AFQ1	AFM1	TOTAL	DNA-Adducts [d]
rCYP3A1	17	62	30	37	27	173	6
rCYP1A1	17	26	20	34	125	222	1
trCYP2K1	34	57	404	39	27	561	131
trCYP1A1	8	47	5	14	12	86	ND

[a] CYPs (0.1 nmol) were reconstituted with rat NADPH P-450 oxidoreductase (0.2 nmol), DLPC (15 μg), SDS (50 μg), and NADPH (0.5 mM) in 50 mM Tris-HCL (pH 8.0) buffer containing EDTA (0.1 mM) and $MgCl_2$ (15 μM) and incubated for 30 min at either 30° or 37 °C. Metabolites were quantified by scintillation counting of fractions co-eluting with standards. Values are in pmol/min/nmol CYP and represent the average of duplicates. [b] Water fraction represents [^{14}C]-AFB1 radioactivity in the soluble fraction containing unidentified AFB1 metabolite(s). [c] Peak 1 is also an unknown early eluting peak containing unidentified AFB1 metabolite(s). [d] DNA adduction was determined using the same reconstitution system but with the addition of 150 μg calf thymus DNA and [^{3}H]-AFB1 as substrate. Data are from Williams and Buhler [58].

In addition to a high rate of CYP2K1 conversion to the AFB1-exo-epoxide, there is evidence in trout of a slow rate of inactivation of the epoxide by liver GST or trapping with other nucleophiles [68]. This factor, plus the slow rate of DNA repair of bulky adducts such as the 8,9-dihydro-8-(N7-guanyl)-9-hydroxyaflatoxin B1, in salmonids enhances the carcinogenic potency of AFB1 [69,70]. The species difference in salmonids (rainbow trout and coho salmon) was attributed solely to the rate of AFB1-8,9-epoxide formation in trout [70]. A log-linear relationship, evident at exposure levels of 0.05–100 μg/kg, between AFB1 dietary dose in trout and HCC, was demonstrated in a 40,000 animal ED001 (effective dose producing 0.1% incidence) tumor study [66]. A log-linear response between AFB1 dose and liver DNA adduction has been demonstrated both in trout and rat [71].

f. Avians (Turkeys, Chickens, Ducks)

Avians, especially turkeys, are extremely sensitive to the toxic effects of AFB1 [72–74]. As discussed in the Introduction, this extreme sensitivity to AFB1 was graphically demonstrated when it was discovered to be the etiological agent of "Turkey X Disease", resulting in widespread deaths of turkeys and other poultry throughout Europe in the 1960s. This event was determined to have been caused by AFB1-contaminated Brazilian peanut meal used for poultry feed [75]. Among avian species, turkeys are considered to be the most susceptible to aflatoxins, quails have intermediate susceptibility, while chickens are considered relatively resistant [72]. Wild turkeys appear to be less susceptible to AFB1 than their domesticated counterparts [76].

In contrast to the abundant data on the role of individual mammalian P450s on AFB1 bioactivation, there is limited information on avian orthologues. Reflecting whole-animal susceptibility differences, turkey liver microsomal AFB1 epoxidation activity was determined to follow a rank order of turkey > quail > chicken [77]. Using P450-orthologue specific substrates, inhibitors, and antisera, CYP1A2, and, to a lesser extent, 3A4, orthologues were postulated to be critical in AFB1 bioactivation in turkey liver [73]. Microsomal AFB1 bioactivation in turkeys is age-related, in that younger birds are more efficient than older birds [78]. The critical role of CYP1A5 in the biological action of AFB1 was further supported by a demonstration that inhibitors of this enzyme alleviate symptoms of aflatoxicosis in poultry exposed to dietary AFB1. Dietary butylated hydroxytoluene (BHT) protects against AFB1-associated symptoms in turkeys, in part, due to its inhibitory effect on P450 1A5, exhibiting Michaelis–Menten competitive inhibition kinetics (K_i = 0.81 μM) [79]. However, these early microsomal metabolic studies were of limited value in identifying, with certainty, AFB1-bioactivating P450 orthologues in avian liver because they relied upon substrates, inhibitors, and antisera validated in mammalian rather than in avian systems.

Confirmation of the central role of avian P450s 1A2 and 3A4 orthologues in AFB1 bioactivation was provided when turkey P450s were cloned and functionally characterized [80]. Turkey liver CYP1A5, the first functional protein amplified from turkeys to be cloned, was predicted to contain 528 amino acids with 94.7% sequence identity to chicken CYP1A5, the structure of which was equivalent to that of human CYP1A1, with seven exons and six intervening sequences. Intron sequences were highly similar to the available chicken sequences (Introns 1 and 4–6), with similarity values of aligned intron and UTR sequences exceeding 91% [80]. Like its human homologue, the *E. coli*-expressed CYP1A5 efficiently bioactivated AFB1 to AFBO, and in addition, produced AFM1. The CYP1A family identity of CYP1A5 was confirmed using specific inhibitors of catalytic activities, and through genetic mapping showing that the structure of the turkey gene was shown to be equivalent to that of the human *CYP1A* genes with seven exons of 38, 858, 127, 90, 124, 87, and 307 bp, and six introns. A single nucleotide polymorphism (SNP) in the 3′ UTR (untranslated region) was used to assign *CYP1A5* to turkey linkage group M16 (equivalent to chicken chromosome 10) [81]. Heterologously expressed CYP1A5 is extremely efficient in AFB1 bioactivation to exo-AFB1 as demonstrated by kinetic values of Km and Vmax of exo-AFBO formation of 65 ± 12 μM and 0.61 ± 0.037 nmol/min/nmol P450, respectively (R^2 = 0.93). Kinetics of AFM1 formation were 34 ± 9 μM and 0.91 ± 0.070 nmol/min/nmol P450, respectively [80].

In a follow-up study, a CYP3A4 orthologue in turkey liver was cloned, heterologously expressed, and functionally characterized, with particular focus on its activity toward AFBO formation. The CYP3A37 gene has an open reading frame (ORF) of 1512 bp, and the protein is predicted to be 504 amino acids with 97% identity to chicken P450 3A37 [82]. These studies showed that the turkey 3A37 was significantly less efficient in AFB1 bioactivation than turkey 1A5, as exemplified by Km and Vmax values for the formation of exo-AFBO of

287 ± 21 μM and 1.45 ± 0.07 nmol/min/nmol P450, respectively [83]. Sequencing of the turkey genome in 2010 enabled a precise comparative assignment of the relative roles of turkey CYPs 1A5 and 3A37 in AFB1 bioactivation [84]. Building on this DNA sequence information, Rawal and Coulombe [85] constructed anti-peptide antibodies directed against P450 1A5 and 3A37 as tools to investigate the role of these enzymes in bioactivation of AFB1 in turkey liver microsomes, especially at relatively low concentrations likely to be achieved in turkey liver in vivo. Anti-peptide antisera are valuable tools for isolating the catalytic contribution of individual AFB1-metabolizing P450s in multi-enzyme systems such as liver microsomes to identify the predominant enzyme. Metabolism in immuno-inhibited microsomes resembled that of individual enzymes. For example, when the contribution of P450 3A37 was immuno-inhibited, microsomes oxidized AFB1 to only two detectable products, exo-AFBO and AFM1, the kinetics of which were characterized by hyperbolic Michaelis–Menten kinetics of tCYP1A5. In incubations where 1A5 was inhibited, 3A37 produced exo-AFBO and AFQ1 following Hill kinetics. At 0.1 μM AFB1, (approximating AFB1 concentrations in livers of exposed animals), 1A5 contributed ~98% of the total exo-AFBO formation (Figure 1). At this concentration, 1A5 accounted for a higher activation: detoxification (50:1, exo-AFBO: AFM1) compared to 3A37 (0.15:1, exo-AFBO:AFQ1), suggesting that 1A5 is high, while 3A4 is the low-affinity enzyme in turkey liver. AFB1 bioactivation by 3A37 at low AFB1 concentrations is minimal. The data support the conclusion that, in turkey liver, CYP1A5 is the dominant enzyme responsible for AFB1 bioactivation and metabolism at environmentally relevant AFB1 concentrations in turkey liver [85]. The CYP3A37 enzyme predominates in AFBO formation but only at high, pharmacologically irrelevant AFB1 (i.e., >100 μM) concentrations (Figure 4).

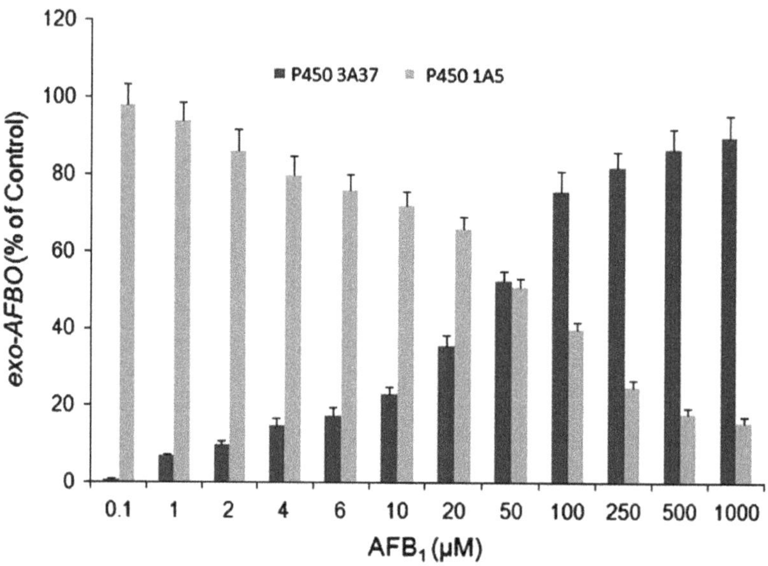

Figure 4. Immuno-inhibition experiments using anti-peptide antiserum against turkey P450s 1A5 and 3A37 demonstrating the relative contribution of P450 1A5 and 3A37 toward AFB1 epoxidation in turkey liver microsomes. Inhibitory effects of anti-P450 1A5 and 3A37 immune serum (5 μg/mL/nmol P450). Initial rates of exo-AFBO formation in the presence of antiserum were calculated as percentage control (treatment with pre-immune serum only). Mean ± SD. (N = 3). From: Rawl and Coulombe, [85]. Reprinted under Open Access Creative Commons Attribution.

2.2. *Step #2 Oxidative Biotransformation of AFB1 to Aflatoxin M1*

In 1963 Allcroft et al. [86,87] proposed that milk from dairy cattle fed AFB-contaminated feed could contain aflatoxin or a toxic metabolite derived from it. Ducklings administered milk from dairy cattle fed aflatoxin-contaminated feed demonstrated toxic symptoms similar to that seen when the ducklings were fed contaminated groundnut meal. Soon after, De Iongh et al. identified the toxin in milk by thin layer chromatography, and proposed calling it Aflatoxin M1 [88]. It is a simple hydroxylation product of AFB1, in the 9a position (Figure 1, reaction #2).

AFM1 is formed in humans following ingestion of dietary AFB1, as indicated by early studies in the Groopman laboratory, where AFM1 was one of several AFB1 metabolites found in human urine by affinity chromatography [17].

Although generally considerably less toxic and carcinogenic than AFB1, AFM1 can be activated to the 8,9-epoxide (AFMO) and thus exhibits similar toxicity to AFB1. The relative carcinogenic potency of AFM1 in Fisher rats is about 2–10% of that of AFB1 [89]. However, Purchase et al. [90] found that AFM1 had similar acute toxicity as AFB1 in 1-day old ducklings. Thus, species differences in the relative toxicity of AFM1 and AFB1 could be important. Because milk is a food staple that can constitute 100% of the diet of infants, the FDA tolerance level for AFM1 in milk is 0.5 ppb, 40 times lower than the tolerance for AFB1 in food (20 ppb) (See: https://www.fda.gov/regulatory-information/search-fda-guidance-documents/guidance-industry-action-levels-poisonous-or-deleterious-substances-human-food-and-animal-feed#afla (accessed on 28 December 2024).

Numerous studies in several species have investigated the carcinogenic effects of AFM1. A comparison of AFB1 with AFM1 in weanling Fisher rats given 25 mg of either AFB1 or AFM1 by gavage for 5 days per week for 8 consecutive weeks found that 100% of the rats given AFB1 had liver tumors at the termination of the experiment, whereas only 1 (3%) rat in the AFM1 group had a liver tumor, although many had preneoplastic lesions [4]. Cullen et al. [91] also compared the relative carcinogenic potency of AFM1 with AFB1 in Fisher rats in a chronic bioassay, and found AFM1 to be carcinogenic in both the liver and intestine, with a potency about 2–10% less than AFB1. AFM1 was also shown to be a potent carcinogen in rainbow trout [92]. Trout hepatocytes exhibit significantly lower DNA adduction in vitro when incubated with AFM1 compared to AFB1 [93]. Hepatic DNA adduction in vivo following injection of trout fry with AFM1 was 11% that of AFB1 and the yield of HCC at 12 months was 8.6% that of AFB1 [94].

As noted above, although AFM1 is often considered a "detoxification" product, it can also undergo activation to the reactive epoxide (AFMO). Studies with human microsomes and lymphoblastoid cells (cell line MCL-5) that were stably transfected with human cDNAs for CYPs 1A2, 2A6, 3A4, and 2E1 together with microsomal epoxide hydrolase were used to evaluate the formation of metabolites of AFM1 [95]. Overall, epoxidation of AFM1 by human liver microsomes was substantially less than seen for AFB1, although some AFM1-dihydrodiol and AFM1-GSH conjugates were evident.

Role of Specific CYP Isoforms in Activating AFB1 to AFM1, by Species

a. Humans

AFM1 was the major AFB1 metabolite in primary cultures of isolated human hepatocytes at a relatively low substrate concentration of 1 μM (Figure 3; [6]), accounting for 57% of overall metabolites.

hCYP1A1 and hCYP1A2 both form AFM1 from AFB1 [18,23,39]. hCYP1A1 forms predominately AFM1, whereas hCYP1A2 forms both AFM1 and AFBO in a ratio of AFM1:AFBO of 1:2.5 [39]. hCYPIA2 produced a higher ratio of activation/ deactivation products (AFBO:AFM1 = 3:1), and the rate of formation of AFBO was about 30-fold higher than that of hCYP1A1. In contrast, hCYP1A1cDNA-expressed microsomes produced >10 times more AFM1 than AFBO [39]. However, hCYP1A1 is not constitutively expressed in human liver, although exposure to AhR ligands found in cigarette smoke and the diet may cause some induction of hCYP1A1 in human liver.

Although human microsomes can form AFMO from AFM1, it is not clear which specific human CYPs are capable of activating AFM1 to the DNA-binding epoxide, or the protein-binding dihydrodiol [95].

Urinary AFM1 has been used as a biomarker of aflatoxin exposure in numerous studies [96–103].

b. Non-human primates

Macaca liver microsomes have a relatively low initial rate of formation of AFM1, similar to humans (Figure 2; [16]. The ratio of AFM1:AFBO in Macaca is 1:10, whereas in humans it is 1:3, largely because the Macaca microsomes are approximately 3 times more active than human microsomes in forming AFBO (Figure 2). Bammler et al. [49] found that liver microsomes from the Marmoset monkey also had a ratio of AFM1:AFBO of about 1:10.

c. Rats

The data in Figure 2 demonstrate that rat liver microsomes are somewhat more efficient at forming AFM1, compared to those of human liver, but the ratio of AFBO:AFM1 is about the same. In isolated rat hepatocytes, AFM1 constituted ~3% of total AFB1 metabolites (Table 1) [50]. However, Gerdemann et al. found that AFM1 accounted for 38% of total AFB1 metabolites after 4 hr of incubation (Figure 3; [6]). Although few, if any, studies have explicitly evaluated specific rodent CYPs for AFM1 formation, it is likely that rat CYP1A isoforms are responsible, as has been described in humans. Gurtoo et al. [104] demonstrated that induction of CYP enzymes in rat liver by the AhR agonist β-naphthoflavone (BNF) substantially increased the formation of AFM1, but also reduced hepatocarcinogenicity of AFB1 by 75%. This is consistent with AFM1 formation via CYP1A1 activity in the rat [39].

d. Mice

Mouse liver microsomes are relatively efficient at forming AFM1, compared to either rat or human microsomes (Figure 2). In primary cultures of mouse hepatocytes at a low substrate concentration of 1 μM, AFM1 accounted for ~3% of total metabolites. However, this increased to 19% at 10 μM (Figure 3; [6]). As with rats, there is no specific Cyp mouse form that has been demonstrated to do this, but it is a reasonable assumption that AFM1 is formed by a mCyp1a isoform. There was little strain differences in formation of AFM1, among eight different strains of mice examined, with the exception of the CD-1 mouse, which had activity about 50% of the activity seen in the other seven strains [105].

e. Fish/Salmonids

Treatment of trout with CYP1A1 inducers such as BNF, PCBs, or indole-3-carbinol prior to or concurrent with AFB1 dosing resulted in a significant reduction in hepatic DNA adduction and subsequent reduced incidence and multiplicity of HCC. Consistent with these results, the metabolic profile of AFB1 both in vitro and in vivo is altered by treatment with BNF, resulting in increased production of AFM1 and a marked reduction in AFL1 [58,69,106,107].

f. Avians (Turkeys, Ducks, Chickens)

As mentioned above, recombinant *E. coli*-expressed CYP1A5, like the human orthologue 1A2, produces AFM1, in addition to efficiently bioactivating AFB1 to AFBO [78]. Otherwise, scant comprehensive data exist on metabolic products of AFB1 in the livers of avian species. But reports of residues of AFB1 metabolites in the tissues of AFB-challenged birds have been reported. For example, in AFB1-fed quail, residues of AFM1, AFB2α, and AFL were detected in eggs [108]. Similarly, AFL and AFM1 was measured in the liver, kidney, and thigh of both male broilers and hens fed AFB1 [109]. Breast meat from laying hens fed AFB1 contained AFL and AFM1 [110].

2.3. Step #3 Oxidative Biotransformation of AFB1 to Aflatoxin P1

Aflatoxin P1 (AFP1) is formed via oxidative demethylation (Figure 1, reaction #3). There appears to be substantial differences among species in the extent of O-demethylation of AFB1 to form AFP1. Based on hepatic microsomal assays, AFP1 was not detected in monkey or human liver microsomes, but was a substantial metabolite produced by rat liver microsomes (Figure 2), and constituted 13% of total oxidative metabolites in isolated rat hepatocytes, of which 93% was found as the glucuronide conjugate, and nearly all of that was exported out of the hepatocytes (Table 1; [50]). Consistent with that observation, the glucuronide conjugate of AFP1 is also a major metabolite of AFB1 in rat bile [111]. However, comparative studies in primary cultures of mouse, rat, and human hepatocytes found that AFP1 was the major oxidative metabolite in mouse hepatocytes, but was a very minor metabolite in rat hepatocytes, and was largely undetectable in human hepatocytes (Figure 3; [6]). Bammler et al. [49] also found no measurable AFP1 formed in microsomal incubations from human, Macaque, and Marmoset monkey livers (N = 3 for each), at 16 μM AFB1 concentration.

Groopman et al. [112] found AFP1 in the urine of human subjects exposed to AFB1 in the diet, although there was no significant correlation between urinary AFP1 levels and estimated dietary intake. In contrast, highly significant correlations were seen between dietary exposure and AFM1 and AFB-N7-Guanine adducts in urine. The authors noted that biliary excretion may be the primary route of elimination of AFP1, and that unconjugated AFP1 in the urine may be highly variable depending on the dose and extent of conjugation, making urinary AFP1 an unreliable biomarker of exposure.

It should be noted that the microsomal enzyme assays typically used to measure AFB1 oxidation may fail to capture the true extent of AFP1 formation. It is possible that AFP1 is rapidly conjugated with glucuronic acid, since UDP-glucuronosyl transferases (UGTs) are also microsomal enzymes and specific membrane transport processes in the endoplasmic reticulum concentrate potential substrates in microsomal membranes [113]. If AFP1 was conjugated after formation in the microsomes, it would not be detected in the HPLC assays used to identify unconjugated AFP1. However, conjugation requires the presence of a significant concentration of uridine diphosphoglucuronic acid (UDPGA), and it is unknown whether residual levels of UDPGA may be present in incubations following isolation of the microsomal fraction.

Role of Specific Isoforms of CYPs in Activating AFB1 to AFP1, by Species

a. Humans

There is relatively little information on which specific CYPs are responsible for the O-demethylation of AFB1 to AFP1 in human liver. Although structurally different than AFB1, the plant toxin aristolochic acid (AA) undergoes a similar O-demethylation of reaction of an anthracene-based O-methyl analog in AA. Stiborova et al. [114] demonstrated that multiple human CYPs contributed to the O-demethylation of AA, but that CYP1A2 was responsible for approximately half of the overall activity, whereas CYP3A4 contributed about 10% of overall activity. Thus, it is reasonable to hypothesize that CYP1A2 contributes to the formation of AFP1 as well as AFBO and AFM1.

b. Non-human primates

As noted above, Bammler et al. [49] compared hepatic microsomal biotransformation of AFB1 in two non-human primate species, *Macaca nemestrina* (Macaque) and *Callithrix jacchus* (Marmoset), with human liver microsomes, and AFP1 formation was below the limit of detection in all six monkey livers (N = 3 for Macaque and Marmoset), as well as in all three human liver microsomal preparations.

No studies were identified that have evaluated specific monkey CYPs for formation of AFP1.

c. Rats

AFP1 is a major oxidative metabolite of AFB1 in rat liver microsomes, as shown in Figure 2. As noted above, Ch'ih et al. [50] also demonstrated that AFP1 is, by far, the dominant hydroxylated AFB1 metabolite formed in isolated rat hepatocytes (Table 1), although Gerdemann et al. [6] found AFP1 to be a minor metabolite in isolated rat hepatocytes. It is unclear whether methodological, and/or rat strain, differences are responsible for this apparent discrepancy. To date, there are no studies that have definitively identified which rat CYP(s) is/are responsible for the formation of AFP1 in the liver.

AFP1 can also undergo a second oxidation reaction for form 4,9a-dihydroxy-AFB1. The same product can be formed via secondary oxidation of AFM1 and appears to be conjugated with glucuronic acid [115].

d. Mice

AFP1 is formed at levels substantially greater than AFQ1 or AFM1 in mouse liver microsomes (Figure 2) and isolated hepatocytes (Figure 3), although, as with rats, there is little information on the specific Cyp form(s) in the mouse that is/are responsible for AFP1 formation.

e. Fish/salmonids

AFB1 O-demethylation to AFP1 is a minor or non-detectable metabolite in trout both in vitro and in vivo. AFP1 has been shown to be a much weaker mutagen and carcinogen in trout [116].

f. Avians (Turkeys, Chickens, Ducks)

AFP1 has not been identified as a significant oxidative metabolite of AFB1 in turkeys or other avian species.

2.4. Step #4 Oxidative Biotransformation of AFB1 to Aflatoxin Q1

Hydroxylation of AFB1 on the cyclopentanone ring gives rise to AFQ1 (Figure 1, reaction #4). In contrast to AFM1, there is little information to suggest that AFQ1 exhibits any significant toxicity, and thus is generally considered a complete detoxification product. The acute toxicity of AFQ1 is only about 5% of AFB1, and in vitro mutagenicity assays found little mutagenic activity for AFQ1 [117,118]. AFQ1 is the predominant in vitro metabolite of AFB1 in human and *Macaque* (monkey) liver microsomes, but is a relatively minor metabolite in rodent (rat, mouse) microsomes (Figure 1) [16,119,120].

Role of Specific Isoforms of CYPs in Activating AFB1 to AFQ1, by Species

a. Humans

There is substantial evidence that hCYP3A4 is the predominant, if not sole, form of hCYP responsible for the formation of AFQ1 in vitro [23,24,33,40,120–122]. As discussed above for AFBO production by human CYPs, CYP3A4 shows unusual non-linear kinetics for AFQ1 formation as well as for AFBO [23]. But even at relatively low concentrations of

AFB1, the relatively high levels of expression of hCYP3A4 in human liver are adequate to form substantial amounts of AFQ1, as suggested by several in vivo studies.

Ezekiel et al. [123] reported that AFQ1 was the predominant aflatoxin metabolite found in urine of infants who were either exclusively breast-fed or non-exclusively breast fed, in a region of the world with notably high mycotoxin exposure (Ogun state, Nigeria). AFQ1 was detected in the urine of 20 out of 23 (87%) exclusively breast-fed infants and 24 of 42 (57%) non-exclusively breast-fed infants. AFM1 was detected in only 6 of the total 65 infant urine samples collected from both cohorts, and the levels of AFM1, where detected, were substantially lower than those of AFQ1. The observation that AFQ1 was present in the urine of infants fed exclusively breast milk demonstrates that AFQ1 was a major metabolite of AFB1 in the nursing mothers and is passed into breast milk. In a study in China, AFQ1 and AFM1 were measured in the urine and feces of 83 young Chinese males selected from a larger population based on the presence of detectable AFM1 in their urine. AFQ1 was measured at levels ~60 and 260 times higher than AFM1 levels in feces and urine, respectively [124].

As noted previously, Gerdemann et al. [6] found AFQ1 was a very minor metabolite at a low (1 μM) AFB1 concentration, but a major metabolite at a higher (10 μM) AFB1 concentration, consistent with the dose-dependent allosteric activation found for AFB1 metabolism to AFBO and AFQ1 by human CYP3A4 [23,39].

b. Non-human primates

Roebuck and Wogan [5] demonstrated that AFQ1 was, by far, the predominant metabolite formed from male rhesus monkey post-mitochondrial supernatant liver preparations (similar to microsomal fractions except that cytosolic enzymes were also present). The formation of AFQ1 in the two monkey liver fractions was higher than that seen for three human liver preparations. Formation of AFQ1 in both rhesus monkey and human liver tissue was >10 times greater than the small quantity of AFQ1 formed in mouse and rat liver fractions. Krieger et al. [118] also demonstrated that AFQ1 was the major metabolite of AFB1 in rhesus monkey liver, with a Vmax about 10 times higher than that for AFM1.

Bammler et al. [49] compared hepatic microsomal biotransformation of AFB1 in two non-human primate species, *Macaca nemestrina* (Macaca) and *Callithrix jacchus* (marmoset), with human liver microsomes, and also found that AFQ1 was, by far, the major oxidative metabolite, with an initial rate of oxidation of ~450 pmol/min/mg protein in both species, 3 times faster than the rate of formation of AFQ1 in human liver microsomes.

No studies using specific CYP enzymes from non-human primates were identified, although it is highly likely that the formation of AFQ1 was mediated by CYP3A64, the rhesus monkey homolog to human CYP3A4, as the deduced amino acid sequence of CYP3A64 is 93% homologous to human CYP3A4, and they have similar activities toward a variety of CYP3A4 substrates [125].

c. Rats

In contrast to primates, rats appear to form less AFQ1 than AFBO (Figure 2), at least at low substrate concentrations (Figure 3; Table 1). In vivo studies support the relatively low rate of AFQ1 formation in rats. For example, Tang et al. [126] administered male F344 rats 250 ug/kg of AFB1 5 days per week for three weeks. Daily urinary AFQ1 levels were 10–50 times lower than AFM1 levels over the 15 days of measurements. No kinetic studies on the oxidative formation of AFQ1 by rat CYP3A2, the ortholog to human CYP3A4, were identified, so it is not clear why rat CYP3A2 (or rat CYP3A1) seems to have much less catalytic activity toward AFQ1 formation, relative to primate CYP3A forms. However, the strong substrate concentration dependence of AFQ1 formation in rat hepatocytes suggests that rat CYP3A2 may follow similar Hill kinetics (allosteric activation), as shown for human CYP3A4 [23,39].

d. Mice

As with rats, mouse liver microsomes seem to have relatively little ability to form AFQ1, as mouse liver microsomes were about 5- and 2-fold less active in forming AFQ1 than human and rat liver microsomes, respectively (Figure 2). No information was identified as to which mouse Cyp(s) is responsible for the relatively small amount of AFQ1 formed, but it would be reasonable to assume that mCyp3a11 was primarily responsible. Cyp1a2 in mouse liver (C57Bl/6 strain) was expressed at about 75% of the level of Cy3a11 [127].

e. Fish/Salmonids

As with mouse and rat, AFQ1 is a minor metabolite in trout, constituting less than 5% of the total metabolites produced by trout liver microsomes [59] (Table 2) and is the weakest mutagen and carcinogen of the primary AFB1 metabolites produced in trout [116].

f. Avians (Turkeys, Ducks, Chickens)

Like human P450 3A4, the *E. coli*-expressed 3A37 biotransformed AFB1 to exo-AFBO and to AFQ1 and possessed nifedipine oxidation activity, both of which were inhibited by the CYP3A4 inhibitor 17α-ethynyl estradiol. The kinetics of oxidation of AFB1 to exo-AFBO followed apparent sigmoidal Hill kinetics, suggestive of an allosteric interaction between the enzyme and the AFB_1 substrate, similar to that described for hCYP3A4 [23]. The Hill coefficient (n) value for tCyp3A37 was 1.9 for exo-AFBO and 1.6 for AFQ1, indicative of positive cooperativity.

3. Phase I Biotransformation of AFB1: Reduction Reactions

Reduction reactions are relatively uncommon in vivo, except in the somewhat anerobic environment of the intestine, where the microbiome readily does both oxidation and reduction reactions. For aflatoxin, there is only one known reduction reaction of AFB1.

Step #5: Reduction of AFB1 to Aflatoxicol (AFL)

Several in vitro studies in a variety of species have demonstrated that the cyclopentanone ring of AFB1 can be reduced to AFL (Figure 1, #5) [128–132]. The reaction is enzymatically mediated via cytosolic reductase(s), but little is known about which specific enzyme(s) is/are involved. Salhab and Edwards [132] compared liver cytosolic fractions from eight species for AFL-forming activity. Rabbit and trout liver formed large quantities of AFL, but the other six species, including human liver cytosol, showed little to no AFL formation. However, once formed, AFL is oxidized back to AFB1 via microsomal dehydrogenases present in the liver. When synthetically prepared AFL was introduced into microsomal fractions from different species (in the presence of carbon monoxide to inhibit CYP oxygenases), liver microsomes from all eight species tested showed some ability to oxidize AFL back to AFB1, with human and hamster liver showing the highest activity [132].

Several studies suggested that AFL was highly toxic to ducklings [133] and mutagenic in different assays [134]. Thus, reduction of AFB1 to AFL may not be a detoxification reaction because it can quickly be oxidized back to AFB1.

Given the relatively small amount of information on the specific reductases and dehydrogenases involved in reduction and oxidation of AFL, we will not detail these reactions by each species. Although early studies suggested that differences in the rate of reductive formation of AFL and its oxidation back to AFB1 may be important in determining species sensitivity [132], very little research on this pathway has been completed in the last 40+ years, with the exception of a 2020 study of poultry liver. Murcia and Diaz [135] evaluated enzyme kinetics for both AFB1 reductase and AFL dehydrogenase activity in 12,000× *g* supernatant fractions of liver from chicken (two different strains), duck, turkey, and quail liver. There were substantial differences in the kinetic characteristics across these four avian species. The authors concluded that "*The ratio AFB1 reductase/AFL dehydrogenase enzyme activity was inversely related to the known in vivo sensitivity to AFB1, being highest for the chicken, lowest for the duck and intermediate for turkeys and quail. Since there is no evidence that AFL is a toxic metabolite of AFB1, these results suggest that AFL production is a detoxication reaction in poultry*".

4. Phase II Biotransformation of AFB1: Hydrolysis, Conjugation and Reduction Reactions

4.1. Step #6 Hydrolysis of AFB1 to Aflatoxin B1-Dihydrodiol

Both the exo- and endo- conformations of AFBO are highly unstable and subject to rapid hydrolysis in the presence of water, giving rise to the dihydrodiol product (Figure 5, reaction #6) (reviewed in [136]).

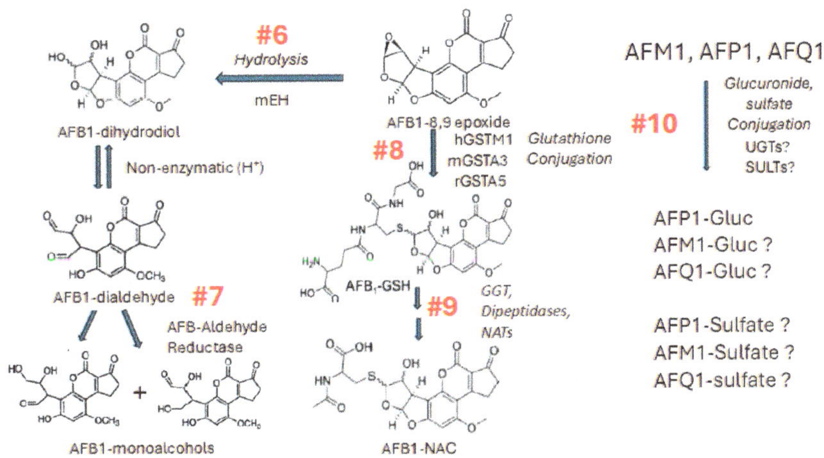

Figure 5. Phase II hydrolysis and conjugation reactions of phase I oxidation products of AFB1 biotransformation.

Although chemically synthesized AFBO is rapidly hydrolyzed in an aqueous environment, the endogenous formation of AFBO in the hydrophobic environment of the endoplasmic reticulum by CYP enzymes must be somewhat protected from spontaneous hydrolysis, because glutathione (GSH) conjugation of the epoxide can occur in the presence of GSH and glutathione-S-transferases (GSTs; discussed in detail in the next section). But hydrolysis of AFBO to the dihydrodiol product does occur, and in the absence of significant GST activity, is a major pathway of elimination for AFBO. Indeed, the half-life of exo-AFBO in an aqueous environment was measured to be approximately 1 s [33]. Because of the high lability of AFBO in an aqueous environment, it was often assumed that hydrolysis was non-enzymatic within the cells.

However, some studies have demonstrated that microsomal Epoxide Hydrolase (mEH) may play an important role in AFBO elimination.

Role of mEH in Hydrolyzing AFBO to AFB-Dihydrodiol, by Species

a. Humans

Guengerich et al. [33,136,137] did not observe any significant effect of purified human EH on the recovery of N7-guanyl-DNA adducts in experiments where synthetic AFBO was mixed with DNA. They did, however, observe a slight increase in the rate of hydrolysis of exo-AFBO (from 0.64/s to 0.78/s) when 19 μM mEH was added to the system [33]. They also used an Ames mutagenesis assay (*Salmonella* strain TA1535) that contained cDNA-expressing hCYP3A4 and varying amounts of purified mEH to evaluate whether mEH could reduce AFB1 mutagenesis. They found a very slight reduction in mutagenesis at high ratios of mEH:CYP3A4 in one purified human mEH sample, but little to no effect with a second. They concluded: "*Further studies are needed to evaluate the role of mEH in the metabolism of aflatoxin-8,9-epoxide*" [33].

Kelly et al. [138] examined the potential role of human mEH in hydrolysis of hCYP1A2-generated AFBO in recombinant yeast, by measuring the effects of co-expression of human mEH in AFB-DNA adduct formation (Figure 6).

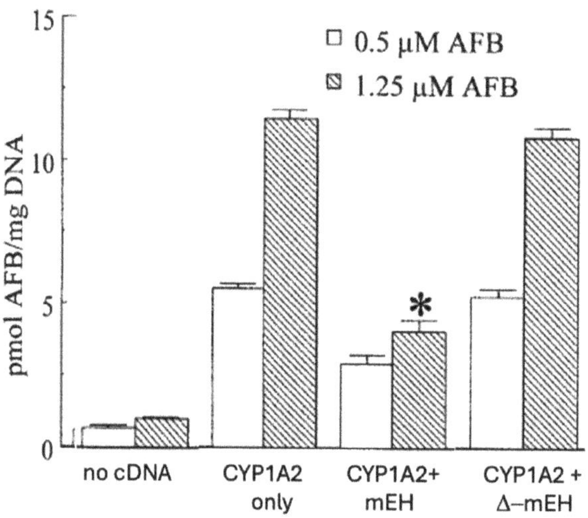

Figure 6. Effects of co-expression of human mEH on AFB-DNA adducts in yeast also co-expressing hCYP1A2 to activate AFB1 to AFBO. Two concentrations of AFB1 were used to expose yeast cells containing human CYP1A2 and mEH cDNAs (adapted from Kelly et al. [138]. * Co-expression of mEH blocked DNA adduction with significant effect ($p < 0.05$) at 1.25 mM AFB. Data are mean 6 SEM from samples analyzed in triplicate. (Figure available under Creative Commons Attribution 4.0 International license).

Co-expression of human mEH with an AFBO-generating system (CYP1A2) resulted in a ~50% decrease in AFB-DNA adducts in the yeast. Insertion of a non-functional mEH cDNA (Δ-mEH) had no protective effect. The yeast strain used was developed for mutagenesis assessment via a *Trp*-reversion assay, so mutagenesis assessment was also completed. Similar to the findings for DNA binding, the rate of AFB-induced mutagenesis was also reduced by about 50%. Finally, they also assessed the impact of co-expression of mEH in the Ames *Salmonella* reversion assay, using hCYP1A2-expressing microsomes as an activation system.

The Gerdemann et al. [6] study of AFB1 biotransformation in isolated human hepatocytes also suggested a potentially important role of mEH in the absence of significant GST activity toward AFBO. AFB1–dihydrodiol represented 65% of total AFB1 metabolites at the higher AFB1 concentration of 10 μM (Figure 3). However, it is not possible to distinguish between enzymatic and non-enzymatic hydrolysis in this study.

b. Non-human primates

No studies were identified that examine the putative protective effects of primate mEH in enzymatic hydrolysis of AFBO.

c. Rats

As discussed above for human mEH, Guengerich et al. [33] assessed the ability of purified rat mEH to reduce mutagenicity in the Ames *Salmonella* assay that utilized hCYP3A4 as an activating system, with 20 μM AFB. Rat mEH reduced AFB1 mutagenesis by about 50%, which was substantially larger than the modest mEH protective effect seen in one of two human mEH samples.

d. Mice

No studies were identified that addressed the potential role of murine mEH in detoxifying AFBO. However, because of the very high AFBO-GST activity presence in mouse liver, it is unlikely that mEH plays a significant role in protecting mouse DNA from damage, given the very high protection afforded by mGSTA3-3 (discussed in detail later). This conclusion is supported by the data in Figure 3, where no AFB-dihydrodiol was detected in mouse hepatocytes exposed to either 1 μM and 10 μM AFB1, where 80–90% of total metabolites were either AFB-GSH or AFP1 [6].

e. Fish/Salmonids

Trout liver has been shown to express both cytosolic and microsomal epoxide hydrolase (EH) activity [139]. However, no studies have documented the contribution of microsomal or cytosolic EH in hydrolysis of AFB1-8,9-exo-epoxide, the major metabolite of AFB1 in this species.

f. Avians (Turkeys, Chickens, Ducks)

Diaz and Murcia [140] demonstrated that microsomes prepared from the livers of ducks, turkeys, and chickens produced AFB-dihydrodiol from AFB1. The authors showed that metabolic activity, as measured by Km, showed significant differences among these avian species: ducks were almost 13 times lower that turkey, 20 times lower than quail, and 30 times lower than the chicken breeds [140]. Activity profiles against prototype inhibitors, substrates, and antibody reactivity in immunoblotting implied the significant involvement of CYP2A6 and CYP1A1 orthologues for the production of AFB-dihydrodiol in microsomes prepared from quail and chicken livers.

4.2. Step #7 Reduction of AFB1–Dihydrodiol to AFB1–Dialdehyde, AFB1–Monoalcohols, and AFB1–Dialcohol

The formation of AFB1–dialdehyde occurs non-enzymatically, resulting in two monoalcohols, (Figure 5, reaction #7). However, the dialdehyde itself is reactive and binds to proteins, particularly lysine residues in albumin, and contributes significantly to the acute toxicity of AFB1 [141,142]. There is, however, an aldehyde reductase enzyme that is effective at reducing AFB-dialdehyde to the monoalcohol, and is commonly referred to as "aflatoxin aldehyde reductase", or AFAR (the *AKR7A1* gene in humans) [141,142]. AFAR reduces AFB-dialdehyde to the C-8, and to a lesser extent, C6a, AFB-monoalcohols. AFAR is also able to further reduce C-8 monoalcohol to AFB-dialcohol [141].

Role of Specific Isoforms of Aldo-Ketoreductases in Reducing AFB1–Dialdehyde, by Species

a. Humans

The human aldo-ketoreductase gene, *AKR7A1*, has been identified as the specific AKR form with activity toward AFB-dialdehyde [143]. Guengerich et al. [141] provided a detailed description of both the non-enzymatic and the enzymatic processes that form and eliminate the reactive AFB1–dialdehyde via AFAR. A second gene coding for a protein with hAFAR-like activity, *AKR7A3*, was cloned and expressed in 1999 [144]. A preliminary comparison of the catalytic properties of the two human AFARs found that hAFAR1 (AKR7a1) was less active than hAFAR2 (AKR7A3) toward AFB1–dialdehyde [141].

b. Non-human primates

No information was identified that addressed specific forms of aldo-ketoreductases in non-human primates that reduce AFB-1-dialdehydre to AFB-alcohols.

c. Rats

A direct comparison of the kinetic characteristics of rat AFAR and human AFAR (AKR7A1) found that the rat form was very similar to the human form. No significant species difference was evident [141].

The rat AFAR1 gene is approximately 8 kb long and comprises seven exons and six introns. It also contains an Antioxidant Response Element (ARE) located in the 5′-regulatory region, and is highly responsive to ARE activators such as ethoxyquin [143]. The substrate specificity of rat AFAR demonstrated that it has broad substrate specificity toward a variety of aldehydes and carbonyls, with highest specific activity toward 9,10-phenanthrenequinone (9,10-PQ). The activity toward 9,10-PQ was ~650 times higher than that of aflatoxin aldehyde [145]. Although the constitutive expression of AFAR in rat liver is low [145], induction of AFAR in vitro has been shown to reduce the acute toxicity of AFB1, and was hypothesized to reduce carcinogenic effects of AFB1, along with the parallel induction of certain GST enzymes [146].

To test the hypothesis that AFAR1 could offer protection against the acute and/or chronic toxicity of AFB1 in vivo in the rat, a liver-specific AKR7A1 transgenic Sprague-Dawley rat was constructed. Two lines, AKR7A1(Tg2) and AKR7A1(Tg5), were found to overexpress AKR7A1 by 18- and 8-fold, respectively. Rates of formation of AFB1 alcohols, as estimated from both in vitro hepatic cytosol assays and in vivo urinary excretion products, were increased in the transgenic lines. However, the substantial over-expression of AKR7A1 in the rat did not provide protection against acute AFB-induced bile duct proliferation (a functional assessment of acute hepatotoxicity by AFB1), nor did it protect against the formation of GST-P positive putative preneoplastic foci as a result of chronic exposure to AFB1 [147,148].

d. Mice

No studies evaluating specific aldo-ketoreductases in mouse were identified, although Ellis and Hayes [145] compared rat AFAR activity toward six other substrates with the mouse aldo-ketoreductase enzymes AR1, AR2, and DD1. The substrate specificity of AFAR was substantially different from any of the three mouse enzymes.

e. Fish/Salmonids

Trout liver cytosol displays slow but detectable aldo-ketoreductase activity toward AFB1 [149], but no information is available on the identity of this AKR or its role in AFB1-induced HCC in this species.

f. Avians (Turkeys, Chickens, Ducks)

Murcia and Diaz [135] reported that hepatic AFAR activity is correlated with acute toxicity of AFB1 in chickens and ducks. These results suggest that AFAR activity is related to resistance to the acute toxic effects of AFB_1 in chickens and ducks, but not in quail and turkey.

4.3. Step #8 Conjugation of AFBO with Glutathione by Glutathione S-Transferases (GSTs)

As discussed above for reaction #1 (Figure 1), the formation of the highly reactive and genotoxic AFBO is an essential step in both acute toxicity and carcinogenesis of AFB1. Although AFBO is highly reactive and unstable in an aqueous environment, it is able to form mutagenic adducts with DNA (discussed in detail later) unless it is either hydrolyzed non-enzymatically, or enzymatically via mEH (Figure 5, reaction #6), or unless it is trapped via reaction with reduced glutathione (GSH; Figure 5, reaction #8). Although some reactive electrophiles can interact with GSH non-enzymatically, little, if any, AFB-GSH conjugate is formed in the absence of GSTs.

Of all the biotransformation pathways characterized for AFB1, the GST-mediated conjugation of AFBO exhibits the largest variability among species, as discussed below. The critical role of GSH in protecting mice from the toxic effects of AFB1 was demonstrated in a comparative study of rats and mice given AFB1. Covalent binding of AFB1 to hepatic DNA in the resistant species, the mouse, was 1.2% of the binding observed in the susceptible species, the rat [150]. The mouse also had 52 times greater in vitro hepatic GST activity toward the AFBO compared to the rat. When GSH was depleted by pretreatment with a combination of buthionine sulfoximine (BSO), an inhibitor of GSH biosynthesis, and diethylmaleate, which depletes existing stores of GSH, AFB-DNA binding in the mouse was increased by 30-fold [150,151].

These and numerous other studies have demonstrated that GST-mediated detoxification of AFBO is a major determinant of species differences in sensitivity to AFB1 hepatotoxicity and hepatocarcinogenesis. Slone et al. [152] evaluated the cytosolic fractions of liver from rats, mice, hamsters, and humans (N = 14) for GST activity toward AFBO, using both synthetic AFBO and microsomally generated AFBO (Table 3).

Table 3. Species comparison of hepatic GST-mediated conjugation of microsomally generated and synthetic AFBO (From Slone et al. [152]. Reprinted with permission from Wolter Kluwers Health, Hagerstown MD, 21741; License #5924970823669, 9 December 2024).

	Synthetic AFBO [a]		Microsomally-Generated AFBO [b]	
Species	**pmol mg^{-1}**	**Normalized to Rat**	**pmol min^{-1}**	**Normalized to Rat**
Human [c]	1.8	0.02	<2 [d]	<0.01 [d]
Rat	88.4	1	140	1
Hamster	103	1.2	930	6.6
Mouse	571	6.5	7080	51

[a] The final concentration of synthetic AFBO was 0.4 mM; [b] 125 μM AFB1 was used in the mouse microsomal AFBO generating System; [c] Equal volumes of 14 human liver cytosols were pooled for this assay; [d] Below the practical detection limit of assay (2 pmol min^{-1} per mg protein).

Activity of cytosolic GSTs from mouse liver were ~50-fold higher than from rat liver. Human liver cytosolic GSTs had little or no measurable activity toward AFBO. A small level of GST activity toward a relatively high concentration (0.4 mM) of synthetic AFBO was detectable in human liver cytosol. Among the 14 different liver samples analyzed, there was a 58-fold variability in AFB-GSH conjugating activity, suggesting that genetic variability may play an important role in determining inter-individual differences in susceptibility to AFB1 toxicity and carcinogenicity [152] (discussed further below).

Kirby et al. [153] also compared cytosolic GST activity toward microsomally generated AFBO in six different species with known or suspected differences in susceptibility to AFB-induced liver tumors. They found that AFB-GST activity in the mouse was 10-fold higher than rat, whereas little or no detectable activity was seen in duck, trout, and human liver cytosolic fractions. The results further demonstrated the large species differences in AFB-GST activity that likely play an important role in determining relative species susceptibility to the carcinogenic effects of AFB1.

Role of Specific Isoforms of GSTs in Conjugation of AFBO, by Species

a. Humans

There are 16 different human genes that code for cytosolic GSTs. Nomenclature has typically classified GST genes into seven classes, using Greek alphabet letters to denote each class: alpha (A), mu (M), omega (O), pi (P), sigma (S), theta (T), and zeta (Z) [154,155]. The alpha class contains five different genes, GSTA1, A2, A3, A4, and A5. As shown in Table 2, human cytosolic GST activity toward AFBO is extremely low—below the limit of detection in assays using microsomally generated AFBO [152].

Buetler et al. [49] evaluated bacterially cDNA-expressed and purified human GSTA1-1 and GSTA2-2 activity toward AFBO generated from mouse liver microsomes and found a little activity, which was detectable, but below the limit of quantitation. Raney et al. [52] measured human GST activity toward synthetic exo- and endo-AFBO with purified human alpha-class GSTs A1-1 and A2-2 and also found measurable, but very low, activity compared to rat alpha-class GSTA1-1. They also measured AFBO-conjugating activity for purified human GSTM1a-1a and GSTP1-1. GSTM1a-1a had measurable activity toward exo-AFBO, whereas GSTP1 had no detectable activity. Johnson et al. [156] performed a comparative kinetic analysis of cDNA-expressed and purified human GSTs A1-1, A2-2, M1-1, P1-1, and T-1-1, as well as rat GSTA5-5. hGSTM1-1 had activity (catalytic efficiency) about 20-fold greater than any of the other human GSTs, but it was ~2000 times lower than the high-activity rGSTA5-5. They did detect a small amount of exo-AFBO activity in recombinant hGSTA1-1 that was ~6-fold lower than GSTM1-1.

The identification of human GSTM1-1 as the only human liver GST with significant activity toward exo-AFBO raises interesting questions regarding potential genetic variability in susceptibility to AFB1, since the human GSTM1 gene is highly polymorphic, with ~50% of the human population homozygous-null for the GSTM1 gene. Several studies have examined this hypothesis. Gross-Steinmeyer et al. [157] measured the extent of AFB-DNA adducts formed in primary human hepatocyte cultures incubated with 0.4 μM ^{3}H-AFB1 for 6 h (Figure 7).

There was a 3-fold reduction in AFB-DNA adducts in hepatocytes from GSTM+ livers, compared to livers that lacked the GSTM1 gene (GSTM1-null) [157].

These and other studies [158,159] provide some evidence to indicate that individuals who are GSTM1-null may be at increased risk of AFB1-induced HCC. However, Stewart et al. [159] evaluated human lung samples for the ability to both activate AFB1 to AFBO and to conjugate AFBO with cytosolic GSTs. At a relatively high in vitro concentration of AFB1 (100 μM), AFB-GSH conjugate was seen in all 10 lung samples, but with very large interindividual variability. They genotyped the samples and found no evidence that GSTM1-null lung samples produced less AFB-GSH. They noted that other GSTM forms (GSTM3, GSTM4) are present in human lung tissue, even in GSTM1-null samples, but there is no information on the relative potential of GSTM3 to conjugate AFBO.

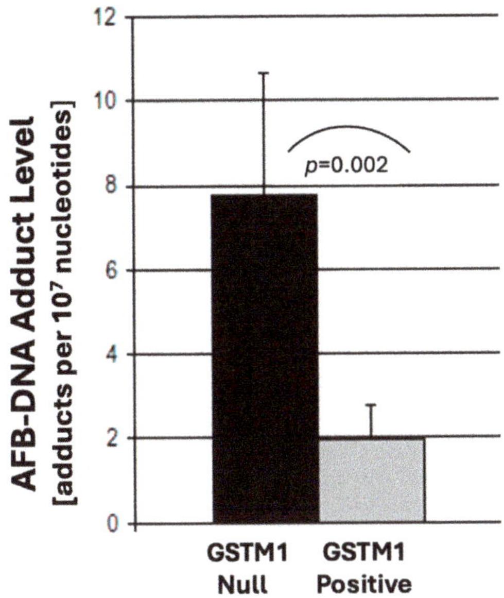

Figure 7. Modulation of AFB-DNA adduct formation in the context of the GSTM1 genotype status. A total of 11 different hepatocyte preparations were examined for AFB-DNA binding. Six of the samples were GSTM1-null and five were GSTM1-positive. AFB-DNA adducts per 10^7 nucleotides were calculated and are shown. Each bar represents the mean and SEM. Statistical significance was determined by unpaired *t*-test with equal variances. Adapted from: Gross-Steinmeyer et al. [157]. Reprinted with permission from Oxford Press, Oxford, UK OX2 6DP; license #5923750542730, 7 December 2024.

b. Non-human primates

Wang et al. [160] purified several hepatic GSTs from the non-human primate, *Macaca fasicularis* (mfaGST) and assessed their ability to conjugate AFBO. Two GSTs exhibited significant AFBO-conjugating activity and were identified by Western blot analysis as belonging to the mu class of GSTs. Similar to those of humans, purified Macaca liver alpha-class GSTs had no detectable AFBO activity. Interestingly, the two Macaca mu-class GSTs differed in their enantioselectivity: one form had higher activity toward the exo-AFBO, and the other had higher activity toward the endo-AFBO. Two cDNA clones of mu-class Macaca GSTs were generated and expressed; one had high activity toward AFBO, and the other had no measurable activity. The high AFBO-activity form shared 86% and 94% sequence homology with hGSTM1a and hGSTM2, respectively. GSTM2 is not expressed significantly in human liver, so does not likely contribute to protection from AFB1. However, the enantioselectivity of the cDNA-expressed mfaGSTM2 was different from the purified mu-class GST, and other differences suggested that the GST protein from the cloned cDNA was not identical to the purified mu-class GST with high AFBO activity. Nevertheless, this paper demonstrated that, like humans, the non-human primate hepatic GST with substantial AFBO activity belongs to the mu-class of GSTs. A subsequent paper cloned and expressed the *Macaca fasicularis* alpha-class GST with homology to human GSTA1 and was shown not to possess any measurable activity toward AFBO [161].

c. Rats

The AFB-GSH conjugate is one of the major metabolites of AFB1 formed in vivo in the rat and is excreted in bile [111,162]. Several studies have evaluated the specific activity of rat GSTs toward AFBO [52,154,163–166]. The major GST expressed constitutively in rat liver is GSTA3-3 [167], but it exhibits less than 0.1% activity toward AFBO compared to mGstA3-3, even though they have similar activity toward the generic GST substrate, 1-chloro-2,4-dinitrobenzene (CDNB) [165,166].

However, another rat GST gene, *GSTA5*, codes for a protein (rGSTA5-5) with high specific activity toward AFBO and is the orthologous rat gene to the mouse *GstA3* gene, which codes for a constitutively expressed protein with extraordinarily high AFBO activity (see discussion below on mouse GSTs). In rats, protection from aflatoxin-induced carcinogenicity may be provided by the induction of rGSTA5 (previously termed rYc2), with high AFBO-conjugation activity [168]. The rGSTA5 subunit shares 91% sequence identity with mGSTA3 and is inducible by ethoxyquin and other antioxidants [169].

Induction of the *rGSTA5* gene with activating ligands for the antioxidant response element pathway (KEAP1/NRF2) greatly reduces AFB-DNA damage in rats, rendering them resistant to the development of preneoplastic lesions and liver tumors [11,170,171].

d. Mice

As discussed above, one specific form of GST in the mouse, mGstA3-3, has been demonstrated to have very high activity towards AFBO and affords extensive protection against AFB1 carcinogenesis in the mouse [172,173]. The mGstA3 gene has been cloned and sequenced [164,174]. The mouse gene is located on chromosome 1, region A3-4, and is encoded by seven exons, spanning approximately 24.6 kb of genomic DNA [175]. A *mGstA3* knockout (KO) mouse has been developed and shows very high sensitivity to AFB-DNA adduct formation, compared to the wild-type, with DNA adduct formation in the KO mouse 112 times greater than in the wild-type (Figure 8) [173].

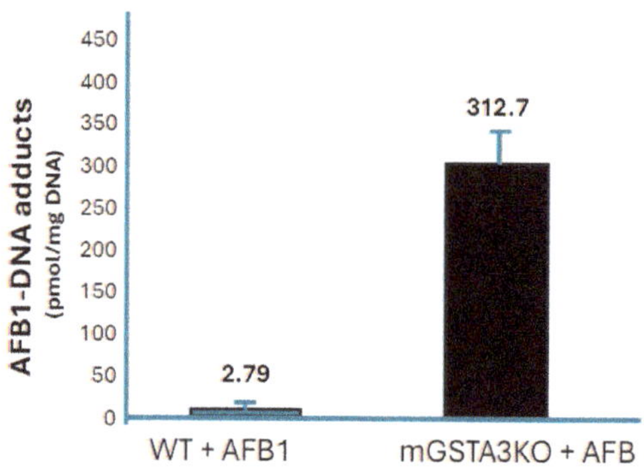

Figure 8. AFB-DNA adduct formation in mGstA3 knockout mice and wild-type. Mice (5 mGstA3 KO and 5 WT, 6 months of age, all males) were injected with a single dose of 5 mg/kg AFB1, dissolved in DMSO, in a volume of 100 μL/30 g of mouse weight, and euthanized 3 h later. Redrawn from: Ilic et al. [173], with permission from Elsevier Press, Berkeley, CA; license # 5923751463839, 7 December 2024.

Amino acid sequence comparison of the high-AFBO-activity mouse GstA3-3 protein with the low-AFBO-activity rat GSTA3-3 protein found only 15 amino acids that are different. Construction of a chimeric rGSTA3 (high AFBO activity) and rGSTA3 (very low AFBO activity) demonstrated that much of the high activity domain of the protein was in the last two-thirds of the protein sequence [165]. Site-directed mutagenesis of the low-activity rGSTA3 gene to different amino acids that were conserved in both the high-AFBO-activity mGstA3-3 and rGSTA5-5 protein identified six amino acids that combine to confer a 2000-fold increase in catalytic activity toward AFBO, approaching that seen in rGSTA5-5, but still 6-fold less than the mGstA3-3 protein (Table 4) [166].

Table 4. Site-directed mutagenesis of rGSTA3 using amino acid substitutions to resemble conserved sites between high AFBO-activity enzymes mGstA3-3 and rGSTA5-5 [a].

Sequence Variant	AFBO-GST Activity	CDNB Activity
(Mutations of fGSTA3 to mGstA3)	nmol/mg/min	mmol/μg/min
mGstA3-3	265.0 ± 11.11 (34)	10.0 ± 0.26 (3)
rGSTA3-3	<0.02 ± 0.0 (9)	18.4 ± 1.04 (9)
rGSTA5-5	57.0 ± 2.32 (12)	9.8 ± 0.79 (6)
hGSTA1-1	<0.02 ± 0.0 (3)	57.1 ± 4.60 (6)
E208D	0.09 ± 0.10 (3)	5.0 ± 0.80 (3)
E208D + H108Y	2.1 ± 0.27 (8)	11.3 ± 1.19 (6)
E208D + H108Y + L207F	5.9 ± 0.56 (12)	48.0 ± 0.90 (9)
E208D + H108Y + L207F + E104I	8.4 ± 0.98 (10)	14.2 ± 0.40 (6)
E208D + H108Y + L207F + E104I + V217K	14 ± 0.62 (23)	23.6 ± 0.64 (6)
E208D + H108Y + L207F + E104I + V217K + Y111H	40 ± 3.09 (9)	8.7 ± 0.31 (9)

[a] Data from Van Ness et al. [166].

One amino acid change, E208D, increased AFBO activity about 100-fold, but additional amino acid changes conferred relatively modest increases, although showing synergistic interactions (Table 3). Surprisingly, adding two additional amino acid changes in the low-activity gene to the high-AFBO sequence (V106Y and Y111H) decreased AFBO-conjugating activity from 40.0 to 2.8 pmol/mg/min [166]. There was no consistent effect on CDNB activity, demonstrating substrate selectivity toward AFBO [166].

Thus, the ~2000-fold differences in AFBO-conjugating activity between the constitutively expressed *mGstA3* gene and the major constitutively expressed alpha-class GST in rats, *rGSTA3*, largely if not completely explains the dramatic difference in sensitivity between mice and rats to the toxic and carcinogenic effects of AFB1.

e. Fish/Salmonids

Conjugation of AFB1-8,9-epoxide with GSH by hepatic GSTs is a minor pathway for AFB1 metabolism in vitro and in vivo [68] and this lack of efficient detoxication is a major factor in the high sensitivity of trout to AFB1-induced HCC.

f. Avians (Turkeys, Chickens, Ducks)

Early studies conducted to determine the biochemical basis for the extreme sensitivity of domesticated turkeys to AFB1 revealed a lack of hepatic cytosolic GST-mediated conjugation activity of exo-AFBO, even in metabolic studies using [^{3}H]-AFB1 as a substrate to enhance sensitivity [73,78] (Figure 9).

Because of the well-established centrality of *GSTs* in species susceptibility, Kim et al. cloned and expressed and functionally characterized six *GSTAs* from the livers of domesticated and wild turkeys [176]. *GSTAs* contained alpha-class conserved domains, signature motifs, and numerous SNPs in their coding regions: *GSTA1.1*, *GSTA1.2*, *GSTA1.3*, *GSTA2*, *GSTA3*, and *GSTA4*. When expressed in *E. coli*, all six *tGSTA* gene products were active toward GST prototype substrates, confirming the catalytic specificity of the GSTA constructs. Activities of cDNA-expressed recombinant GSTAs, as well as their hepatic cytosolic forms, exhibited catalytic activity toward prototype substrates CDNB, DCNB, ECA, and CHP. The highest activity toward CDNB was observed for tGSTA1.2 cloned from domesticated turkey. The GSTA3 allele cloned and expressed from Royal Palm turkeys had substantially higher ECA and CHP activity than all other recombinant GSTs. As we have previously observed in GSTA1.1 from domestic turkey [177], all GSTA1.1 isoforms lack a signature motif (PVxEKVLKxHGxxxL; residues 134–148) in the C-terminal domain. However, this did not appear to discernibly affect the catalytic activity of these recombinant, expressed isoforms. Indeed, the specific enzyme activities of GSTA1.1 were well within the range of that seen from other isoforms.

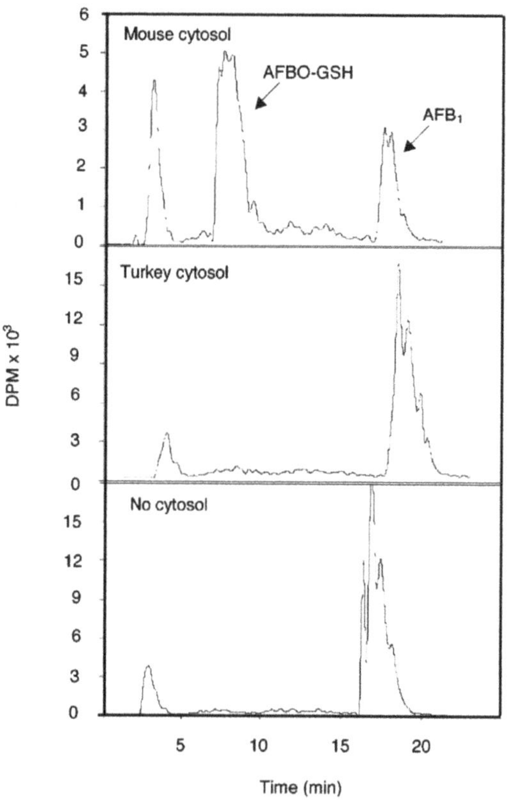

Figure 9. Reverse-phase HPLC radiochromatograms of cytosolic GST conjugation of AFBO in mouse and turkey. The top panel shows [^{3}H]-AFBO-GST activity of BHA-induced mouse liver cytosol (500 mg protein) for comparison. The middle panel show the lack of GST-mediated [^{3}H]-AFBO-conjugating ability of turkey hepatic cytosol (1200 mg protein). A control incubation with no cytosol is also presented (bottom panel). Even when a wide range of turkey cytosolic protein concentrations (400–1200 mg) was used, no GST-mediated trapping was detected [78]. Reprinted with permission from Elsevier Press, Berkeley, CA 94704, license # 5923770700438, 7 December 2024.

Importantly, recombinant GSTAs possessed detoxification activity toward in situ-generated exo-AFBO-reactive intermediate. Recombinant GSTA1.1 and A1.3 from Eastern and Rio Grande wild turkeys appeared to have the highest AFBO-trapping activity. Surprisingly, unlike their hepatic forms, recombinant *E. coli*-expressed *GSTAs* from domesticated turkeys possessed AFBO-trapping activity, on par with that of wild turkeys [178] (Table 5). The observation that recombinant tGSTAs from domesticated turkeys detoxify AFBO, whereas the tGSTs expressed in vivo in the liver do not, implies that the tGST enzymes with AFBO activity are not constitutively expressed and thus must be down-regulated, silenced, or otherwise modified by one or more mechanism(s), possibly epigenetic in nature.

Table 5. Specific GST activity and GST-mediated detoxification of AFBO by unique recombinant alpha-class GSTs and of hepatic cytosolic from domesticated and wild turkeys. Activities obtained from Swiss Webster mouse cytosol are provided for comparison.

	Specific Enzyme Activity (nmol/min/mg Protein)				
	CDNB [1]	DCNB [2]	ECA [3]	CHP [4]	AFB1-GSH [5]
tGST1.1 *	1674.61 ± 48.15 [a]	16.35 ± 0.80 [a]	44.31 ± 2.00 [ab]	451.83 ± 12.41 [ab]	19.54 ± 1.42 [abc]
EWtGSTA1.1	850.45 ± 13.08b [bc]	16.02 ± 0.58 [a]	20.83±0.48 [b]	1977.13 ± 11.45 [de]	26.33 ± 0.89 [de]
rGSTA1.2	7220.94 ± 75.81 [b]	10.85 ± 0.09 [b]	164.51 ± 6.18 [c]	1076.7 ± 11.45 [de]	22.49 ± 1.97 [be]
EWtGSTA1.2	2761 ± 127.16 [e]	5.70 ± 0.16 [c]	48.80 ± 1.37 [ad]	1423 ± 864.02 [ef]	16.59 ± 2.10 [acf]
RGWtGSTA1.2	3137.45 ± 234.93 [f]	8.15 ± 0.61 [d]	69.92 ± 0.96 [d]	2002.85 ± 76.44 [c]	16.62 ± 2.02 [acf]
RPtGSTA1.2	3161.92 ± 15.18 [f]	10.60 ± 0.43 [b]	95.40 ± 7.36 [e]	2769.28 ± 150.69 [g]	21.97 ± 2.54 [be]
tGSTA1.3	1063.48 ± 25.39 [b]	1.46 ± 0.15 [e]	50.58 ± 0.24 [ad]	166.97 ± 68.47 [a]	21.98 ± 2.26 [be]
RGWtGSTA1.3	638.89 ± 12.60 [cg]	1.40 ± 0.05 [e]	23.61 ± 0.51 [b]	1924.87 ± 486.10 [cf]	29.10 ± 1.50 [d]
tGSTA2	3045.23 ± 16.92 [f]	7.55 ± 0.59 [d]	34.49 ± 0.00 [ab]	314.06 ± 7.29 [a]	21.71 ± 0.54 [be]
RGWtGSTA2	1880.01 ± 61.97 [a]	9.31 ± 0.31 [f]	29.58 ± 0.69 [ab]	287.88 ± 7.91 [a]	21.35 ± 0.50 [ab]
RPtGSTA2	1709.40 ± 71.87 [a]	7.23 ± 0.24 [d]	35.85 ± 1.48 [ab]	307.90 ± 8.29 [a]	19.42 ± 0.94 [abc]
tGSTA3	4254.39 ± 37.32 [h]	1.25 ± 0.00 [e]	174.32 ± 1.54 [c]	850.25 ± 59.46 [bd]	18.04 ± 2.67 [abf]
RPtGSTA3	1649.30 ± 53.04 [a]	1.23 ± 0.21 [e]	543.28 ± 24.36 [f]	1934.90 ± 30.79 [cf]	21.42 ± 1.43 [b]
tGSTA4	302.57 ± 44.57 [ij]	0.71 ± 0.28 [e]	21.38 ± 0.98 [b]	27.66 ± 0.45 [a]	20.06 ± 0.33 [abc]
EWtGSTA4	504.92 ± 91.97 [gf]	0.86 ± 0.27 [e]	453.39 ± 15.09 [g]	90.99 ± 3.49 [a]	14.57 ± 1.56 [f]
RGWtGSTA4	251.09 ± 8.98 [j]	1.06 ± 0.42 [e]	365.68 ± 14.88 [h]	91.39 ± 3.52 [a]	16.10 ± 1.29 [cf]
Hepatic GSTs					
DT	1027.20 ± 17.81 [a]	1.51 ± 0.05 [a]	89.58 ± 0.80 [a]	180.87 ± 0.97 [a]	n.d.
EW	714.09 ± 37.10 [b]	2.21 ± 0.30 [a]	90.52 ± 3.75 [a]	209.27 ± 13.56 [a]	0.018 ± 0.004 [a]
RGW	524.14 ± 14.53 [c]	1.59 ± 0.15 [a]	81.06 ± 1.98 [a]	159.56 ± 11.03 [a]	0.028 ± 0.007 [a]
RP	890.18 ± 43.81 [a]	2.61 ± 0.09 [a]	94.78 ± 4.93 [a]	203.91 ± 8.50 [a]	0.017 ± 0.003 [a]
Mouse	2888.69 ± 43.98 [d]	64.55 ± 1.10 [b]	61.10 ± 0.14 [b]	805 ± 43.68 [b]	0.740 ± 0.013 [b]

Under each column, different superscript letters represent significant difference ($p < 0.05$). (A) Recombinant GSTs were analyzed by ANOVA and post hoc LSD was used for mean separation. 1. 1-Chloro-2,4-dinitrobenzene: GSH (1 mM); 2. 1,2-Dichloro-4-nitrobenzene: GSH (5 mM); 3. Ethacrynic acid; GSH (2.5 mM); 4. Cumene Hydroperoxide; GSH (2 mM); 5. AFB1-8,9-epoxide; GSH (5 mM); Mean 6 SD of triplicate determination. * Abbeviations: tGST: domestic turkey; EWtGST: Eastern Wild turkey; RGWtGST: Rio Grande Wild turkey; RPtGST: Royal Palm turkey. From: Kim et al. [178]. Reprinted under Open Access Creative Commons License.

Loss of protective GST alleles in domesticated turkeys through genetic selection for commercially desirable traits is a plausible explanation for their extreme sensitivity compared to wild birds. By comparison, liver cytosol from BHA-induced mice, which expresses high amounts of mGSTA3, the "gold standard" of AFBO-conjugating activity, possessed AFBO-conjugating activity that was 41-, 44-, and 26-fold greater than that in livers from Eastern, Royal Palm, and Rio Grande wild turkeys, respectively. The rate of AFBO conjugation measured in mouse liver [178] was close to that published for similarly BHA-induced Swiss Webster mice [105].

Because human and non-human primate mu-class GSTs have been shown to have catalytic activity toward exo-AFBO [33,156,160], studies were conducted to determine whether GSTM genes in turkeys might also have a role in AFBO detoxification. Livers from domesticated and wild turkeys express two hepatic *mu*-class tGSTs (tGSTMs) which we amplified, cloned, expressed, and functionally characterized [177–179]. These were *tGSTM3* and *tGSTM4* from domesticated turkeys, and a *GSTM4* variant (*ewGSTM4*) from Eastern wild turkeys [179]. The predicted molecular masses of tGSTM3 and two tGSTM4 variants were 25.6 and 25.8 kDa, respectively. Multiple sequence comparisons revealed four GSTM motifs and the mu-loop in both proteins. tGSTM4 has 89% amino acid sequence identity to chicken GSTM2, while tGSTM3 has 73% sequence identity to human GSTM3 (hGSTM3). Specific activities of *E. coli*-expressed tGSTM3 toward CDNB and peroxidase activity toward cumene hydroperoxide were five-fold greater than those of tGSTM4, while tGSTM4 possessed more than three-fold greater activity toward DCNB. The two enzymes displayed equal activity toward ECA. However, unlike the turkey GSTAs, none of the recombinant GSTMs had AFBO detoxification capability. In total, these data indicate that although turkey hepatic GSTMs may contribute to detoxification, they probably play no role in detoxification of AFBO in the liver [179].

4.4. Step #9 Formation of the AFB-NAC Conjugate from AFB-GSH

Once formed, the AFBO-GSH conjugate is subject to transmembrane transport and subsequent enzymatic modifications to the mercapturic acid (Figure 5, reaction #9) [180]. Following conjugation in the hepatocyte, AFB-GSH is transported out of the hepatocyte at the canalicular membrane into the bile. Although no studies were identified that evaluated which of several possible canalicular transporters move AFB-GSH into bile, hydrophobic glutathione conjugates such as AFB-GSH are generally excellent substrates for the multidrug-resistance-associated protein-2 (MRP2) [181,182]. During transport into bile, biliary and/or canalicular γ-glutamyl transferase (γ-GT) removes the y-glutamyl moiety from the AFB-GSH to form a cysteinylglycine S-AFB conjugate (AAFB-Cys-Gly). Moss et al. [183] found that the ratio of AFB-GSH to AFB-Cys-Gly in the bile of rats administered AFB1 intravenously was 5.5:1. They found that inhibition of γ-GT in the rat prior to administration of AFB1 completely eliminated the presence of AFB-Cys-Gly in the bile.

Dipeptidase (DP) present in bile and intestinal tissue then removes the glycine moiety, resulting in a cysteine S-conjugate, which is then absorbed and transported back into the liver [181,182]. In the cytosol, *N*-acetyl transferases create AFB-N-Acetylcysteine (NAC; aka AFB-mercapturic acid), which is more polar and more water soluble than AFB-GSH. AFB-NAC is likely to be non-toxic and excreted from the body through bile or urine.

There is little specific information known about species differences in the formation and excretion of AFB-GSH and its metabolites (AFB-Cys-Gly and AFB-NAC). Since the products of AFB-GSH catabolism are likely of little to no toxicological consequence, we will not discuss this pathway by specific species.

In 1997 the Groopman lab [184] reported on a sensitive LC-ESI/MS method to measure both endo- and exo-AFB-NAC in the urine, with potential use as a biomarker of exposure. After administration of 40 µg of AFB1 for 5 days/week for 8 weeks to rats, urine was collected and analyzed for both endo- and exo-AFB-NAC. About 1% of the administered dose was recovered in urine as AFB-NAC, of which ~90% was the ex-AFB-NAC. Using this assay, Kensler et al. [185] reported the urinary excretion of AFB-NAC was >200-fold higher in wild-type mice compared with single GSTA3 knockout mice, further highlighting the importance of this GST as a key determinant in the resistance of mice to AFB1. An immunoassay for AFB-NAC was also developed [186] and proposed for use as a biomarker of AFB1 exposure. AFB-NAC has been used as a biomarker of AFB1 exposure in several epidemiology studies [126,187]. Wang et al. [187] reported a 2.6-fold increase ($p = 0.017$) in the median rate of AFB-NAC excretion in participants randomized to receive the drug oltipraz daily for 4 weeks compared to placebo. Oltipraz is an effective inhibitor of AFB1 hepatocarcinogenesis in rats, an action likely mediated by induction of GSTs in this species [188]. Perhaps some isoform of human GST can catalyze the conjugation of AFBO under conditions of low ambient AFB1 exposures present in this Chinese study population at the time of the trial. (See also Kensler and Eaton [189] in this *Special Issue* for a discussion of urinary biomarkers of AFB1 exposure.)

Beyond these studies, there is relatively little species-specific information on this pathway.

4.5. Step #10 Glucuronide and Sulfate Conjugation of Hydroxylated AFB1 Metabolites

As noted previously, there is substantial evidence that the glucuronide conjugate of AFP1 is a major biliary metabolite of AFB1 in rats [111,190–192]. AFP1 is a minor oxidative metabolite in humans, and there is little information on which UGT enzyme(s) in humans or other species may form the glucuronide conjugate of AFP1. Several early studies examining the biotransformation of AFB1 reported that the hydroxylated products of AFB1 form glucuronide and sulfate conjugates (Figure 5, reaction #10) [193–197].

Several studies have also shown that direct conjugation of AFB1, or more likely oxidative metabolites of AFB1, with glucuronic acid and sulfate, occurred both in vivo and in hepatocyte cultures [191,192,197–199]. Dalezeos and Wogan [194] reported that AFP1 and its glucuronide and sulfate conjugates were found in the urine of Rhesus monkeys given AFB1. Approximately 50% and 10% were AFP1–glucuronide and AFP1–sulfate, respectively. The balance was unconjugated AFP1.

Wei et al. [192] conducted an extensive analysis to determine the presence of chloroform-extractable and water-soluble AFB1 metabolites in the urine of Rhesus monkey, rat, and mouse given ^{3}H-AFB1. Conjugates of AFM1 were the principal AFB1 metabolites in the urine, accounting for about 20% of total urinary radioactivity, but the hydrolysis procedure used a combination of glucuronidase and sulfatase, so it was not possible to distinguish the contribution of the two. AFP1-conjugate(s) accounted for ~2%, and no AFQ1 conjugate was identified in the urine of monkeys. In rat urine, there was somewhat more AFP1-conjugate(s) than AFM1-conjugate(s), but the fraction of total conjugates was substantially less than seen in either the monkey or mouse urine. Mouse urine contained substantially more water-soluble metabolites, with the distribution of conjugates between AFM1, AFP1, and AFQ1 being similar. There was also a significant quantity of unidentified polar metabolite(s), which may have been the AFB-GSH and AFB-NAC metabolites.

Interestingly, there is some evidence from early studies that AFB1 itself may be subject to glucuronidation and/or sulfation following enol-keto tautomerism of the cyclopentane keto group to a hydroxyl group [192,197]. These authors have suggested that this may contribute to AFB1 toxicity at sites other than the liver, following enzymatic or acid hydrolysis of the conjugate to release AFB1 in other tissues.

Overall, there is relatively little evidence that species differences in glucuronidation and/or sulfation of phase I products of AFB1 metabolism contribute significantly to differences in AFB1 carcinogenicity or other toxic effects.

5. Summary

It is now 65 years on from the discovery of AFB1 as a contaminant of groundnut meal, and identification of its toxic potential. A search of PubMed retrieved 16,741 papers related to aflatoxins between 1960 and the present (Figure 10).

It is evident by the timeline that the scientific world has not lost interest in the public health, veterinary, and agricultural significance of aflatoxins. In the last 5 years, there have been ~750 papers per year, whereas in years prior to 2010, the average number of papers was less than 300 per year. The influence of Professor John D. Groopman's laboratory since he began his training in the laboratory of Dr. Gerald N. Wogan in the late 1970s is illustrated by his publication and citation record (Figure 11). A Web of Science search for Dr. Groopman's publications between 1979 and the present identified 219 publications, with over 7800 papers citing his work (nearly 13,750 total citations). From 1979, when Dr. Groopman published his first paper, to the present, there have been approximately 14,700 publications listed on PubMed on some aspect of aflatoxins.

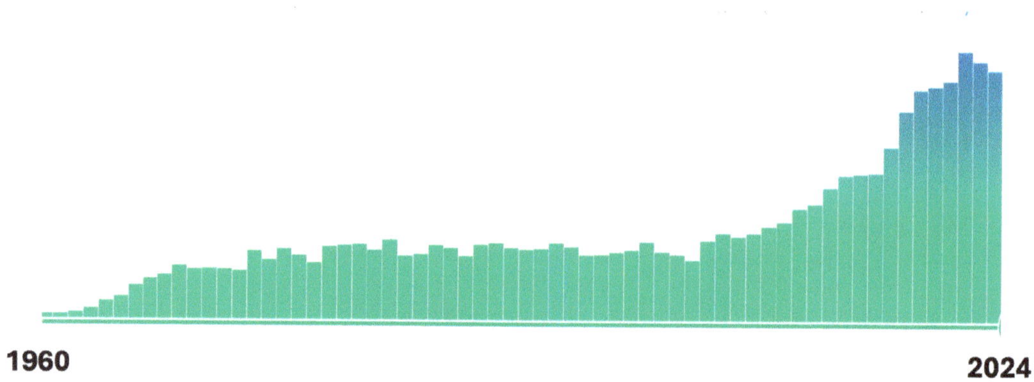

Figure 10. Timeline of research interest in aflatoxins, as indicated by the number of scientific publications each year from 1963 to December 2024. Data from a PubMed search on the term "aflatoxin" or "aflatoxins".

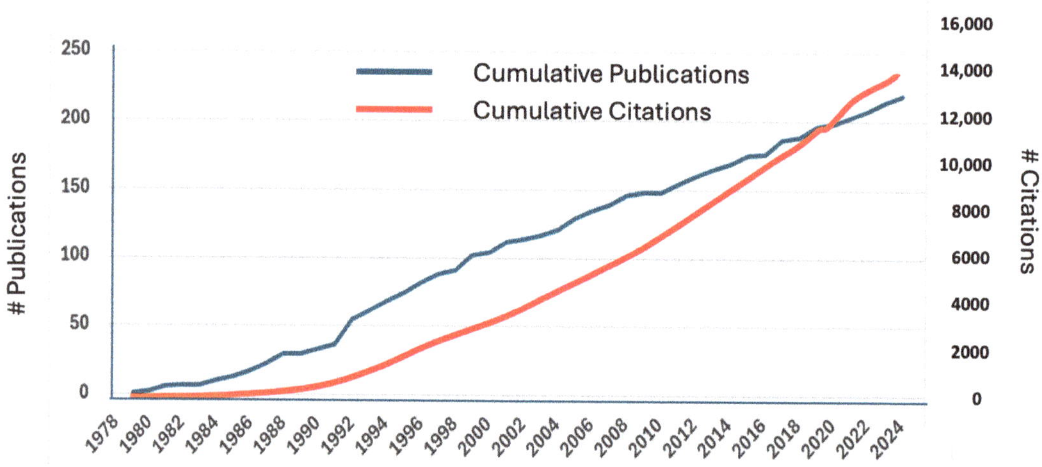

Figure 11. Publication and citation history of Dr. John Groopman's contributions to the past 45 years of aflatoxin research, including many papers related to species differences in biotransformation. (Figure developed from data obtained from a Web of Science citation search on "John D. Groopman" and "aflatoxins").

It is striking to consider that over 50% of these articles (~7800 papers) cited one or more of Dr. Groopman's publications—a tribute to the tremendous impact his work has had on this field.

The importance of species differences in susceptibility to the toxic and carcinogenic effects were recognized almost immediately following early investigations into the effects of aflatoxins on turkeys, ducklings, trout, rats, and mice. It was also evident early on that the biotransformation (referred to as metabolism in most of the older literature) was likely to be the key determinant of species differences in susceptibility to AFB1. Some 60+ years later, the scientific community has largely solved this mystery. We provide here a quick summary of what we now know, by species:

a. Humans and non-human primates

The hepatotoxic and carcinogenic effects, and likely all or nearly all of the other toxic effects, of AFB1 require oxidative biotransformation to AFBO. The exo-conformer of AFBO binds to DNA, causing mutations and cytotoxicity that represent the key molecular initiating event in AFB1 carcinogenesis. Both the endo and the exo conformers form adducts with proteins, which contribute to its hepatotoxicity and likely other toxic effects observed in human populations exposed to AFB1 via the diet. Urinary and blood biomarkers of exposure and effect have been developed by Drs. Groopman and Kensler's laboratories, along with many others across the world [189].

In humans, the formation of both endo- and exo-AFBO is mediated largely, if not exclusively, by two human CYP enzymes. hCYP1A2 forms roughly equivalent amounts of exo- and endo-AFBO, whereas hYP3A4 forms mostly exo-AFBO. However, there are important kinetic differences in the affinity of AFB1 to the active sites of these two CYPs. hCYP1A2 is expressed only in the liver, and in lower amounts than hCYP3A4, and thus has a considerably lower Vmax. Although there is more CYP3A4 enzyme available in the liver (and other tissues) to oxidize AFB1 to AFBO, the enzyme follows Hill kinetics, rather than classic Michaelis–Menten kinetics, and thus exhibits "self-activation" kinetics highly dependent on substrate concentration. At low concentrations in the liver (e.g., less than 0.1 μM), the enzyme is largely inactive toward activation of AFBO. But at concentrations above ~10 μM, it dominates exo-AFBO formation. In contrast, hCYP1A2 follows classic Michaelis–Menten kinetics and exhibits a high affinity (low Km) for AFB1, such that, at the low substrate concentrations that would be seen in human liver following dietary exposure, it dominates AFBO formation.

In addition to AFBO, human CYPs are responsible for the formation of the less toxic AFB1 metabolites, AFM1, AFP1, and AFQ1. AFM1 is formed by both hCYP1A1 and 1A2, but hCYP1A1 is generally expressed at very low levels in human liver, at least in the absence of exposure to AhR inducers, such as numerous polyaromatic hydrocarbon. Thus, it is likely that in most people, AFM1 is formed principally by hCYP1A2. AFM1 is capable of activation to the epoxide, likely via secondary oxidation by hCYP1A2, and thus has some carcinogenic effects, but is about 10-fold less potent than AFB1. AFM1 is the primary AFB1 metabolite found in urine, and has been used by Dr. Groopman and others as a biomarker of exposure in some studies.

AFP1 results from oxidative demethylation in the liver, and appears to be a relatively minor oxidative metabolite in humans, although a major metabolite in rats and mice (see below). It is uncertain which human CYP(s) form AFP1.

AFQ1 is a major oxidative metabolite of AFB1 and is formed largely, if not exclusively, by hCYP3A enzymes. hCYP3A4 is the major form expressed in human liver, and forms approximately 10 times as much AFQ1 as exo-AFBO. In that capacity, hCYP3A4 may serve predominantly as a detoxification pathway. hCYP3A5 is a polymorphic enzyme that is expressed only in a relatively small portion of the population, but does exhibit similar activity toward AFB1 as hCYP3A4. hCYP3A7 is a fetal form and thus found only in fetal tissues, but it, too, seems to have similar activity toward AFB1 as hCY3A4.

There is one reduction pathway involved in AFB1 biotransformation that may occur in humans—reduction of the cyclopentanone moiety to a hydroxyl group, referred to as aflatoxicol (AFL). AFL is capable of undergoing oxidation back to AFB1, so this pathway could potentially serve as a "reservoir" for AFB1, allowing exposure to tissue other than the liver to AFB1 if oxidized back to AFB1. There is relatively little information on the aldo-ketoreductase(s) that is/are responsible for this pathway in humans. It appears that this is a minor pathway, and probably not of great importance in the overall disposition of AFB1 in humans. There is also little information on relative species differences.

AFBO, once formed, is subject to hydrolysis to the AFB1–dihydrodiol. This reaction likely occurs both non-enzymatically through the addition of water across the epoxide bond, but there is some evidence that microsomal Epoxide Hydrolase (mEH) can also mediate this reaction. There are limited data that suggest that human mEH may offer protection against AFBO-DNA damage and mutagenicity.

AFBO is also subject to conjugation with reduced glutathione (GSH). Although exo-AFBO is unstable in an aqueous environment and highly reactive, it does not appear to react non-enzymatically with GSH. The conjugation requires specific glutathione S-transferase (GST) enzymes to detoxify both endo- and exo-AFBO. In humans, all alpha-class GSTs seem to lack catalytic activity toward AFBO. However, hGSTM1-1, a mu-class GST, does have low but measurable activity toward AFBO. This enzyme is polymorphic in the human population, with ~50% of the overall population having a "homozygous null" genotype, and thus no enzyme is produced. There are some data showing that individuals who are GSTM1-null may be at increased susceptibility to AFB1.

The formation of AFB1–dihydrodiol from either enzymatic or non-enzymatic reactions plays an important role in AFB1 toxicity because aldo-keto tautomerization results in the formation of AFB1–dialdehyde, which is reactive and can bind to proteins.

However, two human aldo-ketoreductases, called "aflatoxin aldehyde reductase" or AFAR1 and AFAR2 (from the human genes *AKR7A1* and *AKR7A3*, respectively) can reduce the reactive dialdehyde to AFB1–dialcohol and AFB1–monoalcohol (two forms). Because the alcohols do not bind to proteins, this is considered a detoxification pathway. In the absence of significant GST activity in humans, this pathway may play a significant role in detoxification of AFBO by reducing protein binding.

Relatively little is known about glucuronide and sulfate conjugates of the various hydroxylated AFB1 metabolites, other than some glucuronide conjugates of AFP1 have been identified at low levels in urine. However, with the possible exception of AFM1, the hydroxylated AFB1 metabolites seem not to contribute significantly to AFB1 carcinogenesis and toxicity, and thus potential interindividual and species differences in glucuronidation of aflatoxin metabolites are not likely to contribute significantly to species differences in AFB1 toxicity.

b. Rats

Overall rat hepatic CYP enzymes (microsomal fraction) have about twice the AFBO-forming activity as human liver microsomes. It is less clear which specific CYPs in rats are responsible for AFBO formation, although the rat orthologue of hCYP3A4, rCYP3A2, may be responsible. In contrast to hCYP1A2, rCYP1A2 appears to have little activity toward AFBO formation.

In contrast to humans, rats form relatively large amounts of AFP1, which as the glucuronide conjugate is a major biliary metabolite. At low AFB1 concentrations, AFQ1 is a very minor metabolite in rat hepatocytes, but at higher substrate concentration it accounts for about 20% of total metabolites, suggesting that ratCYP3A enzyme has similar kinetic characteristics to human.

The constitutively expressed GSTs in rat liver (*rGSTA1* and *rGSTA2*) have relatively little ability to detoxify AFBO. However, rGSTA5-5, which is inducible by activating ligands of the KEAP1/NRF2 antioxidant response pathway, has very high activity toward AFBO. Induction of rGSTA5 results in complete inhibition of the carcinogenic effects of aflatoxin. This remarkable protective effect has served as a primary basis for numerous chemoprevention clinical trials.

c. Mice

Mouse liver microsomes have high CYP activity and form AFBO at about twice the rate of rats, and about 5 times that of human liver microsomes. Mouse microsomes form relatively large amounts of AFM1 and AFP1 as well. It is not clear which mouse Cyp enzymes form AFBO, but the limited data available suggest that mCYP3a is likely more important than mCyp1A2.

Although adult mice activate AFB1 to AFBO relatively more rapidly than human or rat microsomes, they are nearly completely resistant to the carcinogenic effects of AFB1. It is now widely recognized that constitutively expressed mGstA3-3 has high activity toward AFBO—at least 10,000-fold higher than human GSTM1-1. mGstA3-3 activity toward AFBO is about 6 times greater than the inducible, highly active form of rats, rGSTA5-5. Studies with m*Gsta3* knockout mice, coupled with studies showing induction of rGSTA5-5, indicate rats, like mice, are resistant to AFB-DNA damage and mutagenesis, confirming that the expression of these two GSTs can account for the gradient in species differences in sensitivity between rodents and then compared to primates.

d. Fish/salmonids

Metabolism of AFB1 plays the key role in determination of species sensitivity to AFB1-dependent HCC. Trout constitutively express a CYP (2K1) with high activity toward production of the exo-epoxide and relatively lower rates of inactivation of the epoxide by conjugation with GSH or production of other phase 1 or phase 2 metabolites. Alteration of this metabolic profile by, for example, BNF or PCBs, induces a CYP1A1-dependent production of AFM1 and markedly reduces AFB1-dependent HCC.

Avians (Turkeys, Chickens, Ducks)

Domesticated turkeys represent an example of an extremely sensitive animal model, owing to, at least in part, to a combination of efficient P4501A5-mediated bioactivation, coupled with deficient GST-mediated detoxification of the AFBO so generated [85]. While domestic turkeys possess constitutive GSTs, none are able to detoxify AFB_1 in vivo or in vitro [73,78,79]. Conversely, wild turkeys, which are relatively AFB_1-resistant compared to their domesticated counterparts [76], possess functional, AFB1-detoxifying hepatic GSTs [178]. As in the case of mammalian species, GST-mediated AFB1 detoxification is the rate-limiting determinant in the sensitivity of various avian species, regardless of the extent of P450-mediated bioactivation [82].

6. Conclusions

To date, appreciation of the well-established species differences in susceptibility to the carcinogenic effects of AFB1 has not altered most risk assessments or regulatory limits on AFB1. Perhaps fortuitously, many relied upon rat liver tumor studies for quantitative assessment for human cancer risk. For example, a recent European Food Safety Authority (EFSA) evaluation of AFB1 carcinogenicity used a BMDL10 of 0.4 μg/kg bw per day for the induction of HCC by AFB1 in male rats as a reference point [200]. However, a Margin of Exposure (MOE) approach, rather than a linear extrapolation of rat liver tumor data, was used, with a 10,000-fold uncertainty factor to adjust for species differences and other uncertainties. They noted that, for more highly exposed populations, MOEs were frequently less than 10,000.

When comparing relative rates of CYP-mediated activation to exo-AFBO, rat and human liver appear similar. However, rats have significant GST-mediated detoxification, and human liver has remarkably little, suggesting that additional uncertainty factors may be warranted when using rat liver tumor data. Indeed, differences in expression and catalytic function of a variety of biotransformation enzymes can explain in large part, if not exclusively, the well-known differences in susceptibility to hepatotoxicity and carcinogenicity of AFB1. Based on the relatively very low level of human GSTs toward AFBO, it would appear that humans should be highly susceptible to AFB1 toxicity. However, studies in isolated perfused liver and human hepatocytes in culture suggest that the hepatic DNA damage from AFBO in humans is more similar to that in rats than would be expected based solely on hepatic AFBO-GST activity. These and other studies suggest that other pathways, perhaps including mEH, play a relatively more important role in protecting human liver cells from AFBO-DNA damage. There is evidence that human mEH may play a significant role in detoxification of AFBO, especially in the presence of limited AFBO-GST activity. It is also possible that human DNA repair processes are more efficient, adding additional protection.

It is notable that there are sex differences in the susceptibility of rats to aflatoxin hepatocarcinogenesis, with males more susceptible than females. In human populations with known exposures to aflatoxins, there are typically 2–3-fold increased rates of liver cancer incidence in males. However, this outcome is not universal, as in regions of Central America no difference by sex is observed. To date, there is little evidence to suggest that differences in aflatoxin biotransformation are likely to account for increased sensitivity of males to carcinogenesis, be it rats or humans.

Finally, there are other well-established interactive risk factors, such as hepatitis B and C virus infections in humans, that greatly potentiate the hepatocarcinogenic activity of AFB1. Conversely, there is a growing body of literature implicating dietary antioxidants as offering some protection against AFBO genotoxicity by either inhibiting CYP-mediated activation or inducing potential protective pathways. Genetic differences in AFB1 biotransformation pathways (such as the GSTM1 genotype) further complicate the quantitative extrapolation of laboratory animal data to human liver cancer risk. Yet, despite all of these uncertainties, it appears that the rat has been a useful surrogate for risk assessment of aflatoxin carcinogenicity in humans given the dominant role of overall metabolism as the determinant of susceptibility with generally similar activation activity. Although GST-mediated detoxification is much lower in humans than in rats, it appears that alternative detoxification pathways, perhaps including human mEH, compensate for the relative lack of GST activity, giving rise to a relatively similar overall activation: detoxification profile between humans and rats. The remarkable sensitivities of turkeys and rainbow trout provide further demonstration that biotransformation pathways are the major determinants of species susceptibility to AFB1 hepatoxicity and carcinogenesis.

Author Contributions: D.L.E. developed the conceptualization, and organization of the manuscript, and project administration. D.L.E., D.E.W. and R.A.C. contributed writing, review and editing. All authors have read and agreed to the published version of the manuscript.

Funding: This review received no external funding.

Institutional Review Board Statement: Not applicable.

Informed Consent Statement: Not applicable.

Data Availability Statement: No new data were created or analyzed in this study.

Acknowledgments: The authors thank our mentors, Groopman and Kensler, along with theirs and our students, fellows and other collaborators for the aflatoxin journeys we have all undertaken. We thank the National Institutes of Health (NIEHS, NCI and NIGMS) and the United States Department of Agriculture (NIFA, Animal Genome Project), for decades of support for our research on aflatoxin and related topics.

Conflicts of Interest: The authors declare no conflicts of interest.

References

1. Ayres, J.L.; Lee, D.J.; Wales, J.H.; Sinnhuber, R.O. Aflatoxin structure and hepatocarcinogenicity in rainbow trout (*Salmo gairdneri*). *J. Natl. Cancer Inst.* **1971**, *46*, 561–564.
2. Lee, D.J.; Wales, J.H.; Sinnhuber, R.O. Promotion of aflatoxin-induced hepatoma growth in trout by methyl malvalate and sterculate. *Cancer Res.* **1971**, *31*, 960–963. [PubMed]
3. Wogan, G.N.; Newberne, P.M. Dose-response characteristics of aflatoxin B1 carcinogenesis in the rat. *Cancer Res.* **1967**, *27*, 2370–2376. [PubMed]
4. Wogan, G.N.; Paglialunga, S.; Newberne, P.M. Carcinogenic effects of low dietary levels of aflatoxin B1 in rats. *Food Cosmet. Toxicol.* **1974**, *12*, 681–685. [CrossRef] [PubMed]
5. Roebuck, B.D.; Wogan, G.N. Species comparison of in vitro metabolism of aflatoxin B1. *Cancer Res.* **1977**, *37*, 1649–1656.
6. Gerdemann, A.; Cramer, B.; Degen, G.H.; Veerkamp, J.; Gunther, G.; Albrecht, W.; Behrens, M.; Esselen, M.; Ghallab, A.; Hengstler, J.G.; et al. Comparative metabolism of aflatoxin B(1) in mouse, rat and human primary hepatocytes using HPLC-MS/MS. *Arch. Toxicol.* **2023**, *97*, 3179–3196. [CrossRef] [PubMed]
7. Cao, W.; Yu, P.; Yang, K.; Cao, D. Aflatoxin B1: Metabolism, toxicology, and its involvement in oxidative stress and cancer development. *Toxicol. Mech. Methods* **2022**, *32*, 395–419. [CrossRef] [PubMed]
8. Pickova, D.; Ostry, V.; Toman, J.; Malir, F. Aflatoxins: History, significant milestones, recent data on their toxicity and ways to mitigation. *Toxins* **2021**, *13*, 399. [CrossRef] [PubMed]
9. Rushing, B.R.; Selim, M.I. Aflatoxin B1: A review on metabolism, toxicity, occurrence in food, occupational exposure, and detoxification methods. *Food Chem. Toxicol.* **2019**, *124*, 81–100. [CrossRef]
10. Wogan, G.N.; Kensler, T.W.; Groopman, J.D. Present and future directions of translational research on aflatoxin and hepatocellular carcinoma. A review. *Food Addit. Contam. Part A Chem. Anal. Control. Expo. Risk Assess.* **2012**, *29*, 249–257. [CrossRef]
11. Kensler, T.W.; Roebuck, B.D.; Wogan, G.N.; Groopman, J.D. Aflatoxin: A 50-year odyssey of mechanistic and translational toxicology. *Toxicol. Sci.* **2011**, *120* (Suppl. 1), S28–S48. [CrossRef] [PubMed]
12. Guengerich, F.P.; Johnson, W.W.; Shimada, T.; Ueng, Y.F.; Yamazaki, H.; Langouet, S. Activation and detoxication of aflatoxin B1. *Mutat. Res.* **1998**, *402*, 121–128. [CrossRef]
13. Eaton, D.L.; Gallagher, E.P. Mechanisms of aflatoxin carcinogenesis. *Annu. Rev. Pharmacol. Toxicol.* **1994**, *34*, 135–172. [CrossRef] [PubMed]
14. Eaton, D.L.; Groopman, J.D. *The Toxicology of Aflatoxins: Human Health, Veterinary, and Agricultural Significance*; Academic Press: Boston, MA, USA, 1994.
15. IARC. *Some Naturally Occurring Substances: Food Items and Constituents, Heterocyclic Aromatic Amines and Mycotoxins*; IARC Press: Lyon, France, 1993; Volume 56.
16. Ramsdell, H.S.; Eaton, D.L. Species susceptibility to aflatoxin B1 carcinogenesis: Comparative kinetics of microsomal biotransformation. *Cancer Res.* **1990**, *50*, 615–620. [PubMed]
17. Groopman, J.D.; Donahue, P.R.; Zhu, J.Q.; Chen, J.S.; Wogan, G.N. Aflatoxin metabolism in humans: Detection of metabolites and nucleic acid adducts in urine by affinity chromatography. *Proc. Natl. Acad. Sci. USA* **1985**, *82*, 6492–6496. [CrossRef]
18. Ueng, Y.F.; Shimada, T.; Yamazaki, H.; Guengerich, F.P. Oxidation of aflatoxin B1 by bacterial recombinant human cytochrome P450 enzymes. *Chem. Res. Toxicol.* **1995**, *8*, 218–225. [CrossRef]
19. Groopman, J.D.; Fowler, K.W.; Busby, W.F., Jr.; Wogan, G.N. Interaction of aflatoxin B2 with rat liver DNA and histones in vivo. *Carcinogenesis* **1981**, *2*, 1371–1373. [CrossRef]
20. Gross-Steinmeyer, K.; Stapleton, P.L.; Tracy, J.H.; Bammler, T.K.; Lehman, T.; Strom, S.C.; Eaton, D.L. Influence of Matrigel-overlay on constitutive and inducible expression of nine genes encoding drug-metabolizing enzymes in primary human hepatocytes. *Xenobiotica* **2005**, *35*, 419–438. [CrossRef]
21. Gross-Steinmeyer, K.; Stapleton, P.L.; Tracy, J.H.; Bammler, T.K.; Strom, S.C.; Buhler, D.R.; Eaton, D.L. Modulation of aflatoxin B1-mediated genotoxicity in primary cultures of human hepatocytes by diindolylmethane, curcumin, and xanthohumols. *Toxicol. Sci.* **2009**, *112*, 303–310. [CrossRef]
22. Aoyama, T.; Yamano, S.; Guzelian, P.S.; Gelboin, H.V.; Gonzalez, F.J. Five of 12 forms of vaccinia virus-expressed human hepatic cytochrome P450 metabolically activate aflatoxin B1. *Proc. Natl. Acad. Sci. USA* **1990**, *87*, 4790–4793. [CrossRef] [PubMed]
23. Gallagher, E.P.; Kunze, K.L.; Stapleton, P.L.; Eaton, D.L. The kinetics of aflatoxin B1 oxidation by human cDNA-expressed and human liver microsomal cytochromes P450 1A2 and 3A4. *Toxicol. Appl. Pharmacol.* **1996**, *141*, 595–606. [CrossRef] [PubMed]
24. Kamdem, L.K.; Meineke, I.; Godtel-Armbrust, U.; Brockmoller, J.; Wojnowski, L. Dominant contribution of P450 3A4 to the hepatic carcinogenic activation of aflatoxin B1. *Chem. Res. Toxicol.* **2006**, *19*, 577–586. [CrossRef]
25. Zhang, Z.; Yang, X.; Wang, Y.; Wang, X.; Lu, H.; Zhang, X.; Xiao, X.; Li, S.; Wang, X.; Wang, S.L. Cytochrome P450 2A13 is an efficient enzyme in metabolic activation of aflatoxin G1 in human bronchial epithelial cells. *Arch. Toxicol.* **2013**, *87*, 1697–1707. [CrossRef] [PubMed]

26. Kitada, M.; Taneda, M.; Ohi, H.; Komori, M.; Itahashi, K.; Nagao, M.; Kamataki, T. Mutagenic activation of aflatoxin B1 by P-450 HFLa in human fetal livers. *Mutat. Res.* **1989**, *227*, 53–58. [CrossRef] [PubMed]
27. Kitada, M.; Taneda, M.; Ohta, K.; Nagashima, K.; Itahashi, K.; Kamataki, T. Metabolic activation of aflatoxin B1 and 2-amino-3-methylimidazo[4,5-f]-quinoline by human adult and fetal livers. *Cancer Res.* **1990**, *50*, 2641–2645. [PubMed]
28. Fanni, D.; Fanos, V.; Ambu, R.; Lai, F.; Gerosa, C.; Pampaloni, P.; Van Eyken, P.; Senes, G.; Castagnola, M.; Faa, G. Overlapping between CYP3A4 and CYP3A7 expression in the fetal human liver during development. *J. Matern.-Fetal Neonatal Med.* **2015**, *28*, 1291–1295. [CrossRef] [PubMed]
29. Wild, C.P.; Rasheed, F.N.; Jawla, M.F.; Hall, A.J.; Jansen, L.A.; Montesano, R. In-utero exposure to aflatoxin in west Africa. *Lancet* **1991**, *337*, 1602. [CrossRef] [PubMed]
30. Wang, H.; Dick, R.; Yin, H.; Licad-Coles, E.; Kroetz, D.L.; Szklarz, G.; Harlow, G.; Halpert, J.R.; Correia, M.A. Structure-function relationships of human liver cytochromes P450 3A: Aflatoxin B1 metabolism as a probe. *Biochemistry* **1998**, *37*, 12536–12545. [CrossRef]
31. Krishna, D.R.; Shekar, M.S. Cytochrome P450 3A: Genetic polymorphisms and inter-ethnic differences. *Methods Find. Exp. Clin. Pharmacol.* **2005**, *27*, 559–567. [CrossRef] [PubMed]
32. Johnson, W.W.; Guengerich, F.P. Reaction of aflatoxin B1 exo-8,9-epoxide with DNA: Kinetic analysis of covalent binding and DNA-induced hydrolysis. *Proc. Natl. Acad. Sci. USA* **1997**, *94*, 6121–6125. [CrossRef] [PubMed]
33. Guengerich, F.P.; Johnson, W.W.; Ueng, Y.F.; Yamazaki, H.; Shimada, T. Involvement of cytochrome P450, glutathione S-transferase, and epoxide hydrolase in the metabolism of aflatoxin B1 and relevance to risk of human liver cancer. *Environ. Health Perspect.* **1996**, *104* (Suppl. 3), 557–562. [CrossRef] [PubMed]
34. Ekins, S.; Ring, B.J.; Binkley, S.N.; Hall, S.D.; Wrighton, S.A. Autoactivation and activation of the cytochrome P450s. *Int. J. Clin. Pharmacol. Ther.* **1998**, *36*, 642–651. [PubMed]
35. Houston, J.B.; Galetin, A. Modelling atypical CYP3A4 kinetics: Principles and pragmatism. *Arch. Biochem. Biophys.* **2005**, *433*, 351–360. [CrossRef]
36. Kenworthy, K.E.; Clarke, S.E.; Andrews, J.; Houston, J.B. Multisite kinetic models for CYP3A4: Simultaneous activation and inhibition of diazepam and testosterone metabolism. *Drug Metab. Dispos.* **2001**, *29*, 1644–1651. [PubMed]
37. Muller, C.S.; Knehans, T.; Davydov, D.R.; Bounds, P.L.; von Mandach, U.; Halpert, J.R.; Caflisch, A.; Koppenol, W.H. Concurrent cooperativity and substrate inhibition in the epoxidation of carbamazepine by cytochrome P450 3A4 active site mutants inspired by molecular dynamics simulations. *Biochemistry* **2015**, *54*, 711–721. [CrossRef] [PubMed]
38. Ueng, Y.F.; Kuwabara, T.; Chun, Y.J.; Guengerich, F.P. Cooperativity in oxidations catalyzed by cytochrome P450 3A4. *Biochemistry* **1997**, *36*, 370–381. [CrossRef]
39. Gallagher, E.P.; Stapleton, P.L.; Kunze, K.L.; Eaton, D.L. Aflatoxin B1 oxidation in human CYP1A1 and CYP1A2 cDNA-expressed microsomes. *Int. Toxicol. VII Int. Congr. Toxicol.* **1995**, *7*, 34.
40. Gallagher, E.P.; Wienkers, L.C.; Stapleton, P.L.; Kunze, K.L.; Eaton, D.L. Role of human microsomal and human complementary DNA-expressed cytochromes P4501A2 and P4503A4 in the bioactivation of aflatoxin B1. *Cancer Res.* **1994**, *54*, 101–108.
41. Putt, D.A.; Ding, X.; Coon, M.J.; Hollenberg, P.F. Metabolism of aflatoxin B1 by rabbit and rat nasal mucosa microsomes and purified cytochrome P450, including isoforms 2A10 and 2A11. *Carcinogenesis* **1995**, *16*, 1411–1417. [CrossRef] [PubMed]
42. Kranendonk, M.; Carreira, F.; Theisen, P.; Laires, A.; Fisher, C.W.; Rueff, J.; Estabrook, R.W.; Vermeulen, N.P. Escherichia coli MTC, a human NADPH P450 reductase competent mutagenicity tester strain for the expression of human cytochrome P450 isoforms 1A1, 1A2, 2A6, 3A4, or 3A5: Catalytic activities and mutagenicity studies. *Mutat. Res.* **1999**, *441*, 73–83. [CrossRef]
43. Kelly, J.D.; Eaton, D.L.; Guengerich, F.P.; Coulombe, R.A., Jr. Aflatoxin B1 activation in human lung. *Toxicol. Appl. Pharmacol.* **1997**, *144*, 88–95. [CrossRef]
44. Marcelloni, A.M.; Pigini, D.; Chiominto, A.; Gioffre, A.; Paba, E. Exposure to airborne mycotoxins: The riskiest working environments and tasks. *Ann. Work. Expo. Health* **2024**, *68*, 19–35. [CrossRef]
45. Hayes, R.B.; van Nieuwenhuize, J.P.; Raatgever, J.W.; ten Kate, F.J. Aflatoxin exposures in the industrial setting: An epidemiological study of mortality. *Food Chem. Toxicol.* **1984**, *22*, 39–43. [CrossRef] [PubMed]
46. Berggren, S.; Gall, C.; Wollnitz, N.; Ekelund, M.; Karlbom, U.; Hoogstraate, J.; Schrenk, D.; Lennernas, H. Gene and protein expression of P-glycoprotein, MRP1, MRP2, and CYP3A4 in the small and large human intestine. *Mol. Pharm.* **2007**, *4*, 252–257. [CrossRef] [PubMed]
47. Ding, X.; Kaminsky, L.S. Human extrahepatic cytochromes P450: Function in xenobiotic metabolism and tissue-selective chemical toxicity in the respiratory and gastrointestinal tracts. *Annu. Rev. Pharmacol. Toxicol.* **2003**, *43*, 149–173. [CrossRef] [PubMed]
48. Harrison, J.C.; Carvajal, M.; Garner, R.C. Does aflatoxin exposure in the United Kingdom constitute a cancer risk? *Environ. Health Perspect.* **1993**, *99*, 99–105. [CrossRef] [PubMed]
49. Bammler, T.K.; Slone, D.H.; Eaton, D.L. Effects of dietary oltipraz and ethoxyquin on aflatoxin B1 biotransformation in non-human primates. *Toxicol. Sci.* **2000**, *54*, 30–41. [CrossRef] [PubMed]

50. Ch'ih, J.J.; Biedrzycka, D.W.; Devlin, T.M. Isolated hepatocytes are capable of excreting aflatoxin metabolites. *Biochem. Biophys. Res. Commun.* **1991**, *178*, 1002–1007. [CrossRef] [PubMed]
51. Halvorson, M.R.; Safe, S.H.; Parkinson, A.; Phillips, T.D. Aflatoxin B1 hydroxylation by the pregnenolone-16 alpha-carbonitrile-inducible form of rat liver microsomal cytochrome P-450. *Carcinogenesis* **1988**, *9*, 2103–2108. [CrossRef]
52. Raney, K.D.; Meyer, D.J.; Ketterer, B.; Harris, T.M.; Guengerich, F.P. Glutathione conjugation of aflatoxin B1 exo- and endo-epoxides by rat and human glutathione S-transferases. *Chem. Res. Toxicol.* **1992**, *5*, 470–478. [CrossRef]
53. Buetler, T.M.; Bammler, T.K.; Hayes, J.D.; Eaton, D.L. Oltipraz-mediated changes in aflatoxin B(1) biotransformation in rat liver: Implications for human chemointervention. *Cancer Res.* **1996**, *56*, 2306–2313. [PubMed]
54. Yanagimoto, T.; Itoh, S.; Sawada, M.; Kamataki, T. Mouse cytochrome P450 (Cyp3a11): Predominant expression in liver and capacity to activate aflatoxin B1. *Arch. Biochem. Biophys.* **1997**, *340*, 215–218. [CrossRef] [PubMed]
55. Yanagimoto, T.; Itoh, S.; Sawada, M.; Hashimoto, H.; Kamataki, T. Molecular cloning and functional expression of a mouse cytochrome P-450 (Cyp3a-13): Examination of Cyp3a-13 enzyme to activate aflatoxin B1 (AFB1). *Biochim. Biophys. Acta* **1994**, *1201*, 405–410. [CrossRef] [PubMed]
56. Kirby, G.M.; Chemin, I.; Montesano, R.; Chisari, F.V.; Lang, M.A.; Wild, C.P. Induction of specific cytochrome P450s involved in aflatoxin B1 metabolism in hepatitis B virus transgenic mice. *Mol. Carcinog.* **1994**, *11*, 74–80. [CrossRef] [PubMed]
57. Sun, B.; Fukuhara, M. Effects of co-administration of butylated hydroxytoluene, butylated hydroxyanisole and flavonoids on the activation of mutagens and drug-metabolizing enzymes in mice. *Toxicology* **1997**, *122*, 61–72. [CrossRef] [PubMed]
58. Williams, D.E.; Buhler, D.R. Purified form of cytochrome P-450 from rainbow trout with high activity toward conversion of aflatoxin B1 to aflatoxin B1-2,3-epoxide. *Cancer Res.* **1983**, *43*, 4752–4756.
59. Williams, D.E.; Buhler, D.R. Purification of cytochromes P-448 from beta-naphthoflavone-treated rainbow trout. *Biochim. Biophys. Acta* **1982**, *717*, 398–404. [CrossRef] [PubMed]
60. Williams, D.E.; Buhler, D.R. Benzo[a]pyrene-hydroxylase catalyzed by purified isozymes of cytochrome P-450 from beta-naphthoflavone-fed rainbow trout. *Biochem. Pharmacol.* **1984**, *33*, 3743–3753. [CrossRef]
61. Williams, D.E.; Bender, R.C.; Morrissey, M.T.; Selivonchick, D.P.; Buhler, D.R. Cytochrome P-450 isozymes in salmonds determined with antibodies to purifed forms of P-450 from rainbow trout. *Mar. Environ. Res.* **1984**, *14*, 13–21. [CrossRef]
62. Buhler, D.R.; Yang, Y.H.; Dreher, T.W.; Miranda, C.L.; Wang, J.L. Cloning and sequencing of the major rainbow trout constitutive cytochrome P450 (CYP2K1): Identification of a new cytochrome P450 gene subfamily and its expression in mature rainbow trout liver and trunk kidney. *Arch. Biochem. Biophys.* **1994**, *312*, 45–51. [CrossRef]
63. Williams, D.E.; Okita, R.T.; Buhler, D.R.; Masters, B.S. Regiospecific hydroxylation of lauric acid at the (omega-1) position by hepatic and kidney microsomal cytochromes P-450 from rainbow trout. *Arch. Biochem. Biophys.* **1984**, *231*, 503–510. [CrossRef]
64. Yang, Y.H.; Miranda, C.L.; Henderson, M.C.; Wang-Buhler, J.L.; Buhler, D.R. Heterologous expression of CYP2K1 and identification of the expressed protein (BV-CYP2K1) as lauric acid (omega-1)-hydroxylase and aflatoxin B1 exo-epoxidase. *Drug Metab. Dispos.* **2000**, *28*, 1279–1283. [CrossRef] [PubMed]
65. Troxel, C.M.; Reddy, A.P.; O'Neal, P.E.; Hendricks, J.D.; Bailey, G.S. In vivo aflatoxin B1 metabolism and hepatic DNA adduction in zebrafish (Danio rerio). *Toxicol. Appl. Pharmacol.* **1997**, *143*, 213–220. [CrossRef] [PubMed]
66. Williams, D.E. The rainbow trout liver cancer model: Response to environmental chemicals and studies on promotion and chemoprevention. *Comp. Biochem. Physiol. C Toxicol. Pharmacol.* **2012**, *155*, 121–127. [CrossRef] [PubMed]
67. Wang-Buhler, J.L.; Lee, S.J.; Chung, W.G.; Stevens, J.F.; Tseng, H.P.; Hseu, T.H.; Hu, C.H.; Westerfield, M.; Yang, Y.H.; Miranda, C.L.; et al. CYP2K6 from zebrafish (Danio rerio): Cloning, mapping, developmental/tissue expression, and aflatoxin B1 activation by baculovirus expressed enzyme. *Comp. Biochem. Physiol. C Toxicol. Pharmacol.* **2005**, *140*, 207–219. [CrossRef] [PubMed]
68. Valsta, L.M.; Hendricks, J.D.; Bailey, G.S. The significance of glutathione conjugation for aflatoxin B1 metabolism in rainbow trout and coho salmon. *Food Chem. Toxicol.* **1988**, *26*, 129–135. [CrossRef] [PubMed]
69. Bailey, G.; Selivonchick, D.; Hendricks, J. Initiation, promotion, and inhibition of carcinogenesis in rainbow trout. *Environ. Health Perspect.* **1987**, *71*, 147–153. [CrossRef] [PubMed]
70. Bailey, G.S.; Williams, D.E.; Wilcox, J.S.; Loveland, P.M.; Coulombe, R.A.; Hendricks, J.D. Aflatoxin B1 carcinogenesis and its relation to DNA adduct formation and adduct persistence in sensitive and resistant salmonid fish. *Carcinogenesis* **1988**, *9*, 1919–1926. [CrossRef] [PubMed]
71. Bechtel, D.H. Molecular dosimetry of hepatic aflatoxin B1-DNA adducts: Linear correlation with hepatic cancer risk. *Regul. Toxicol. Pharmacol.* **1989**, *10*, 74–81. [CrossRef]
72. Arafa, A.S.; Bloomer, R.J.; Wilson, H.R.; Simpson, C.F.; Harms, R.H. Susceptibility of various poultry species to dietary aflatoxin. *Br. Poult. Sci.* **1981**, *22*, 431–436. [CrossRef] [PubMed]
73. Klein, P.J.; Buckner, R.; Kelly, J.; Coulombe, R.A., Jr. Biochemical basis for the extreme sensitivity of turkeys to aflatoxin B(1). *Toxicol. Appl. Pharmacol.* **2000**, *165*, 45–52. [CrossRef] [PubMed]

74. Kubena, L.F.; Edrington, T.S.; Kamps-Holtzapple, C.; Harvey, R.B.; Elissalde, M.H.; Rottinghaus, G.E. Effects of feeding fumonisin B1 present in Fusarium moniliforme culture material and aflatoxin singly and in combination to turkey poults. *Poult. Sci.* **1995**, *74*, 1295–1303. [CrossRef]
75. Blount, W.P. Turkey "X" Disease. *J. Br. Turk. Fed.* **1961**, *9*, 55–58.
76. Quist, C.F.; Bounous, D.I.; Kilburn, J.V.; Nettles, V.F.; Wyatt, R.D. The effect of dietary aflatoxin on wild turkey poults. *J. Wildl. Dis.* **2000**, *36*, 436–444. [CrossRef]
77. Lozano, M.C.; Diaz, G.J. Microsomal and cytosolic biotransformation of aflatoxin B1 in four poultry species. *Br. Poult. Sci.* **2006**, *47*, 734–741. [CrossRef] [PubMed]
78. Klein, P.J.; Van Vleet, T.R.; Hall, J.O.; Coulombe, R.A., Jr. Biochemical factors underlying the age-related sensitivity of turkeys to aflatoxin B(1). *Comp. Biochem. Physiol. C Toxicol. Pharmacol.* **2002**, *132*, 193–201. [CrossRef] [PubMed]
79. Guarisco, J.A.; Hall, J.O.; Coulombe, R.A., Jr. Mechanisms of butylated hydroxytoluene chemoprevention of aflatoxicosis—Inhibition of aflatoxin B1 metabolism. *Toxicol. Appl. Pharmacol.* **2008**, *227*, 339–346. [CrossRef] [PubMed]
80. Yip, S.S.; Coulombe, R.A., Jr. Molecular cloning and expression of a novel cytochrome p450 from turkey liver with aflatoxin b1 oxidizing activity. *Chem. Res. Toxicol.* **2006**, *19*, 30–37. [CrossRef] [PubMed]
81. Reed, K.M.; Mendoza, K.M.; Coulombe, R.A., Jr. Structure and genetic mapping of the Cytochrome P450 gene (CYP1A5) in the turkey (Meleagris gallopavo). *Cytogenet. Genome Res.* **2007**, *116*, 104–109. [CrossRef]
82. Rawal, S.; Kim, J.E.; Coulombe, R., Jr. Aflatoxin B1 in poultry: Toxicology, metabolism and prevention. *Res. Vet. Sci.* **2010**, *89*, 325–331. [CrossRef] [PubMed]
83. Rawal, S.; Yip, S.S.; Coulombe, R.A., Jr. Cloning, expression and functional characterization of cytochrome P450 3A37 from turkey liver with high aflatoxin B1 epoxidation activity. *Chem. Res. Toxicol.* **2010**, *23*, 1322–1329. [CrossRef] [PubMed]
84. Dalloul, R.A.; Long, J.A.; Zimin, A.V.; Aslam, L.; Beal, K.; Blomberg Le, A.; Bouffard, P.; Burt, D.W.; Crasta, O.; Crooijmans, R.P.; et al. Multi-platform next-generation sequencing of the domestic turkey (Meleagris gallopavo): Genome assembly and analysis. *PLoS Biol.* **2010**, *8*, e1000475. [CrossRef]
85. Rawal, S.; Coulombe, R.A., Jr. Metabolism of aflatoxin B1 in turkey liver microsomes: The relative roles of cytochromes P450 1A5 and 3A37. *Toxicol. Appl. Pharmacol.* **2011**, *254*, 349–354. [CrossRef] [PubMed]
86. Allcroft, R.; Caarnaghhan, R.B.A. Groundnut toxicity: An examination for toxin in human food products from animals fed toxic groundnut meal. *Vet. Rec.* **1963**, *75*, 259–263.
87. Allcroft, R.; Carnaghan, R.B.A. Toxic Products in Groundnuts. Biological Effects. *Chem. Ind.* **1963**, *2*, 50–53.
88. De Iongh, H.; Vles, R.O.; Van, P. Milk of Mammals Fed an Aflatoxin-Containing Diet. *Nature* **1964**, *202*, 466–467. [CrossRef]
89. Hsieh, D.P.; Cullen, J.M.; Hsieh, L.S.; Shao, Y.; Ruebner, B.H. Cancer risks posed by aflatoxin M1. *Princess Takamatsu Symp.* **1985**, *16*, 57–65. [PubMed]
90. Purchase, I.F. Acute toxicity of aflatoxins M1 and M2 in one-day-old ducklings. *Food Cosmet. Toxicol.* **1967**, *5*, 339–342. [CrossRef] [PubMed]
91. Cullen, J.M.; Ruebner, B.H.; Hsieh, L.S.; Hyde, D.M.; Hsieh, D.P. Carcinogenicity of dietary aflatoxin M1 in male Fischer rats compared to aflatoxin B1. *Cancer Res.* **1987**, *47*, 1913–1917. [PubMed]
92. Sinnhuber, R.O.; Lee, D.J.; Wales, J.H.; Landers, M.K.; Keyl, A.C. Hepatic carcinogenesis of aflatoxin M1 in rainbow trout (Salmo gairdneri) and its enchancement by cyclopropene fatty acids. *J. Natl. Cancer Inst.* **1974**, *53*, 1285–1288. [CrossRef]
93. Loveland, P.M.; Wilcox, J.S.; Hendricks, J.D.; Bailey, G.S. Comparative metabolism and DNA binding of aflatoxin B1, aflatoxin M1, aflatoxicol and aflatoxicol-M1 in hepatocytes from rainbow trout (*Salmo gairdneri*). *Carcinogenesis* **1988**, *9*, 441–446. [CrossRef] [PubMed]
94. Bailey, G.S.; Dashwood, R.; Loveland, P.M.; Pereira, C.; Hendricks, J.D. Molecular dosimetry in fish: Quantitative target organ DNA adduction and hepatocarcinogenicity for four aflatoxins by two exposure routes in rainbow trout. *Mutat. Res.* **1998**, *399*, 233–244. [CrossRef] [PubMed]
95. Neal, G.E.; Eaton, D.L.; Judah, D.J.; Verma, A. Metabolism and toxicity of aflatoxins M1 and B1 in human-derived in vitro systems. *Toxicol. Appl. Pharmacol.* **1998**, *151*, 152–158. [CrossRef]
96. Ali, N.; Habib, A.; Mahmud, F.; Tuba, H.R.; Degen, G.H. Aflatoxin M(1) Analysis in Urine of Mill Workers in Bangladesh: A Pilot Study. *Toxins* **2024**, *16*, 45. [CrossRef] [PubMed]
97. Ali, N.; Manirujjaman, M.; Rana, S.; Degen, G.H. Determination of aflatoxin M(1) and deoxynivalenol biomarkers in infants and children urines from Bangladesh. *Arch. Toxicol.* **2020**, *94*, 3775–3786. [CrossRef] [PubMed]
98. Apolinario, L.A.; Ramalho, L.N.Z.; Moosavi, M.H.; Jager, A.V.; Augusto, M.J.; Trotta, M.R.; Petta, T.; Khaneghah, A.M.; Oliveira, C.A.F.; Ramalho, F.S. Oncogenic and tumor suppressor pathways in subchronic aflatoxicosis in rats: Association with serum and urinary aflatoxin exposure biomarkers. *Food Chem. Toxicol.* **2021**, *153*, 112263. [CrossRef] [PubMed]
99. Ashraf, W.; Rehman, A.; Ahmad, M.U.; Rabbani, M.; Mushtaq, M.H.; Aamir, K.; Akhtar, F.; Wang, J.S. Assessment of aflatoxin M(1) exposure and associated determinants in children from Lahore, Pakistan. *Food Addit. Contam. Part A Chem. Anal. Control Expo. Risk Assess.* **2023**, *40*, 121–133. [CrossRef] [PubMed]

100. Ndaw, S.; Remy, A.; Jargot, D.; Antoine, G.; Denis, F.; Robert, A. Mycotoxins exposure of French grain elevator workers: Biomonitoring and airborne measurements. *Toxins* **2021**, *13*, 382. [CrossRef]
101. Qian, G.S.; Ross, R.K.; Yu, M.C.; Yuan, J.M.; Gao, Y.T.; Henderson, B.E.; Wogan, G.N.; Groopman, J.D. A follow-up study of urinary markers of aflatoxin exposure and liver cancer risk in Shanghai, People's Republic of China. *Cancer Epidemiol. Biomark. Prev.* **1994**, *3*, 3–10.
102. Sanchez, E.M.; Diaz, G.J. Frequency and levels of aflatoxin M(1) in urine of children in Bogota, Colombia. *Mycotoxin Res.* **2019**, *35*, 271–278. [CrossRef]
103. Sulaiman, S.H.; Jamaluddin, R.; Sabran, M.R. Association between urinary aflatoxin (AFM(1)) and dietary Intake among adults in Hulu Langat district, Selangor, Malaysia. *Nutrients* **2018**, *10*, 460. [CrossRef] [PubMed]
104. Gurtoo, H.L.; Koser, P.L.; Bansal, S.K.; Fox, H.W.; Sharma, S.D.; Mulhern, A.I.; Pavelic, Z.P. Inhibition of aflatoxin B1-hepatocarcinogenesis in rats by beta-naphthoflavone. *Carcinogenesis* **1985**, *6*, 675–678. [CrossRef]
105. Borroz, K.I.; Ramsdell, H.S.; Eaton, D.L. Mouse strain differences in glutathione S-transferase activity and aflatoxin B1 biotransformation. *Toxicol. Lett.* **1991**, *58*, 97–105. [CrossRef]
106. Goeger, D.E.; Shelton, D.W.; Hendricks, J.D.; Pereira, C.; Bailey, G.S. Comparative effect of dietary butylated hydroxyanisole and beta-naphthoflavone on aflatoxin B1 metabolism, DNA adduct formation, and carcinogenesis in rainbow trout. *Carcinogenesis* **1988**, *9*, 1793–1800. [CrossRef] [PubMed]
107. Loveland, P.M.; Coulombe, R.A.; Libbey, L.M.; Pawlowski, N.E.; Sinnhuber, R.O.; Nixon, J.E.; Bailey, G.S. Identification and mutagenicity of aflatoxicol-M1 produced by metabolism of aflatoxin B1 and aflatoxicol by liver fractions from rainbow trout (Salmo gairdneri) fed beta-naphthoflavone. *Food Chem. Toxicol.* **1983**, *21*, 557–562. [CrossRef] [PubMed]
108. Oliveira, C.A.; Rosmaninho, J.F.; Castro, A.L.; Butkeraitis, P.; Reis, T.A.; Correa, B. Aflatoxin residues in eggs of laying Japanese quail after long-term administration of rations containing low levels of aflatoxin B1. *Food Addit. Contam.* **2003**, *20*, 648–653. [CrossRef] [PubMed]
109. Micco, C.; Miraglia, M.; Onori, R.; Brera, C.; Mantovani, A.; Ioppolo, A.; Stasolla, D. Long-term administration of low doses of mycotoxins to poultry. 1. Residues of aflatoxin B1 and its metabolites in broilers and laying hens. *Food Addit. Contam.* **1988**, *5*, 303–308. [CrossRef]
110. Diaz-Zaragoza, M.; Carvajal-Moreno, M.; Mendez-Ramirez, I.; Chilpa-Galvan, N.C.; Avila-Gonzalez, E.; Flores-Ortiz, C.M. Aflatoxins, hydroxylated metabolites, and aflatoxicol from breast muscle of laying hens. *Poult. Sci.* **2014**, *93*, 3152–3162. [CrossRef] [PubMed]
111. Holeski, C.J.; Eaton, D.L.; Monroe, D.H.; Bellamy, G.M. Effects of phenobarbital on the biliary excretion of aflatoxin P1-glucuronide and aflatoxin B1-S-glutathione in the rat. *Xenobiotica* **1987**, *17*, 139–153. [CrossRef]
112. Groopman, J.D.; Hasler, J.A.; Trudel, L.J.; Pikul, A.; Donahue, P.R.; Wogan, G.N. Molecular dosimetry in rat urine of aflatoxin-N7-guanine and other aflatoxin metabolites by multiple monoclonal antibody affinity chromatography and immunoaffinity/high performance liquid chromatography. *Cancer Res.* **1992**, *52*, 267–274.
113. Rowland, A.; Mackenzie, P.I.; Miners, J.O. Transporter-mediated uptake of UDP-glucuronic acid by human liver microsomes: Assay conditions, kinetics, and inhibition. *Drug Metab. Dispos.* **2015**, *43*, 147–153. [CrossRef]
114. Stiborova, M.; Barta, F.; Levova, K.; Hodek, P.; Schmeiser, H.H.; Arlt, V.M.; Martinek, V. A Mechanism of O-demethylation of aristolochic acid I by cytochromes P450 and their contributions to this reaction in human and rat livers: Experimental and theoretical approaches. *Int. J. Mol. Sci.* **2015**, *16*, 27561–27575. [CrossRef] [PubMed]
115. Eaton, D.L.; Monroe, D.H.; Bellamy, G.; Kalman, D.A. Identification of a novel dihydroxy metabolite of aflatoxin B1 produced in vitro and in vivo in rats and mice. *Chem. Res. Toxicol.* **1988**, *1*, 108–114. [CrossRef]
116. Coulombe, R.A.; Shelton, D.W.; Sinnhuber, R.O.; Nixon, J.E. Comparative mutagenicity of aflatoxins using a Salmonella/trout hepatic enzyme activation system. *Carcinogenesis* **1982**, *3*, 1261–1264. [CrossRef] [PubMed]
117. Ames, B.N.; Durston, W.E.; Yamasaki, E.; Lee, F.D. Carcinogens are mutagens: A simple test system combining liver homogenates for activation and bacteria for detection. *Proc. Natl. Acad. Sci. USA* **1973**, *70*, 2281–2285. [CrossRef]
118. Krieger, R.I.; Salhab, A.S.; Dalezios, J.I.; Hsieh, D.P. Aflaxation B1 hydroxylation by hepatic microsomal preparations from the rhesus monkey. *Food Cosmet. Toxicol.* **1975**, *13*, 211–219. [CrossRef] [PubMed]
119. Hsieh, D.P.; Dalezios, J.I.; Krieger, R.I.; Masri, M.S.; Haddon, W.F. Use of monkey liver microsomes in production of aflatoxin Q1. *J. Agric. Food Chem.* **1974**, *22*, 515–517. [CrossRef] [PubMed]
120. Raney, K.D.; Shimada, T.; Kim, D.H.; Groopman, J.D.; Harris, T.M.; Guengerich, F.P. Oxidation of aflatoxins and sterigmatocystin by human liver microsomes: Significance of aflatoxin Q1 as a detoxication product of aflatoxin B1. *Chem. Res. Toxicol.* **1992**, *5*, 202–210. [CrossRef] [PubMed]
121. Forrester, L.M.; Neal, G.E.; Judah, D.J.; Glancey, M.J.; Wolf, C.R. Evidence for involvement of multiple forms of cytochrome P-450 in aflatoxin B1 metabolism in human liver. *Proc. Natl. Acad. Sci. USA* **1990**, *87*, 8306–8310. [CrossRef]
122. Ramsdell, H.S.; Parkinson, A.; Eddy, A.C.; Eaton, D.L. Bioactivation of aflatoxin B1 by human liver microsomes: Role of cytochrome P450 IIIA enzymes. *Toxicol. Appl. Pharmacol.* **1991**, *108*, 436–447. [CrossRef] [PubMed]

123. Ezekiel, C.N.; Abia, W.A.; Braun, D.; Sarkanj, B.; Ayeni, K.I.; Oyedele, O.A.; Michael-Chikezie, E.C.; Ezekiel, V.C.; Mark, B.N.; Ahuchaogu, C.P.; et al. Mycotoxin exposure biomonitoring in breastfed and non-exclusively breastfed Nigerian children. *Environ. Int.* **2022**, *158*, 106996. [CrossRef] [PubMed]
124. Mykkanen, H.; Zhu, H.; Salminen, E.; Juvonen, R.O.; Ling, W.; Ma, J.; Polychronaki, N.; Kemilainen, H.; Mykkanen, O.; Salminen, S.; et al. Fecal and urinary excretion of aflatoxin B1 metabolites (AFQ1, AFM1 and AFB-N7-guanine) in young Chinese males. *Int. J. Cancer* **2005**, *115*, 879–884. [CrossRef] [PubMed]
125. Carr, B.; Norcross, R.; Fang, Y.; Lu, P.; Rodrigues, A.D.; Shou, M.; Rushmore, T.; Booth-Genthe, C. Characterization of the rhesus monkey CYP3A64 enzyme: Species comparisons of CYP3A substrate specificity and kinetics using baculovirus-expressed recombinant enzymes. *Drug Metab. Dispos.* **2006**, *34*, 1703–1712. [CrossRef] [PubMed]
126. Tang, L.; Guan, H.; Ding, X.; Wang, J.S. Modulation of aflatoxin toxicity and biomarkers by lycopene in F344 rats. *Toxicol. Appl. Pharmacol.* **2007**, *219*, 10–17. [CrossRef] [PubMed]
127. Renaud, H.J.; Cui, J.Y.; Khan, M.; Klaassen, C.D. Tissue distribution and gender-divergent expression of 78 cytochrome P450 mRNAs in mice. *Toxicol. Sci.* **2011**, *124*, 261–277. [CrossRef] [PubMed]
128. Edwards, G.S.; Rintel, T.D.; Parker, C.M. Aflatoxicol as a possible predictor for species sensitivity to aflatoxin B1 (AFB1). *Cancer Res.* **1975**, *16*, 133.
129. Garner, R.C.; Miller, E.C.; Miller, J.A. Liver microsomal metabolism of aflatoxin B 1 to a reactive derivative toxic to Salmonella typhimurium TA 1530. *Cancer Res* **1972**, *32*, 2058–2066. [PubMed]
130. Patterson, D.S. Hydroxylation and toxicity of aflatoxins. *Biochem. J.* **1971**, *125*, 19P–20P. [CrossRef] [PubMed]
131. Patterson, D.S.P. Metabolism as a factor in determining the toxic action of the aflatoxins in different animal species. *Food Cosmet. Toxicol.* **1973**, *11*, 287–294.
132. Salhab, A.S.; Edwards, G.S. Comparative in vitro metabolism of aflatoxicol by liver preparations from animals and humans. *Cancer Res.* **1977**, *37*, 1016–1021. [PubMed]
133. Campbell, T.C.; Hayes, J.R. The role of aflatoxin metabolism in its toxic lesion. *Toxicol. Appl. Pharmacol.* **1976**, *35*, 199–222. [CrossRef] [PubMed]
134. Stich, H.F.; Laishes, B.A. The response of Xeroderma pigmentosum cells and controls to the activated mycotoxins, aflatoxins and sterigmatocystin. *Int. J. Cancer* **1975**, *16*, 266–274. [CrossRef]
135. Murcia, H.; Diaz, G.J. Dealing with aflatoxin B1 dihydrodiol acute effects: Impact of aflatoxin B1-aldehyde reductase enzyme activity in poultry species tolerant to AFB1 toxic effects. *PLoS ONE* **2020**, *15*, e0235061. [CrossRef] [PubMed]
136. Guengerich, F.P.; Johnson, W.W. Kinetics of hydrolysis and reaction of aflatoxin B1 exo-8,9-epoxide and relevance to toxicity and detoxication. *Drug Metab. Rev.* **1999**, *31*, 141–158. [CrossRef] [PubMed]
137. Johnson, W.W.; Yamazaki, H.; Shimada, T.; Ueng, Y.F.; Guengerich, F.P. Aflatoxin B1 8,9-epoxide hydrolysis in the presence of rat and human epoxide hydrolase. *Chem. Res. Toxicol.* **1997**, *10*, 672–676. [CrossRef] [PubMed]
138. Kelly, E.J.; Erickson, K.E.; Sengstag, C.; Eaton, D.L. Expression of human microsomal epoxide hydrolase in Saccharomyces cerevisiae reveals a functional role in aflatoxin B1 detoxification. *Toxicol. Sci.* **2002**, *65*, 35–42. [CrossRef]
139. Andersson, T.; Pesonen, M.; Johansson, C. Differential induction of cytochrome P-450-dependent monooxygenase, epoxide hydrolase, glutathione transferase and UDP glucuronosyl transferase activities in the liver of the rainbow trout by beta-naphthoflavone or Clophen A50. *Biochem. Pharmacol.* **1985**, *34*, 3309–3314. [CrossRef] [PubMed]
140. Diaz, G.J.; Murcia, H.W. An unusually high production of hepatic aflatoxin B(1)-dihydrodiol, the possible explanation for the high susceptibility of ducks to aflatoxin B(1). *Sci. Rep.* **2019**, *9*, 8010. [CrossRef]
141. Guengerich, F.P.; Cai, H.; McMahon, M.; Hayes, J.D.; Sutter, T.R.; Groopman, J.D.; Deng, Z.; Harris, T.M. Reduction of aflatoxin B1 dialdehyde by rat and human aldo-keto reductases. *Chem. Res. Toxicol.* **2001**, *14*, 727–737. [CrossRef] [PubMed]
142. Judah, D.J.; Hayes, J.D.; Yang, J.C.; Lian, L.Y.; Roberts, G.C.; Farmer, P.B.; Lamb, J.H.; Neal, G.E. A novel aldehyde reductase with activity towards a metabolite of aflatoxin B1 is expressed in rat liver during carcinogenesis and following the administration of an anti-oxidant. *Biochem. J.* **1993**, *292*, 13–18. [CrossRef]
143. Ellis, E.M.; Slattery, C.M.; Hayes, J.D. Characterization of the rat aflatoxin B1 aldehyde reductase gene, AKR7A1. Structure and chromosomal localization of AKR7A1 as well as identification of antioxidant response elements in the gene promoter. *Carcinogenesis* **2003**, *24*, 727–737. [CrossRef] [PubMed]
144. Knight, L.P.; Primiano, T.; Groopman, J.D.; Kensler, T.W.; Sutter, T.R. cDNA cloning, expression and activity of a second human aflatoxin B1-metabolizing member of the aldo-keto reductase superfamily, AKR7A3. *Carcinogenesis* **1999**, *20*, 1215–1223. [CrossRef] [PubMed]
145. Ellis, E.M.; Hayes, J.D. Substrate specificity of an aflatoxin-metabolizing aldehyde reductase. *Biochem. J.* **1995**, *312*, 535–541. [CrossRef] [PubMed]
146. Judah, D.J.; Davies, R.; Hayes, J.D.; McLellan, L.I.; Neal, G.E. The primary and secondary metabolism of aflatoxin B1 by rat hepatocytes cultured on matrigel. *Toxicol. Appl. Pharmacol.* **1994**, *125*, 27–33. [CrossRef]

147. Johnson, D.N.; Egner, P.A.; Obrian, G.; Glassbrook, N.; Roebuck, B.D.; Sutter, T.R.; Payne, G.A.; Kensler, T.W.; Groopman, J.D. Quantification of urinary aflatoxin B1 dialdehyde metabolites formed by aflatoxin aldehyde reductase using isotope dilution tandem mass spectrometry. *Chem. Res. Toxicol.* **2008**, *21*, 752–760. [CrossRef]
148. Roebuck, B.D.; Johnson, D.N.; Sutter, C.H.; Egner, P.A.; Scholl, P.F.; Friesen, M.D.; Baumgartner, K.J.; Ware, N.M.; Bodreddigari, S.; Groopman, J.D.; et al. Transgenic expression of aflatoxin aldehyde reductase (AKR7A1) modulates aflatoxin B1 metabolism but not hepatic carcinogenesis in the rat. *Toxicol. Sci.* **2009**, *109*, 41–49. [CrossRef] [PubMed]
149. Tulayakul, P.; Sakuda, S.; Dong, K.S.; Kumagai, S. Comparative activities of glutathione-S-transferase and dialdehyde reductase toward aflatoxin B1 in livers of experimental and farm animals. *Toxicon* **2005**, *46*, 204–209. [CrossRef]
150. Monroe, D.H.; Eaton, D.L. Comparative effects of butylated hydroxyanisole on hepatic in vivo DNA binding and in vitro biotransformation of aflatoxin B1 in the rat and mouse. *Toxicol. Appl. Pharmacol.* **1987**, *90*, 401–409. [CrossRef]
151. Monroe, D.H.; Eaton, D.L. Effects of modulation of hepatic glutathione on biotransformation and covalent binding of aflatoxin B1 to DNA in the mouse. *Toxicol. Appl. Pharmacol.* **1988**, *94*, 118–127. [CrossRef] [PubMed]
152. Slone, D.H.; Gallagher, E.P.; Ramsdell, H.S.; Rettie, A.E.; Stapleton, P.L.; Berlad, L.G.; Eaton, D.L. Human variability in hepatic glutathione S-transferase-mediated conjugation of aflatoxin B1-epoxide and other substrates. *Pharmacogenetics* **1995**, *5*, 224–233. [CrossRef] [PubMed]
153. Kirby, G.M.; Wolf, C.R.; Neal, G.E.; Judah, D.J.; Henderson, C.J.; Srivatanakul, P.; Wild, C.P. In vitro metabolism of aflatoxin B1 by normal and tumorous liver tissue from Thailand. *Carcinogenesis* **1993**, *14*, 2613–2620. [CrossRef] [PubMed]
154. Eaton, D.L.; Bammler, T.K. Concise review of the glutathione S-transferases and their significance to toxicology. *Toxicol. Sci.* **1999**, *49*, 156–164. [CrossRef] [PubMed]
155. Hayes, J.D.; Pulford, D.J. The glutathione S-transferase supergene family: Regulation of GST and the contribution of the isoenzymes to cancer chemoprotection and drug resistance. *Crit. Rev. Biochem. Mol. Biol.* **1995**, *30*, 445–600. [CrossRef] [PubMed]
156. Johnson, W.W.; Ueng, Y.F.; Widersten, M.; Mannervik, B.; Hayes, J.D.; Sherratt, P.J.; Ketterer, B.; Guengerich, F.P. Conjugation of highly reactive aflatoxin B1 exo-8,9-epoxide catalyzed by rat and human glutathione transferases: Estimation of kinetic parameters. *Biochemistry* **1997**, *36*, 3056–3060. [CrossRef] [PubMed]
157. Gross-Steinmeyer, K.; Stapleton, P.L.; Tracy, J.H.; Bammler, T.K.; Strom, S.C.; Eaton, D.L. Sulforaphane- and phenethyl isothiocyanate-induced inhibition of aflatoxin B1-mediated genotoxicity in human hepatocytes: Role of GSTM1 genotype and CYP3A4 gene expression. *Toxicol. Sci.* **2010**, *116*, 422–432. [CrossRef]
158. McGlynn, K.A.; Rosvold, E.A.; Lustbader, E.D.; Hu, Y.; Clapper, M.L.; Zhou, T.; Wild, C.P.; Xia, X.L.; Baffoe-Bonnie, A.; Ofori-Adjei, D.; et al. Susceptibility to hepatocellular carcinoma is associated with genetic variation in the enzymatic detoxification of aflatoxin B1. *Proc. Natl. Acad. Sci. USA* **1995**, *92*, 2384–2387. [CrossRef]
159. Stewart, R.K.; Smith, G.B.; Donnelly, P.J.; Reid, K.R.; Petsikas, D.; Conlan, A.A.; Massey, T.E. Glutathione S-transferase-catalyzed conjugation of bioactivated aflatoxin B(1) in human lung: Differential cellular distribution and lack of significance of the GSTM1 genetic polymorphism. *Carcinogenesis* **1999**, *20*, 1971–1977. [CrossRef] [PubMed]
160. Wang, C.; Bammler, T.K.; Guo, Y.; Kelly, E.J.; Eaton, D.L. Mu-class GSTs are responsible for aflatoxin B(1)-8, 9-epoxide-conjugating activity in the nonhuman primate macaca fascicularis liver. *Toxicol. Sci.* **2000**, *56*, 26–36. [CrossRef]
161. Wang, C.; Bammler, T.K.; Eaton, D.L. Complementary DNA cloning, protein expression, and characterization of alpha-class GSTs from Macaca fascicularis liver. *Toxicol. Sci.* **2002**, *70*, 20–26. [CrossRef]
162. Degen, G.H.; Neumann, H.G. The major metabolite of aflatoxin B1 in the rat is a glutathione conjugate. *Chem. Biol. Interact.* **1978**, *22*, 239–255. [CrossRef]
163. Eaton, D.L.; Ramsdell, H.S.; Neal, G.E. Biotransformation of Aflatoxins. In *The Toxicology of Aflatoxins: Human Health, Veterinary and Agricultural Significance*; Eaton, D.L., Groopman, J.D., Eds.; Academic Press: Boston, MA, USA, 1995; pp. 45–72.
164. Pulford, D.J.; Hayes, J.D. Characterization of the rat glutathione S-transferase Yc2 subunit gene, GSTA5: Identification of a putative antioxidant-responsive element in the 5′-flanking region of rat GSTA5 that may mediate chemoprotection against aflatoxin B1. *Biochem. J.* **1996**, *318*, 75–84. [CrossRef] [PubMed]
165. Van Ness, K.P.; Buetler, T.M.; Eaton, D.L. Enzymatic characteristics of chimeric mYc/rYc1 glutathione S-transferases. *Cancer Res.* **1994**, *54*, 4573–4575. [PubMed]
166. Van Ness, K.P.; McHugh, T.E.; Bammler, T.K.; Eaton, D.L. Identification of amino acid residues essential for high aflatoxin B1-8,9-epoxide conjugation activity in alpha class glutathione S-transferases through site-directed mutagenesis. *Toxicol. Appl. Pharmacol.* **1998**, *152*, 166–174. [CrossRef] [PubMed]
167. Hayes, J.D.; Nguyen, T.; Judah, D.J.; Petersson, D.G.; Neal, G.E. Cloning of cDNAs from fetal rat liver encoding glutathione S-transferase Yc polypeptides. The Yc2 subunit is expressed in adult rat liver resistant to the hepatocarcinogen aflatoxin B1. *J. Biol. Chem.* **1994**, *269*, 20707–20717. [CrossRef] [PubMed]
168. Hayes, J.D.; Judah, D.J.; Neal, G.E. Resistance to aflatoxin B1 is associated with the expression of a novel aldo-keto reductase which has catalytic activity towards a cytotoxic aldehyde-containing metabolite of the toxin. *Cancer Res.* **1993**, *53*, 3887–3894.

169. Hayes, J.D.; Judah, D.J.; McLellan, L.I.; Neal, G.E. Contribution of the glutathione S-transferases to the mechanisms of resistance to aflatoxin B1. *Pharmacol. Ther.* **1991**, *50*, 443–472. [CrossRef] [PubMed]
170. Kensler, T.W.; Groopman, J.D.; Eaton, D.L.; Curphey, T.J.; Roebuck, B.D. Potent inhibition of aflatoxin-induced hepatic tumorigenesis by the monofunctional enzyme inducer 1,2-dithiole-3-thione. *Carcinogenesis* **1992**, *13*, 95–100. [CrossRef]
171. Yates, M.S.; Kwak, M.K.; Egner, P.A.; Groopman, J.D.; Bodreddigari, S.; Sutter, T.R.; Baumgartner, K.J.; Roebuck, B.D.; Liby, K.T.; Yore, M.M.; et al. Potent protection against aflatoxin-induced tumorigenesis through induction of Nrf2-regulated pathways by the triterpenoid 1-[2-cyano-3-,12-dioxooleana-1,9(11)-dien-28-oyl]imidazole. *Cancer Res.* **2006**, *66*, 2488–2494. [CrossRef] [PubMed]
172. Crawford, D.R.; Ilic, Z.; Guest, I.; Milne, G.L.; Hayes, J.D.; Sell, S. Characterization of liver injury, oval cell proliferation and cholangiocarcinogenesis in glutathione S-transferase A3 knockout mice. *Carcinogenesis* **2017**, *38*, 717–727. [CrossRef] [PubMed]
173. Ilic, Z.; Crawford, D.; Vakharia, D.; Egner, P.A.; Sell, S. Glutathione-S-transferase A3 knockout mice are sensitive to acute cytotoxic and genotoxic effects of aflatoxin B1. *Toxicol. Appl. Pharmacol.* **2010**, *242*, 241–246. [CrossRef] [PubMed]
174. Buetler, T.M.; Eaton, D.L. Complementary DNA cloning, messenger RNA expression, and induction of alpha-class glutathione S-transferases in mouse tissues. *Cancer Res.* **1992**, *52*, 314–318. [PubMed]
175. Jowsey, I.R.; Jiang, Q.; Itoh, K.; Yamamoto, M.; Hayes, J.D. Expression of the aflatoxin B1-8,9-epoxide-metabolizing murine glutathione S-transferase A3 subunit is regulated by the Nrf2 transcription factor through an antioxidant response element. *Mol. Pharmacol.* **2003**, *64*, 1018–1028. [CrossRef] [PubMed]
176. Kim, J.E.; Bauer, M.M.; Mendoza, K.M.; Reed, K.M.; Coulombe, R.A., Jr. Comparative genomics identifies new alpha class genes within the avian glutathione S-transferase gene cluster. *Gene* **2010**, *452*, 45–53. [CrossRef]
177. Kim, J.E.; Bunderson, B.R.; Croasdell, A.; Coulombe, R.A., Jr. Functional characterization of alpha-class glutathione s-transferases from the Turkey (*Meleagris gallopavo*). *Toxicol. Sci.* **2011**, *124*, 45–53. [CrossRef] [PubMed]
178. Kim, J.E.; Bunderson, B.R.; Croasdell, A.; Reed, K.M.; Coulombe, R.A., Jr. Alpha-class glutathione S-transferases in wild turkeys (*Meleagris gallopavo*): Characterization and role in resistance to the carcinogenic mycotoxin aflatoxin B1. *PLoS ONE* **2013**, *8*, e60662. [CrossRef] [PubMed]
179. Bunderson, B.R.; Kim, J.E.; Croasdell, A.; Mendoza, K.M.; Reed, K.M.; Coulombe, R.A., Jr. Heterologous expression and functional characterization of avian mu-class glutathione S-transferases. *Comp. Biochem. Physiol. C Toxicol. Pharmacol.* **2013**, *158*, 109–116. [CrossRef] [PubMed]
180. Moss, E.J.; Neal, G.E.; Judah, D.J. The mercapturic acid pathway metabolites of a glutathione conjugate of aflatoxin B1. *Chem. Biol. Interact.* **1985**, *55*, 139–155. [CrossRef] [PubMed]
181. Klaassen, C.D.; Aleksunes, L.M. Xenobiotic, bile acid, and cholesterol transporters: Function and regulation. *Pharmacol. Rev.* **2010**, *62*, 1–96. [CrossRef]
182. Lee, T.K.; Li, L.; Ballatori, N. Hepatic glutathione and glutathione S-conjugate transport mechanisms. *Yale J. Biol. Med.* **1997**, *70*, 287–300. [PubMed]
183. Moss, E.J.; Manson, M.M.; Neal, G.E. Effect of manipulation of gamma-glutamyl transpeptidase levels on biliary excretion of aflatoxin B1 conjugates. *Carcinogenesis* **1984**, *5*, 869–874. [CrossRef]
184. Scholl, P.F.; Musser, S.M.; Groopman, J.D. Synthesis and characterization of aflatoxin B1 mercapturic acids and their identification in rat urine. *Chem. Res. Toxicol.* **1997**, *10*, 1144–1151. [CrossRef] [PubMed]
185. Kensler, K.H.; Slocum, S.L.; Chartoumpekis, D.V.; Dolan, P.M.; Johnson, N.M.; Ilic, Z.; Crawford, D.R.; Sell, S.; Groopman, J.D.; Kensler, T.W.; et al. Genetic or pharmacologic activation of Nrf2 signaling fails to protect against aflatoxin genotoxicity in hypersensitive GSTA3 knockout mice. *Toxicol. Sci.* **2014**, *139*, 293–300. [CrossRef] [PubMed]
186. Nayak, S.; Tanuja, P.; Sashidhar, R.B. Synthesis and characterization of mercapturic acid (N-acetyl-L-cysteine)-aflatoxin B1 adduct and its quantitation in rat urine by an enzyme immunoassay. *J. AOAC Int.* **2009**, *92*, 487–495. [CrossRef]
187. Wang, J.S.; Shen, X.; He, X.; Zhu, Y.R.; Zhang, B.C.; Wang, J.B.; Qian, G.S.; Kuang, S.Y.; Zarba, A.; Egner, P.A.; et al. Protective alterations in phase 1 and 2 metabolism of aflatoxin B1 by oltipraz in residents of Qidong, People's Republic of China. *J. Natl. Cancer Inst.* **1999**, *91*, 347–354. [CrossRef] [PubMed]
188. Roebuck, B.D.; Liu, Y.L.; Rogers, A.E.; Groopman, J.D.; Kensler, T.W. Protection against aflatoxin B1-induced hepatocarcinogenesis in F344 rats by 5-(2-pyrazinyl)-4-methyl-1,2-dithiole-3-thione (oltipraz): Predictive role for short-term molecular dosimetry. *Cancer Res.* **1991**, *51*, 5501–5506. [PubMed]
189. Kensler, T.W.; Eaton, D.L. 65 Years on-Aflatoxin Biomarkers Blossoming: Whither Next? *Toxins* **2024**, *16*, 496. [CrossRef] [PubMed]
190. Ehrich, M.; Huckle, W.R.; Larsen, C. Increase in glucuronide conjugation of aflatoxin P1 after pretreatment with microsomal enzyme inducers. *Toxicology* **1984**, *32*, 145–152. [CrossRef] [PubMed]
191. Wei, C.I.; Hsieh, D.P. Characterization of water-soluble glucuronide and sulphate conjugates of aflatoxin B_1. 2. Studies in primary cultures of rat hepatocytes. *Food Chem. Toxicol.* **1985**, *23*, 821–825. [CrossRef]
192. Wei, C.I.; Marshall, M.R.; Hsieh, D.P. Characterization of water-soluble glucuronide and sulphate conjugates of aflatoxin B_1. 1. Urinary excretion in monkey, rat and mouse. *Food Chem. Toxicol.* **1985**, *23*, 809–819. [CrossRef] [PubMed]

193. Chipley, J.R.; Mabee, M.S.; Alegate, K.L.; Dreyfuss, M.S. Further characterization of tissue distribution and metabolism of (14C)aflatoxin B1 in chickens. *Appl. Microbiol.* **1974**, *28*, 1027–1029. [CrossRef]
194. Dalezios, J.; Wogan, G.N.; Weinreb, S.M. Aflatoxin P-1: A new aflatoxin metabolite in monkeys. *Science* **1971**, *171*, 584–585. [CrossRef] [PubMed]
195. Dalezios, J.I.; Hsieh, D.P.; Wogan, G.N. Excretion and metabolism of orally administered aflatoxin B1 by rhesus monkeys. *Food Cosmet. Toxicol.* **1973**, *11*, 605–616. [CrossRef] [PubMed]
196. Dalezios, J.I.; Wogan, G.N. Metabolism of aflatoxin B 1 in rhesus monkeys. *Cancer Res.* **1972**, *32*, 2297–2303. [PubMed]
197. Gregory, J.F., 3rd; Goldstein, S.L.; Edds, G.T. Metabolite distribution and rate of residue clearance in turkeys fed a diet containing aflatoxin B1. *Food Chem. Toxicol.* **1983**, *21*, 463–467. [CrossRef]
198. Gregory, J.F., 3rd; Edds, G.T. Effect of dietary selenium on the metabolism of aflatoxin B1 in turkeys. *Food Chem. Toxicol.* **1984**, *22*, 637–642. [CrossRef] [PubMed]
199. Wei, C.I.; Decad, G.M.; Wong, Z.A.; Byard, J.L.; Hsieh, D.P.H. Characterization and mutagenciity of water-soluble conjugates of aflatoxin B1. *Toxicol. Appl. Pharmacol.* **1978**, *45*, 45–52.
200. EFSA Panel on Contaminants in the Food Chain (CONTAM); Schrenk, D.; Bignami, M.; Bodin, L.; Chipman, J.K.; Del Mazo, J.; Grasl-Kraupp, B.; Hogstrand, C.; Hoogenboom, L.R.; Leblanc, J.C.; et al. Risk assessment of aflatoxins in food. *EFSA J.* **2020**, *18*, e06040. [CrossRef]

toxins

MDPI

Article

Structurally Similar Mycotoxins Aflatoxin B_1 and Sterigmatocystin Trigger Different and Distinctive High-Resolution Mutational Spectra in Mammalian Cells

Pennapa Thongararm [1,2,*], Marisa Chancharoen [2,3], Nutchapong Suwanwong [4], Somsak Ruchirawat [4,5,6], Mathuros Ruchirawat [1,5], Bogdan I. Fedeles [2], Robert G. Croy [2] and John M. Essigmann [2,*]

1 Laboratory of Environmental Toxicology, Chulabhorn Research Institute, Bangkok 10210, Thailand; mathuros@cri.or.th
2 Department of Biological Engineering, Department of Chemistry, and Center for Environmental Health Sciences, Massachusetts Institute of Technology, Cambridge, MA 02139, USA; marisa@cgi.ac.th (M.C.); bogdan@mit.edu (B.I.F.); rgcroy@mit.edu (R.G.C.)
3 Program in Applied Biological Sciences, Chulabhorn Graduate Institute, Bangkok 10210, Thailand
4 Program in Chemical Sciences, Chulabhorn Graduate Institute, Bangkok 10210, Thailand; nutchapongs@cgi.ac.th (N.S.); somsak@cri.or.th (S.R.)
5 Center of Excellence on Environmental Health and Toxicology (EHT), OPS, Ministry of Higher Education, Science, Research and Innovation, Bangkok 10400, Thailand
6 Laboratory of Medicinal Chemistry, Chulabhorn Research Institute, Bangkok 10210, Thailand
* Correspondence: pennapa@cri.or.th (P.T.); jessig@mit.edu (J.M.E.)

Abstract: Aflatoxin B_1 (AFB_1) and sterigmatocystin (ST) are mycotoxins that pose significant threats to human and animal health owing to their mutagenic, carcinogenic, and toxic properties. They are structurally similar and widely believed to exert their biological effects via the generation of DNA-damaging epoxides at their respective terminal furan rings. Despite structural identity in the warhead portion of each toxin, this work shows that distal parts of each molecule are responsible for the distinctive mutational fingerprints seen in *gpt*Δ C57BL/6J mouse embryo fibroblasts (MEFs). The two toxins differ structurally in the puckered cyclopentenone ring of AFB_1 and in the planar xanthone functionality of ST. While both toxins mainly induce GC→TA mutations, the aforementioned differences in structure apparently trigger unique patterns of mutations, as revealed by high-resolution duplex sequencing of MEF genomes. AFB_1 is more mutagenic than ST and displays its transversion mutations in a pattern with primary and secondary hotspots (underscored) in 5′-C<u>G</u>C-3′ and 5′-C<u>G</u>G-3′ contexts, respectively. ST displays a modest 5′-C<u>G</u>G-3′ hotspot while its other GC→TA transversions are more uniformly distributed in a pattern resembling established oxidative stress mutational spectra. This research delineates the mutational spectra of AFB_1 and ST, establishing these patterns as possible early-onset biomarkers of exposure.

Keywords: mycotoxins; high-resolution mutational spectra; mutagenesis; biomarkers; mammalian cells

Key Contribution: This study elucidates the mutational spectra generated by metabolically activated aflatoxin B_1 and sterigmatocystin in mouse embryo fibroblasts. This cell culture system is much easier to use and more efficient than classical intact animal models. Despite the structural similarities between the toxins, their mutational spectra are characteristic and easily distinguished from one another. The findings are also in accord with a growing literature showing that the mutational fingerprints of toxic agents can be potential early biomarkers of environmental exposure, advancing our understanding of their health risks.

1. Introduction

Mycotoxins represent one of the most significant global threats to public health and food safety, with aflatoxin B_1 (AFB_1) and sterigmatocystin (ST) standing out as two toxicologically relevant examples [1–8]. Produced by several species of *Aspergillus* molds, these secondary metabolites have raised considerable concern due to their prevalence in agricultural products, particularly in areas of the world with inadequate food storage practices [9,10]. The urgency of addressing the risks posed by AFB_1 and ST has been heightened by the effects of climate change. Warming temperatures and shifting environmental conditions have created favorable habitats for heat-tolerant *Aspergillus* species, leading to increased contamination of staple crops, including maize, peanuts, and grains [11,12]. These environmental changes disproportionately impact developing regions, where agricultural practices often lack the infrastructure for effective mitigation. Consequently, the contamination of food supplies by AFB_1 and ST has become not only a food safety issue but also a major public health concern, contributing to long-term health risks associated with liver damage, cancer, and immune suppression [13,14]. Understanding the biochemical pathways and the genetic mechanisms underlying the toxicity of these compounds is therefore critical for developing effective early disease detection and preventive strategies, and appropriate regulatory frameworks.

AFB_1 and ST (Figure 1) are mycotoxins synthesized via a shared biosynthetic pathway involving approximately 20 enzymatic steps [15]. Late in the pathway, the xanthone ring of ST is converted to the coumarin–cyclopentenone product, AFB_1. Figure 1 has differential coloration to show the differences between the two toxins. Both toxins originate from a common polyketide precursor that undergoes enzymatic cyclization and modifications, culminating in the formation of the difuranocoumarin core [16,17]; this structural motif underpins many of their toxicological effects, as it facilitates bioactivation into reactive intermediates that can interact with cellular macromolecules [18,19]. Despite their structural similarities, AFB_1 and ST exhibit distinct toxicological profiles, partly due to differences in their metabolic activation and interaction with cellular targets. AFB_1 is bioactivated primarily by cytochrome P450 enzymes, specifically CYP1A2 and CYP3A4 in humans, to generate the highly reactive *exo*-AFB_1-8,9-epoxide [19–27]. This epoxide intermediate forms covalent DNA adducts, most notably 8,9-dihydro-8-(N7-guanyl-9-hydroxyaflatoxin B_1 (AFB_1-N7-Gua) [20] and its imidazole ring-hydrolyzed derivatives, the AFB_1 formamidopyrimidines (FAPYs) [27]. These DNA adducts disrupt normal base-pairing during replication, leading to mutations that can initiate carcinogenesis [4,21,28–36]. The mutational spectrum induced by AFB_1 is well-characterized, with hallmark mutations frequently identified in the *TP53* tumor suppressor gene in hepatocellular carcinoma (HCC) patients [37–39]. Epidemiological evidence underscores the strong correlation between chronic AFB_1 exposure and liver cancer, particularly in populations co-infected with hepatitis B virus, where a powerful synergistic interaction amplifies disease risk [40,41].

ST undergoes a similar metabolic activation, yielding the epoxide intermediate *exo*-ST-1,2-epoxide. This metabolite also forms DNA adducts, predominantly 1,2-dihydro-2-(N7-guanyl)-1-hydroxysterigmatocystin (ST-N7-Gua) [22,42,43], but its mutagenic effects appear to be less pronounced than those of AFB_1 [44,45]. While the cytotoxicity and DNA-binding capacity of ST are well-documented [43,44,46,47], its mutational spectrum remains uncharacterized, complicating efforts to associate its mutagenic profile with possible downstream cancers. Regulatory agencies have responded to these uncertainties with varying levels of oversight, with AFB_1 subject to strict limits, such as 20 $\mu g/kg$ in food products set by the U.S. Food and Drug Administration [48] and even lower thresholds established by the European Union [49]. In contrast, ST is less stringently regulated, reflecting the limited data on its long-term health impacts.

Despite extensive research on AFB_1, significant gaps remain in our understanding of its precise molecular mechanisms and its interactions with other environmental and genetic factors. Recent technological advancements have provided new tools for addressing these challenges. High-resolution DNA sequencing has emerged as a powerful approach for delineating the detailed context-dependent mutational patterns induced by mycotoxins. These patterns offer valuable insights into the molecular origins of cancer and provide a basis for comparing experimental models to human malignancies [34,50]. In parallel, bioinformatic analyses have enabled the identification of mutational signatures associated with specific environmental exposures, enhancing our ability to link experimental findings to epidemiological data [51]. In this study, we leverage these recent advances to investigate the cytotoxic and mutagenic effects of AFB_1 and ST using mouse embryo fibroblasts (MEFs) derived from the *gpt*Δ C57BL/6J mouse, an animal model that is widely used in regulatory toxicology. This model, previously validated for studying DNA alkylation [50,52] and oxidative stress [53], provides a robust platform for exploring the mechanisms underlying mycotoxin-induced DNA damage. To account for the requirement of metabolic activation, we incorporate in the present work a microsomal activation system, enabling the formation of reactive intermediates. We also employ bioinformatic tools to compare the mutational patterns observed in our model to those found in human cancers, providing a translational link between experimental and clinical findings.

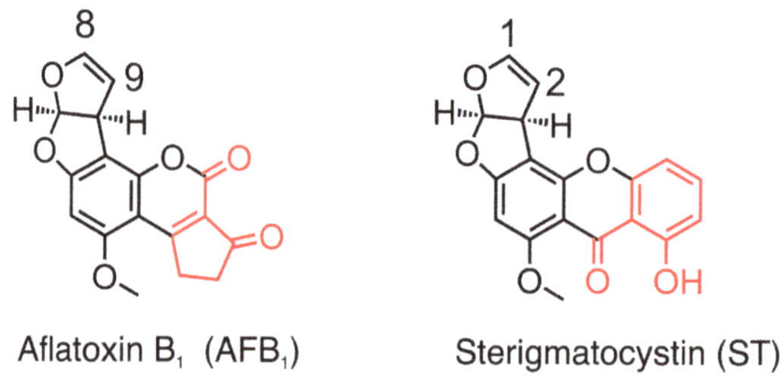

Figure 1. Comparison of the chemical structures of AFB_1 and ST. Both molecules share a similar core structure (black) that includes a difuran moiety that has a double bond between the 8 and 9 carbons of AFB_1 and the 1 and 2 carbons of ST. Differences between the structures of AFB_1 and ST are highlighted in red.

The findings from this study might have significant implications for public health and food safety. By elucidating the mechanisms through which AFB_1 and ST induce DNA damage and mutations, we aim to provide a clearer understanding of their relative risks and inform strategies for mitigating their impact. Such strategies are particularly important in regions of the world where contamination of food by these toxins is pervasive and regulatory enforcement is limited. Improved detection methods, coupled with enhanced storage practices, could play critical roles in reducing exposure. Moreover, our work highlights the need for a more nuanced approach to the regulation of mycotoxins. While the stringent limits on AFB_1 contamination reflect its well-documented risks, the relative lack of regulation for ST may underestimate its potential health impacts. A more comprehensive assessment of ST, informed by advanced toxicological and epidemiological studies, could provide the basis for updated regulatory guidelines.

2. Results

2.1. Metabolic Activation Distinguishes the Cytotoxicity Profiles of AFB_1 and ST in MEFs

Figure 2 depicts the experimental workflow of this study. The cytotoxic effects of AFB_1 and ST on MEFs were significantly influenced by metabolic activation, which substantially increased the toxicity of the toxins to the cell culture model (Figure 3A,B). Without metabolic activation, AFB_1 exhibited minimal cytotoxicity, with cell viability exceeding 90% even at the highest concentration tested (1 μM). Interestingly, however, even without metabolic activation ST demonstrated enhanced dose-dependent baseline toxicity, making it more toxic than aflatoxin at any given dose. Upon activation with the S9 fraction and NADPH, both compounds showed markedly enhanced toxicity, but the effect was more pronounced for AFB_1, which led to near-complete inhibition of cell growth at 1 μM. This result is in line with the expected conclusion that AFB_1 strongly relies on enzymatic bioactivation to produce reactive metabolites responsible for triggering its potent cytotoxicity. While ST also became significantly more toxic following S9 activation, its intrinsic cytotoxicity in the absence of metabolism underscores fundamental differences between it and AFB_1 in their toxicological profiles.

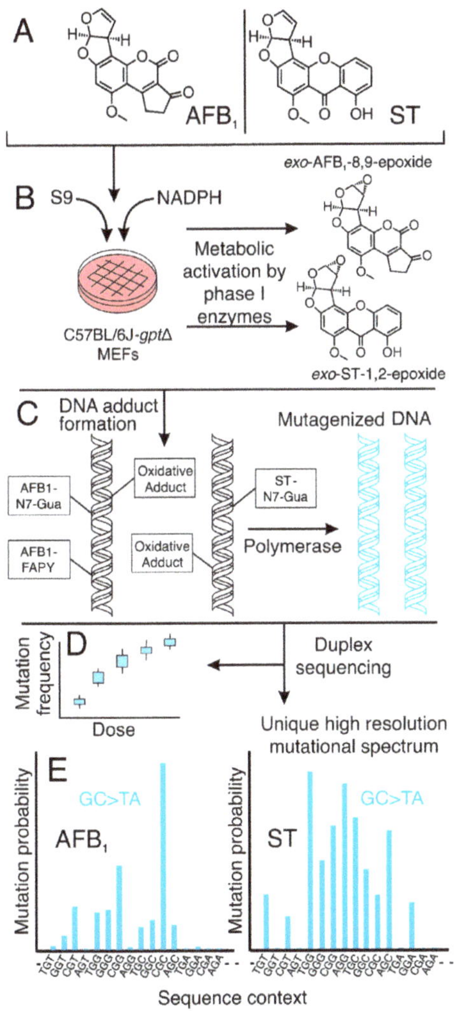

Figure 2. Schematic overview of experimental workflow for determining mutagenic signatures of AFB_1 and ST. (**A**,**B**) The carcinogenic mycotoxins AFB_1 and ST undergo metabolic activation to form highly reactive epoxide intermediates capable of covalently bonding to DNA. Mouse embryo fibroblasts derived from *gpt*Δ C57BL/6J mice were treated with AFB_1 or ST in the presence of S9 metabolic activation and NADPH. Phase I metabolism converts the parent compounds into their

respective electrophilic species: exo-AFB_1-8,9-epoxide and exo-ST-1,2-epoxide. (**C**) Reactive epoxide metabolites form DNA adducts, such as AFB_1-N7-Gua, AFB_1-FAPY, and ST-N7-Gua, which disrupt DNA structure and informational integrity. These adducts lead to mutations following bypass by error-prone DNA polymerases or failed repair. (**D**) Mutational frequency was quantified across multiple toxin doses using a highly sensitive *gpt* assay. (**E**) High-resolution mutational spectra were generated using duplex DNA sequencing, enabling precise characterization of the mutation profiles induced by AFB_1 and ST. GC→TA transversions emerged as the hallmark mutation type for both compounds, with distinct sequence-context dependencies reflected in unique mutational fingerprints.

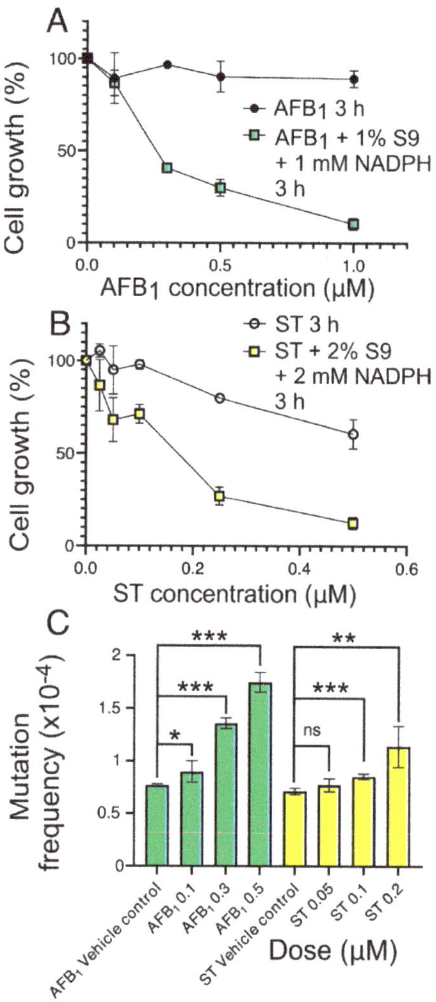

Figure 3. Cytotoxicity and mutagenicity of AFB_1 and ST in MEFs with and without S9 metabolic activation. (**A**) Percent cell growth in MEFs treated with AFB_1 for 3 h, depicted as a comparison between conditions without S9 (black circles) and with S9 metabolic activation (green squares; 1% S9 and 1 mM NADPH). (**B**) Percent cell growth in MEFs treated with ST for 3 h, shown without S9 (open circles) and with S9 metabolic activation (yellow squares; 2% S9 and 2 mM NADPH). (**C**) Mutation frequency induced by AFB_1 and ST under S9 metabolic activation at selected concentrations, with dose-dependent effects evident for AFB_1. Data are expressed as mean ± SD, with statistical significance denoted as * $p < 0.05$, ** $p < 0.01$, *** $p < 0.001$, and ns = not significant.

2.2. *Differential Mutagenic Potentials of AFB_1 and ST in MEFs*

The mutational frequency analysis of AFB_1 and ST in MEFs with S9 metabolic activation (Figure 3C) revealed striking differences in their mutagenic capacity, reflecting their distinct metabolic and mutagenicity profiles (vide infra). AFB_1 exhibited a strong, dose-dependent increase in mutation frequency, with the highest concentration (0.5 μM) showing a pronounced elevation as compared to lower doses (0.1 and 0.3 μM). This result highlights the potent mutagenic capacity of AFB_1's reactive metabolites generated through bioactivation.

In contrast, ST displayed only a modest increase in mutation frequency, with no clear dose-dependent trend observed across the tested concentrations (0, 0.05, 0.1, and 0.2 μM). The selected doses for this study were based on prior cytotoxicity assessments, ensuring sufficient cell viability to capture the mutagenic effects of the mycotoxins. AFB_1 consistently demonstrated a significantly higher mutagenic activity than ST. While both AFB_1 and ST depend on metabolic activation for their genotoxic effects, AFB_1 appears to be metabolized more readily into its reactive form, contributing to its stronger mutagenic potential.

2.3. *Unique Mutational Spectra of Metabolically Activated AFB_1 and ST*

Both AFB_1 and ST exhibited mutational profiles dominated by GC→TA transversions (Table 1 and blue bars in Figure 4A). While some features of the mutational patterns look similar, for the most part, the patterns are distinct, with a cosine similarity of only ~0.4 between the background-subtracted spectra (see Figure S2 for the background spectra and Figure S3 for the clustering analysis). Given the nearly exclusive propensity of both toxins to damage guanines, we assume that the G→T mutations originate from the polymerase-mediated insertion of adenines opposite the adducted guanines. This mechanism of mutagenesis, termed the "A-rule", is seen when individual adducts of aflatoxin, as well as many bulky or helix-distorting mutagens, are replicated in vitro and inside living cells [30]. Figure 4B shows a model explaining the pathway underlying the G→T mutations observed from both AFB_1 and ST. In this model, the guanine of an undamaged GC base pair (in the upper yellow box) becomes an AFB_1 or ST adduct (the blue lollipops). Replication of the strands containing each lesion results in an adenine being put in opposite the respective adducts; further rounds of replication reveal the emergence of GC→TA mutations (lower yellow box).

Both compounds demonstrated strong sequence-context biases in their mutational patterns, with GC-rich trinucleotide motifs prominently targeted (Figure 4A,C). Interestingly, AFB_1 displayed a heightened preference for mutation at 5′-C$\underline{G}$C-3′ sequences (the underscored $\underline{G}$ indicates the position in the 3-base context where mutations occur), likely indicative of a unique binding interaction with DNA that precedes alkylation. This characteristic hotspot for G→T mutations was previously observed in the livers of mice treated with AFB_1 [34]. While ST also predominantly induced G→T mutations, its G→T mutations are much more uniformly distributed among all 16 3-base sequence contexts (Figure 4A, top panel). Moreover, ST induced a more diverse spectrum of base substitutions, with additional contributions evident in GC→CG (black bars), AT→GC (green bars), and GC→AT (red bars) domains, suggesting concomitant oxidative stress or alternative DNA repair pathways.

Table 1. Relative frequencies of point mutation types in mutational spectra corresponding to AFB_1-treated and ST-treated MEFs with metabolic activation (spectra shown in Figure 4), and corresponding vehicle controls (spectra shown in Supplementary Materials, Figure S2). Both AFB_1 and ST data reflect background-subtracted spectra. An expanded version of this Table is in Supplementary Materials (Table S1).

Substitution Type	AFB_1 (%)	AFB_1-Control (%)	ST (%)	ST-Control (%)
		Transitions		
GC→AT	10.3	27.9	9.6	26.7
AT→GC	0.0	11.6	5.9	11.6
		Transversions		
GC→TA	74.0	32.4	60.8	30.4
GC→CG	14.3	9.8	19.1	10.3
AT→CG	0.5	9.6	1.4	10.2
AT→TA	0.8	8.7	3.1	10.8
Percentage of all substitutions	100	100	100	100

Probability LOGO (pLOGO) analysis further refined the sequence context distributions around the guanines targeted by both mycotoxins, which become the sites for the G→T mutations (Figure 4C). This analysis provides statistical data on the sequence-specific preferences for mutation by looking at an expanded window of sequences (+/−7 bases) around the site of each mutation. The results recapitulate well the patterns observed in the trinucleotide mutational spectra (Figure 4A), highlighting the different sequence biases for the two mycotoxins. For AFB_1, the G→T mutations occur most often in C<u>G</u>C and C<u>G</u>G sequence contexts, whereas for ST, the G→T mutations are mildly enriched in N<u>G</u>G sequence contexts (where N = any base). No longer range (beyond the immediate flanking bases) sequence context preferences were observed for either compound. Moreover, no significantly enriched sequence contexts were found in the pLOGO analysis on control spectra (Figure S4).

Unsupervised clustering using the cosine similarity metric (Figure 5 and Figure S3) aligned the mutational signature of AFB_1 with COSMIC signature SBS24, which is characteristic of aflatoxin-induced mutagenesis; this signature is enriched for G→T substitutions in certain guanine-rich trinucleotide contexts. AFB_1 showed a strong concordance with SBS24 (cosine similarity = 0.90–0.93), underscoring its potent guanine-directed mutagenic activity. ST correlated only weakly with SBS24 (cosine similarity = 0.60) and, indeed, shared a higher similarity to the COSMIC signatures SBS18, SBS4, and SBS29 (cosine similarity = 0.79). SBS18 is associated with oxidative damage, whereas SBS4 and SBS29 are both linked to tobacco exposure (smoking and chewing, respectively). Interestingly, ST has been identified as a fungal contaminant in dried tobacco leaves [54,55], and therefore, it is conceivable that the tobacco-associated mutational signatures may reflect an ST-induced mutational process.

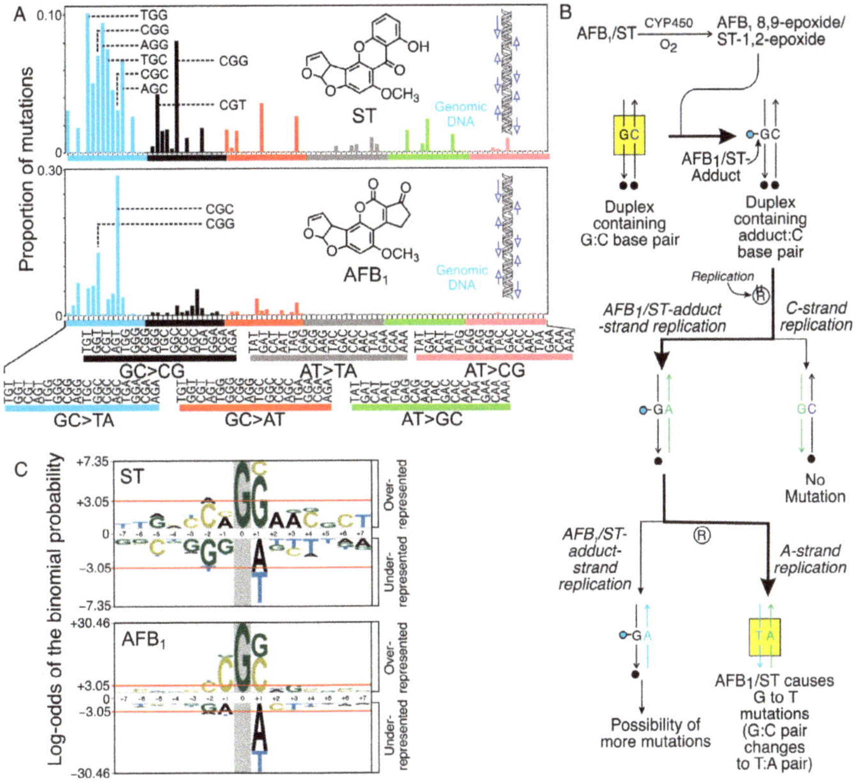

Figure 4. Mutational spectra, a proposed mutational pathway and sequence context preferences of AFB_1 and ST for mutagenesis. Mutational spectra and probability LOGO (pLOGO) analyses of AFB_1 (0.5 μM) and ST (0.2 μM) reveal their distinct mutagenic properties. (A) Proportion of mutations caused by AFB_1 (bottom) and ST (top) across the interrogated areas of the genome. Shown here are background-subtracted mutational spectra. Background spectra are included in Supplementary Material, Figure S2. AFB_1 predominantly induced GC→TA transversions in specific GC-rich contexts, while ST showed a lower mutation frequency and a broader range of GC→TA 3-base mutation contexts and mutation types. (**B**) Mutation logic diagram of AFB_1 and ST. CYP450 enzymes convert AFB_1 and ST into their epoxide forms, which form covalent adducts (shown as blue lollipops) with guanine bases in GC base pairs (a GC pair undergoing adduction is shown in the yellow box). During replication, these adducts can mispair; predominant mispairing is guanine with adenine, resulting in GC→TA transversions. Bold arrows show the main pathway to GC→TA mutations. Parental duplexes are black and marked with black circles under the duplexes. Upon replication (encircled "R" character), strands separate into black/green hybrids, where green denotes the nascent strand. A subsequent round of replication yields a green/blue hybrid, which contains an AT pair (in lower yellow box); this mutation occurs at the site of the original GC pair in the parental (black strands) genome. Alternative pairings may lead to other mutation types. (C) pLOGO analyses of the 15mer sequence contexts surrounding G→T mutations reveal sequence-specific preferences. Both compounds target guanine at the central mutation site (the large G at position 0), with overrepresented flanking nucleotide sequences suggesting unique interaction patterns with DNA. AFB_1 displays a sharper sequence context bias compared to ST, underscoring its higher mutagenic potency and specificity. Statistical significance thresholds ($p < 0.05$) are indicated by red horizontal lines.

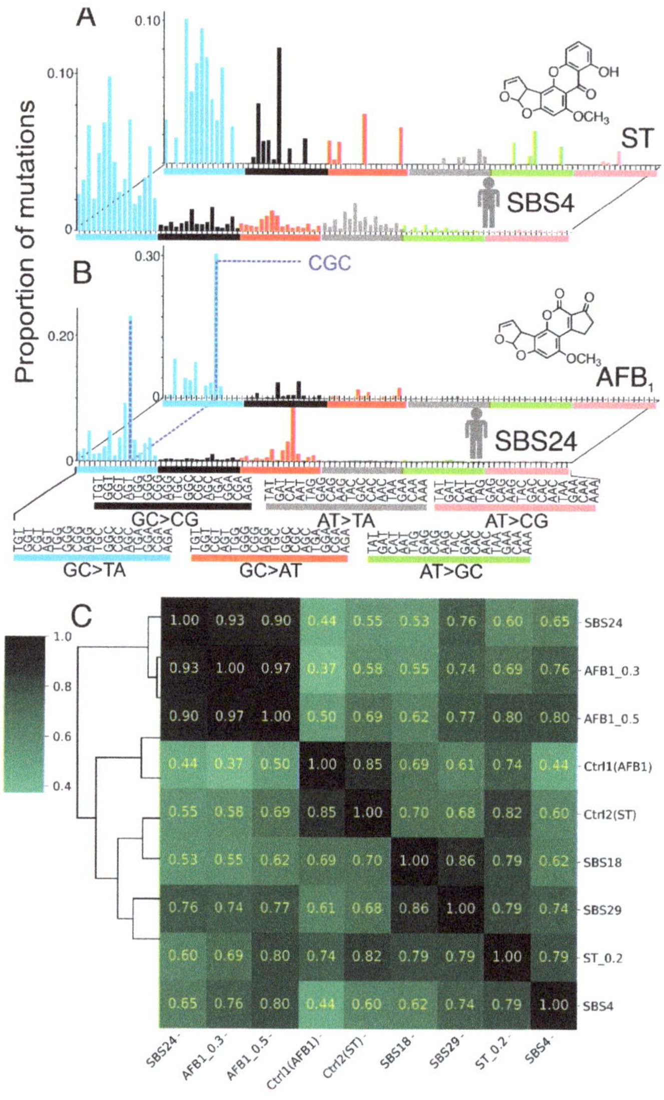

Figure 5. Comparison of mutational spectra of AFB_1 and ST with computationally derived mutational signatures of human cancers. (**A**) Comparison of mutational spectrum of ST from present work with human mutational signature SBS4, which is common in tobacco-associated cancers. Cosine similarity of these two spectra is 0.79. (**B**) Similar comparison with mutational spectrum of AFB_1 with human SBS24, which is seen in hepatocellular carcinomas of people from areas of the world where exposure to aflatoxin was likely. (**C**) Cosine similarity matrix comparing the data from present work on ST and AFB_1 with control spectra (background from vehicle-treated MEFs), human SBS18, human SBS29, human SBS24, and human SBS4. As one example, AFB_1 at 0.5 μM shows a cosine similarity of 0.9 with hepatocellular carcinoma signature SBS24. The intensity of the green color in each square reflects the level of similarity among elements in the matrix.

3. Discussion

AFB_1 and ST are structurally related toxins, both derived from fungal species. They share a common furofuran motif that is principally responsible for the biological activity of their electrophilic metabolites. Both are known to be potent mutagens and carcinogens, capable of forming bulky DNA adducts that disrupt normal DNA replication and repair processes, ultimately promoting genomic instability and cancer [28,30,42,56–58]. While both compounds are activated by epoxidation of their terminal furan rings, this study has revealed several differences in their toxicological properties that suggest that, in the case of ST, features not related to epoxidation contribute significantly to its toxic and genetic effects [4,28,30,59]. This work explored these differences in depth and projects implications for cancer etiology, mutational profiling, and potential public health interventions.

AFB_1 and ST both require bioactivation via Phase I metabolic enzymes, predominantly cytochrome P450s, to exert their mutagenic effects [18,42]. This activation results in the formation of highly electrophilic intermediates, the AFB_1-8,9-epoxide and ST-1,2-epoxide, that covalently bond to nucleophilic sites in DNA, particularly guanine residues [43]. It is noteworthy that the biological effects of each epoxide can be mitigated in vivo by Phase II enzymes, including glutathione transferases and epoxide hydrolases [60]. If the aflatoxin epoxide evades destruction, it will react with guanine residues to form its initial adduct, AFB_1-N7-Gua. This adduct can spontaneously depurinate [61] and its presence in the urine of exposed individuals has become a powerful biomarker of aflatoxin exposure [62]. An alternative fate of DNA-bound AFB_1-N7-Gua involves hydrolysis of its imidazole ring to form the AFB_1-FAPY adducts (several isomers exist). Formation of the FAPY adducts, particularly the *Ra* atropisomer where the deoxyglycosidic bond is in the β configuration [27] (often referred to as FAPY-I or FAPY-minor) is the principal pathway to AFB_1-induced mutations, resulting in the well-documented emergence of guanine-to-thymine ($G \rightarrow T$) transversions [28,30,33]. The AFB_1-FAPY adducts, which are relatively refractory to repair and hence persist for long times in the genome, are likely to be the principal source of aflatoxin's replication errors [30].

ST shares many of aflatoxin's properties but exhibits lower reactivity toward guanine residues, likely due to differences in the structure of its reactive intermediates, which lead to the formation of fewer and less stable DNA adducts compared to AFB_1 [22]. As a result, ST-induced DNA adducts are less abundant, and their $G \rightarrow T$ mutagenic effects are comparatively moderate. However, ST compensates for this lower efficiency by inducing broader types of mutagenic DNA damage, including oxidative lesions mediated by reactive oxygen species (ROS) [46,47]. This dual mechanism of direct DNA damage and oxidative stress probably contributes to the more diverse mutational spectrum of ST, which includes not only $G \rightarrow T$ transversions but also thymine-to-cytosine ($T \rightarrow C$) and cytosine-to-thymine ($C \rightarrow T$) transitions (Table 1). The interplay among these mechanisms underscores the complexity of ST's biological activity and highlights its potential to cause diverse mutagenic outcomes.

The cytotoxicity profiles of AFB_1 and ST provide further insights into their distinct biological behaviors. ST is intrinsically more cytotoxic than AFB_1, likely due to its ability to affect cellular processes beyond those triggered solely by covalent DNA damage [46]. For example, ST's strong association with ROS generation, as indicated above, provides a clue that oxidative stress may play a significant role in its cytotoxicity. ROS can damage cellular membranes, proteins, and other macromolecules in addition to DNA, leading to widespread cellular dysfunction [47,63,64]. This broader cytotoxic activity may explain why ST causes greater inhibition of cell proliferation at equivalent concentrations compared to AFB_1, even in the absence of S9.

With regard to mutagenicity, AFB_1 exhibited a higher dose-dependent mutagenicity than ST, likely driven by its high efficiency in forming guanine adducts that evade repair mechanisms. The persistence of AFB_1-FAPY adducts through multiple replication cycles makes them highly mutagenic [28,30,36]. Analysis of AFB_1-induced high-resolution mutational spectra reveals a striking enrichment of G→T transversions, particularly in the guanine-rich trinucleotide contexts CGG and CGC (where the underscored base is the site of mutation). This specificity is likely owed to the property of the AFB_1 epoxide to interact preferentially with guanines in the underscored 3-base contexts. The specific mutational patterns observed for aflatoxin have repeatedly been observed in different mammalian systems, including mouse liver in vivo [34], human HepG2 and HepaRG liver cell lines [35], and human-induced pluripotent stem cells (hiPSCs) [65]. There is remarkable concordance among the results of these genetic studies, which paint a strikingly consistent picture of the mechanism of aflatoxin-induced mutations and cancer.

ST-induced mutations, on the other hand, lack such pronounced context-specificity. While G→T transversions are prominent in ST's mutational profile, they are accompanied by a broader spectrum of other substitutions, including T→C and C→T. One factor leading to a broader mutational pattern might be the propensity of ST to induce oxidative DNA lesions in cells [64], in addition to covalent ST-base adducts, thus leading to a multifaceted mechanism of action [66]. Oxidative stress by ST could lead to oxidative lesions such as 7,8-dihydro-8-oxodeoxyguanosine (8-oxo-dG), which mispairs with adenine during replication [46,47,67]. Moreover, oxidative damage to thymine [68] as well as adenine deamination can lead to T→C substitutions [69], mutations that are also seen in ST's mutational spectrum (Figure 4A). In addition to adverse genetic effects, oxidative stress induced by ST could activate cellular signaling pathways involved in inflammation, apoptosis, and stress responses, further amplifying ST's cytotoxic and mutagenic effects. These secondary effects may also play a role in the broader range of cancers associated with ST exposure, including colorectal and gastric malignancies [46,47].

An interesting feature of the data may shed light on the mechanism underlying the differences between the respective mutagenicities and toxicities of ST and AFB_1. As indicated above, ST (without metabolic activation) is more toxic than AFB_1 in our model system. A straightforward explanation could be its more efficient penetration into the cells. Another intriguing hypothesis, however, is that ST may interact with DNA more favorably than aflatoxin as an intercalating agent. ST (as well as its epoxide) has a completely planar xanthone ring system (Figure 1) that is responsible for its potent ability to intercalate into DNA. If the intercalation event, which precedes the covalent reaction with guanine in the case of the ST-epoxide, is not very sequence-specific, one would expect that ST would form adducts with guanine residues in many different sequence contexts. Supporting this notion, Gopalakrishnan et al. provided evidence to show that the xanthone ring system is intercalated in the solution structure of ST-N7-Gua in DNA [70]; moreover, the bases 5′ and 3′ to the adducted guanine do not appear to affect eventual binding. Based on that result, one would expect that ST would bond with guanines in a relatively context-independent manner, resulting in a relatively uniform distribution of G→T mutations as seen in Figure 4A. Aflatoxin, by contrast, has a cyclopentenone ring, lacking in ST, that is puckered by two adjacent sp^3 centers. Because AFB_1, or more appropriately the AFB_1-8,9-epoxide, is less planar than ST, one could speculate that it is more discriminating in the sequence contexts into which it will intercalate. The hotspots in which we see AFB_1 mutations are 5′-CGC-3′ and 5′-CGG-3; these contexts are suggested to be hotspots for binding, which would result in the observed mutational pattern favoring mutations at the underscored guanines in vivo.

The integration of high-resolution mutational spectra with COSMIC mutational signatures provides a valuable framework for understanding the carcinogenic potential of AFB_1 and ST. AFB_1's mutational profile characterized by G→T transversions in guanine-rich contexts that are strongly aligned with COSMIC signature SBS24 makes it likely that human SBS24 is due to environmental exposure to aflatoxin [30,34,65]. This alignment underscores AFB_1's specificity as a guanine-targeted mutagen and its well-established role in the etiology of hepatocellular carcinoma [31,71,72].

The ST spectrum shares some similarities with SBS24 but also exhibits stronger features that align with COSMIC signature SBS18, which is associated with oxidative stress-related mutagenesis [73]. This overlap highlights ST's dual mechanisms of mutagenicity, combining direct adduct formation with ROS-mediated damage. The partial alignment of both AFB_1 and ST with COSMIC signature SBS4 (Figure 5C), linked to bulky DNA adducts formed by environmental carcinogens such as tobacco, further emphasizes their shared pathways of adduct-induced mutagenesis [65,73]. These findings provide important insights into both the distinct and overlapping mechanisms of AFB_1 and ST and their relevance to human cancers.

Lastly, this study was motivated by two issues. First, AFB_1 and ST are important environmental toxins, and it was timely to use recently developed tools to delve deeply into their genetic effects. Second, however, we saw the opportunity to compare the genetic effects of two natural products that differ in from one another in subtle ways. In the interest of further mechanistically informative structure–activity studies, the aflatoxin family of molecules offers many opportunities for detailed study. As a few examples, aflatoxins M_1, G_1, Q_1, and P_1 have structural features that likely would affect the interaction of their respective epoxides with DNA, and they would possibly display distinctive mutational spectra.

4. Conclusions

The research described here defined the distinct mutagenic landscapes of structurally similar mycotoxins, AFB_1 and ST. Through high-resolution mutation analysis, unique genomic fingerprints were established, and these fingerprints could be future biomarkers aiding the fields of risk assessment and cancer prevention. The increasing pressures from climate change and global food contamination further highlight the need for improved mechanistically-informed public health policies. While the carcinogenic properties of AFB_1 are well recognized and closely regulated, ST and other members of the aflatoxin family are markedly less governed, underscoring a possible lack of sufficient awareness regarding their dangers. Modern genomic technologies will help further refine toxicological model systems and support the precision prevention strategies. Lastly, AFB_1 and ST serve as critical models for understanding the interplay among DNA adduct formation, oxidative damage, and mutagenesis.

Dedication: We are pleased to have this paper included in the series honoring the many contributions of our colleague, Professor John D. Groopman, to mycotoxin research. His work, especially in the biomarker, cancer epidemiology, and chemo-prevention fields, serves as a model and inspiration for future generations of toxicologists.

5. Materials and Methods

5.1. Cell Culture and Growth Inhibition Assay

*Gpt*Δ C57BL/6J MEFs, confirmed mycoplasma-free by PCR, were established and maintained as previously described [52]. The effects of AFB_1 (Sigma-Aldrich, St. Louis, MO, USA) and ST (kindly provided by George H. Buchi (MIT)), with purity confirmed by NMR as shown in the Supplementary materials Figure S1 on cell growth inhibition, were assessed. For both compounds, 2.5×10^4 cells per well were seeded in 6-well plates containing growth media (high glucose DMEM containing GlutaMAX (Life Technologies, Carlsbad, CA, USA) supplemented with 10% FBS (VWR Scientific Products, Pittsburgh, PA, USA), 100 IU/mL penicillin, 100 μg/mL streptomycin (Sigma-Aldrich, St. Louis, MO, USA), and 1 mM sodium pyruvate (Life Technologies, Carlsbad, CA, USA)) and incubated overnight in a humidified atmosphere containing 5% CO_2. The cells were then treated with either 0–1 μM AFB_1, 1% *v*/*v* Aroclor 1254-induced S9 fraction (Fisher Scientific, Pittsburgh, PA, USA), and 1 mM NADPH (Sigma-Aldrich, St. Louis, MO, USA), or 0–0.5 μM ST with 2% *v*/*v* Aroclor 1254-induced S9 and 2 mM NADPH in 1X HBSS (Life Technologies, Carlsbad, CA, USA), and incubated for 3 h, after which the cells were washed with 1X PBS (pH 7.4, Life Technologies, Carlsbad, CA, USA) before fresh growth media was added. Following a 48 h recovery period in the incubator, cell growth was assessed by trypsinizing the MEFs and counting them using the Vi-CELL XR cell viability analyzer (Beckman Coulter, Brea, CA, USA).

5.2. *Gpt Mutation Assay*

MEFs were seeded in 100-mm tissue culture plates at a density of 5×10^5 cells per plate and allowed to adhere overnight. Following this incubation, the growth medium was replaced with treatment 1X HBSS solutions containing either 0–0.2 μM AFB_1 combined with 1% *v*/*v* Aroclor 1254-induced S9 fraction and 1 mM NADPH, or 0–0.5 μM ST with 2% S9 and 2 mM NADPH. The MEFs were exposed to these treatments for 3 h, after which they were washed with 1X PBS to remove the treatment solution and subsequently allowed to recover in fresh growth media for 48 h, following the established growth inhibition assay protocol. After the recovery period, the cells were harvested and washed twice with 1X PBS. Genomic DNA was isolated from 2×10^6 cells per treatment group using the RecoverEase DNA Isolation Kit (Agilent Technologies, Santa Clara, CA, USA). The λ-EG10 phage was then packaged in vitro from the extracted genomic DNA using the Transpack Packaging Extract (Agilent Technologies, Santa Clara, CA, USA) and transfected into *Escherichia coli* YG6020, which expresses Cre-recombinase, thereby generating a 6.4 kb plasmid encoding both the *gpt* and chloramphenicol acetyltransferase genes. The transfected *E. coli* were cultured on selective media containing 25 μg/mL chloramphenicol (CHL, Sigma-Aldrich, St. Louis, MO, USA) and 25 μg/mL 6-thioguanine (6-TG, Sigma-Aldrich, St. Louis, MO, USA), or on media containing only CHL. Confirmation of 6-TG resistance was achieved through the regrowth of colonies on plates supplemented with both CHL and 6-TG. The mutational frequency for each treatment group was subsequently calculated as the ratio of total 6-TG-resistant colonies to the average number of CHL-resistant colonies, consistent with methodologies outlined in prior studies [50,52,53].

5.3. *Duplex Sequencing (High-Resolution Mutational Spectrometry)*

Genomic DNA for duplex sequencing (DS) libraries was extracted from MEFs that had been treated with AFB_1 or ST using the same treatment protocol as in the *gpt* assay. The DNA extraction was carried out using the dNeasy Blood and Tissue Kit (Qiagen, Valencia, CA, USA), following the manufacturer's instructions. Approximately 1 μg of purified genomic DNA was then utilized to construct the DS libraries with the Mouse Mutagenesis Kit (TwinStrand Biosciences, Seattle, WA, USA). This kit employs specially designed probes that hybridize to 20 distinct genomic regions, each measuring 2.4 kb, strategically chosen to encompass intronic and intergenic areas, thereby minimizing selection bias. Sequencing was conducted on an Illumina NovaSeq 6000 DNA sequencer with an S4 flow cell, utilizing a 150 bp paired-end protocol, supported by the MIT BioMicro Center. Detailed genomic coordinates for the targeted regions can be found in the Supplementary Materials, Table S2.

5.4. *Data Processing*

The data generated from the TwinStrand DuplexSeq assay were processed using the TwinStrand DuplexSeq Mutagenesis App (v4.5.0) via the DNANexus platform. Mutation-position files (.mut) produced by this pipeline were further analyzed using custom Python scripts available on GitHub (see Data Availability Statement). For each sample, a unique list of mutations was compiled, ensuring that a mutation at any specific genomic location was counted only once. Using this list, trinucleotide mutational spectra were constructed and normalized by dividing the observed mutation frequency for each trinucleotide context by the frequency of that context within the target genomic sequence (Figure S5). To compare the mutational spectra, cosine similarity was calculated against spectra generated within this study and the single base substitution (SBS) mutational signatures from the COSMIC v3.4 repository. Additionally, pLOGO plots were generated by extracting 15mer sequence contexts (7 bases upstream and downstream of each G→T mutation) and analyzing them with the Schwartz pLOGO tool (https://plogo.uconn.edu/; version accessed on 7 February 2025).

5.5. Statistical Analysis

All data are presented as mean ± standard deviation. Statistical analyses were performed using GraphPad Prism 8. Differences between groups were evaluated using the two-tailed Student's *t*-test. Statistical significance was defined as a p-value < 0.05. Each experiment was conducted in triplicate to ensure reproducibility, and the results were subjected to rigorous statistical validation to confirm reliability and accuracy.

Supplementary Materials: The following supporting information can be downloaded at: https://www.mdpi.com/article/10.3390/toxins17030112/s1, Figure S1: ^{1}H-NMR and ^{13}C-NMR spectra of sterigmatocystin in DMSO-d_6 [74,75]; Figure S2: Mutational spectra of vehicle controls; Figure S3: Unsupervised clustering and cosine similarity matrix of background-subtracted spectra of AFB_1 and ST; Figure S4: pLOGO probability distribution of G→T mutations in control spectra; Figure S5: Trinucleotide frequencies for sequences covered by TwinStrand mouse probes; Table S1: Relative frequencies of point mutation types in mutational spectra; Table S2: Genomic coordinates of hybrid-captured regions analyzed by TwinStrand protocol.

Author Contributions: Conceptualization, P.T. and J.M.E.; Methodology, P.T., M.C., N.S., B.I.F. and R.G.C.; Software, B.I.F. and R.G.C.; Validation, P.T., M.C., B.I.F. and R.G.C.; Formal Analysis, P.T., M.C., B.I.F. and R.G.C.; Investigation, P.T., M.C., N.S. and B.I.F.; Resources, P.T. and J.M.E.; Data Curation, P.T., B.I.F., R.G.C. and J.M.E.; Writing—Original Draft Preparation, P.T., B.I.F. and J.M.E.; Writing—Review & Editing, P.T., M.C., N.S., B.I.F., R.G.C. and J.M.E.; Visualization, P.T., M.C., B.I.F., R.G.C. and J.M.E.; Supervision, S.R., M.R., R.G.C. and J.M.E.; Project Administration, J.M.E.; Funding Acquisition, P.T., M.R., B.I.F. and J.M.E. All authors have read and agreed to the published version of the manuscript.

Funding: This work was financially supported by the U.S. National Institutes of Health grants R01-CA080024, R21-ES036341, the CEHS core center grant P30-ES002109 and the Thailand Science Research and Innovation (TSRI) program, Chulabhorn Research Institute: Grant No. 49892/4759805.

Institutional Review Board Statement: Not applicable.

Informed Consent Statement: Not applicable.

Data Availability Statement: The sequencing data files referenced in the present work have been uploaded to the Sequence Read Archive (SRA) repository of the National Center for Biotechnology Information (NCBI) as the BioProject PRJNA1217835 (http://www.ncbi.nlm.nih.gov/bioproject/1217835). The data analysis and visualization Python scripts are available on GitHub (https://github.com/essigmannlab/AFB1_ST_spectra/).

Acknowledgments: The authors acknowledge the Massachusetts Institute of Technology BioMicro Facilities Core for DNA sequencing, the Department of Chemistry Instrumentation Core for NMR facilities, and the Center for Environmental Health Sciences for analytical support.

Conflicts of Interest: The authors declare no conflicts of interest.

References

1. Busby, W.F.; Wogan, G.N. Aflatoxins. In *Chemical Carcinogen*; Searle, C.E., Ed.; American Chemical Society: Washington, DC, USA, 1984; pp. 945–1136.
2. Groopman, J.D.; Cain, L.G. Interactions of Fungal and Plant Toxins with DNA: Aflatoxins, Sterigmatocystin, Safrole, Cycasin, and Pyrrolizidine Alkaloids. In *Chemical Carcinogenesis and Mutagenesis I*; Cooper, C.S., Grover, P.L., Eds.; Springer: Berlin/Heidelberg, Germany, 1990; pp. 373–407.
3. Wild, C.P.; Turner, P.C. The toxicology of aflatoxins as a basis for public health decisions. *Mutagenesis* **2002**, *17*, 471–481. [CrossRef]
4. Kensler, T.W.; Roebuck, B.D.; Wogan, G.N.; Groopman, J.D. Aflatoxin: A 50-year odyssey of mechanistic and translational toxicology. *Toxicol. Sci.* **2011**, *120*, S28–S48. [CrossRef] [PubMed]
5. Ostry, V.; Malir, F.; Toman, J.; Grosse, Y. Mycotoxins as human carcinogens-the IARC monographs classification. *Mycotoxin Res.* **2017**, *33*, 65–73. [CrossRef]
6. McCullough, A.K.; Lloyd, R.S. Mechanisms underlying aflatoxin-associated mutagenesis—Implications in carcinogenesis. *DNA Repair.* **2019**, *77*, 76–86. [CrossRef] [PubMed]
7. Pickova, D.; Ostry, V.; Toman, J.; Malir, F. Aflatoxins: History, significant milestones, recent data on their toxicity and ways to mitigation. *Toxins* **2021**, *13*, 399. [CrossRef]
8. Kensler, T.W.; Eaton, D.L. 65 years on-aflatoxin biomarkers blossoming: Whither next? *Toxins* **2024**, *16*, 496. [CrossRef] [PubMed]
9. Wild, C.P.; Gong, Y.Y. Mycotoxins and human disease: A largely ignored global health issue. *Carcinogenesis* **2010**, *31*, 71–82. [CrossRef]
10. Alonso-Jauregui, M.; López de Cerain, A.; Azqueta, A.; Rodriguez-Garraus, A.; Gil, A.G.; González-Peñas, E.; Vettorazzi, A. In vivo genotoxicity and toxicity assessment of sterigmatocystin individually and in mixture with aflatoxin B_1. *Toxins* **2023**, *15*, 491. [CrossRef]
11. Zingales, V.; Taroncher, M.; Martino, P.A.; Ruiz, M.J.; Caloni, F. Climate change and effects on molds and mycotoxins. *Toxins* **2022**, *14*, 445. [CrossRef] [PubMed]
12. Muñoz-Solano, B.; Lizarraga Pérez, E.; González-Peñas, E. Monitoring mycotoxin exposure in food-producing animals (cattle, pig, poultry, and sheep). *Toxins* **2024**, *16*, 218. [CrossRef] [PubMed]
13. Bondy, G.S.; Pestka, J.J. Immunomodulation by fungal toxins. *J. Toxicol. Environ. Health B Crit. Rev.* **2000**, *3*, 109–143. [PubMed]
14. Ekwomadu, T.; Mwanza, M.; Musekiwa, A. Mycotoxin-linked mutations and cancer risk: A global health issue. *Int. J. Environ. Res. Public. Health* **2022**, *19*, 7754. [CrossRef]
15. Minto, R.E.; Townsend, C.A. Enzymology and molecular biology of aflatoxin biosynthesis. *Chem. Rev.* **1997**, *97*, 2537–2556. [CrossRef]
16. Iram, W.; Anjum, T.; Iqbal, M.; Ghaffar, A.; Abbas, M.; Khan, A.H. Structural analysis and biological toxicity of aflatoxins B_1 and B_2 degradation products following detoxification by *Ocimum basilicum* and *Cassia fistula* aqueous extracts. *Front. Microbiol.* **2016**, *7*, 1105. [CrossRef] [PubMed]
17. Wang, Y.; Zhang, H.; Yan, H.; Chen, Y.; Liu, Y.; Xu, Q.; Liu, X.; Zhang, Z. Effective biodegradation of aflatoxin B_1 using the *Bacillus licheniformis* (BL010) strain. *Toxins* **2018**, *10*, 497. [CrossRef]
18. Forrester, L.M.; Neal, G.E.; Judah, D.J.; Glancey, M.J.; Wolf, C.R. Evidence for involvement of multiple forms of cytochrome P-450 in aflatoxin B_1 metabolism in human liver. *Proc. Natl. Acad. Sci. USA* **1990**, *87*, 8306–8310. [CrossRef] [PubMed]
19. Guengerich, F.P.; Johnson, W.W.; Shimada, T.; Ueng, Y.F.; Yamazaki, H.; Langouët, S. Activation and detoxication of aflatoxin B_1. *Mutat. Res.-Fundam. Mol. Mech. Mutagen.* **1998**, *402*, 121–128. [CrossRef]
20. Essigmann, J.M.; Croy, R.G.; Nadzan, A.M.; Busby, W.F.; Reinhold, V.N.; Büchi, G.; Wogan, G.N. Structural identification of the major DNA adduct formed by aflatoxin B_1 in vitro. *Proc. Natl. Acad. Sci. USA* **1977**, *74*, 1870–1874. [CrossRef]
21. Croy, R.G.; Essigmann, J.M.; Reinhold, V.N.; Wogan, G.N. Identification of the principal aflatoxin B_1-DNA adduct formed in vivo in rat liver. *Proc. Natl. Acad. Sci. USA* **1978**, *75*, 1745–1749. [CrossRef] [PubMed]
22. Baertschi, S.W.; Raney, K.D.; Shimada, T.; Harris, T.M.; Guengerich, F.P. Comparison of rates of enzymatic oxidation of aflatoxin B_1, aflatoxin G_1, and sterigmatocystin and activities of the epoxides in forming guanyl-N7 adducts and inducing different genetic responses. *Chem. Res. Toxicol.* **1989**, *2*, 112–114.
23. Raney, V.M.; Harris, T.M.; Stone, M.P. DNA conformation mediates aflatoxin B_1-DNA binding and the formation of guanine N7 adducts by aflatoxin B_1 8,9-*exo*-epoxide. *Chem. Res. Toxicol.* **1993**, *6*, 64–68. [CrossRef]
24. Guengerich, F.P.; Johnson, W.W.; Ueng, Y.F.; Yamazaki, H.; Shimada, T. Involvement of cytochrome P450, glutathione S-transferase, and epoxide hydrolase in the metabolism of aflatoxin B_1 and relevance to risk of human liver cancer. *Environ. Health Perspect.* **1996**, *104*, 557–562. [CrossRef]
25. Johnson, W.W.; Yamazaki, H.; Shimada, T.; Ueng, Y.F.; Guengerich, F.P. Aflatoxin B_1 8,9-epoxide hydrolysis in the presence of rat and human epoxide hydrolase. *Chem. Res. Toxicol.* **1997**, *10*, 672–676. [CrossRef] [PubMed]
26. Johnson, W.W.; Guengerich, F.P. Reaction of aflatoxin B_1 *exo* -8,9-epoxide with DNA: Kinetic analysis of covalent binding and DNA-induced hydrolysis. *Proc. Natl. Acad. Sci. USA* **1997**, *94*, 6121–6125. [CrossRef] [PubMed]

27. Brown, K.L.; Deng, J.Z.; Iyer, R.S.; Iyer, L.G.; Voehler, M.W.; Stone, M.P.; Harris, C.M.; Harris, T.M. Unraveling the aflatoxin−FAPY conundrum: Structural basis for differential replicative processing of isomeric forms of the formamidopyrimidine-type DNA adduct of aflatoxin B_1. *J. Am. Chem. Soc.* **2006**, *128*, 15188–15199. [CrossRef]
28. Bailey, E.A.; Iyer, R.S.; Stone, M.P.; Harris, T.M.; Essigmann, J.M. Mutational properties of the primary aflatoxin B_1-DNA adduct. *Proc. Natl. Acad. Sci. USA* **1996**, *93*, 1535–1539. [CrossRef] [PubMed]
29. Giri, I.; Jenkins, M.; Schnetz-Boutaud, N.; Stone, M.P. Structural refinement of the 8,9-dihydro-8-(N7-guanyl)-9-hydroxy-aflatoxin B_1 adduct in a 5′-CpAFBG-3′ sequence. *Chem. Res. Toxicol.* **2002**, *15*, 638–647. [CrossRef] [PubMed]
30. Smela, M.E.; Hamm, M.L.; Henderson, P.T.; Harris, C.M.; Harris, T.M.; Essigmann, J.M. The aflatoxin B_1 formamidopyrimidine adduct plays a major role in causing the types of mutations observed in human hepatocellular carcinoma. *Proc. Natl. Acad. Sci. USA* **2002**, *99*, 6655–6660. [CrossRef] [PubMed]
31. Hamid, A.S.; Tesfamariam, I.G.; Zhang, Y.; Zhang, Z.G. Aflatoxin B_1-induced hepatocellular carcinoma in developing countries: Geographical distribution, mechanism of action and prevention. *Oncol. Lett.* **2013**, *5*, 1087–1092. [CrossRef] [PubMed]
32. Lin, Y.C.; Li, L.; Makarova, A.V.; Burgers, P.M.; Stone, M.P.; Lloyd, R.S. Error-prone replication bypass of the primary aflatoxin B_1 DNA adduct, AFB_1-N7-Gua. *J. Biol. Chem.* **2014**, *289*, 18497–18506. [CrossRef]
33. Lin, Y.C.; Li, L.; Makarova, A.V.; Burgers, P.M.; Stone, M.P.; Lloyd, R.S. Molecular basis of aflatoxin-induced mutagenesis—Role of the aflatoxin B_1-formamidopyrimidine adduct. *Carcinogenesis* **2014**, *35*, 1461–1468. [CrossRef] [PubMed]
34. Chawanthayatham, S.; Valentine, C.C.; Fedeles, B.I.; Fox, E.J.; Loeb, L.A.; Levine, S.S.; Slocum, S.L.; Wogan, G.N.; Croy, R.G.; Essigmann, J.M. Mutational spectra of aflatoxin B_1 in vivo establish biomarkers of exposure for human hepatocellular carcinoma. *Proc. Natl. Acad. Sci. USA* **2017**, *114*, E3101–E3109. [CrossRef]
35. Huang, M.N.; Yu, W.; Teoh, W.W.; Ardin, M.; Jusakul, A.; Ng, A.W.T.; Boot, A.; Abedi-Ardekani, B.; Villar, S.; Myint, S.S.; et al. Genome-scale mutational signatures of aflatoxin in cells, mice, and human tumors. *Genome Res.* **2017**, *27*, 1475–1486. [CrossRef] [PubMed]
36. Minko, I.G.; Kellum, A.H.; Stone, M.P.; Lloyd, R.S. The aflatoxin B_1-induced imidazole ring-opened guanine adduct: High mutagenic potential that is minimally affected by sequence context. *Environ. Mol. Mutagen.* **2024**, *65* (Suppl. S1), 9–13. [CrossRef] [PubMed]
37. Bressac, B.; Kew, M.; Wands, J.; Ozturk, M. Selective G to T mutations of *P53* gene in hepatocellular carcinoma from Southern Africa. *Nature* **1991**, *350*, 429–431. [CrossRef]
38. Scorsone, K.A.; Zhou, Y.Z.; Butel, J.S.; Slagle, B.L. *P53* mutations cluster at codon 249 in hepatitis B virus-positive hepatocellular carcinomas from China. *Cancer Res.* **1992**, *52*, 1635–1638. [PubMed]
39. Jiao, J.; Niu, W.; Wang, Y.; Baggerly, K.; Ye, Y.; Wu, X.; Davenport, D.; Almeda, J.L.; Betancourt-Garcia, M.M.; Forse, R.A.; et al. Prevalence of aflatoxin-associated *TP53R249S* mutation in hepatocellular carcinoma in hispanics in South Texas. *Cancer Prev. Res. (Phila)* **2018**, *11*, 103–112. [CrossRef]
40. Groopman, J.D.; Kensler, T.W. Role of metabolism and viruses in aflatoxin-induced liver cancer. *Toxicol. Appl. Pharmacol.* **2005**, *206*, 131–137. [CrossRef] [PubMed]
41. Han, C.; Yu, T.; Qin, W.; Liao, X.; Huang, J.; Liu, Z.; Yu, L.; Liu, X.; Chen, Z.; Yang, C.; et al. Genome-wide association study of the *TP53 R249S* mutation in hepatocellular carcinoma with aflatoxin B_1 exposure and infection with hepatitis B virus. *J. Gastrointest. Oncol.* **2020**, *11*, 1333–1349. [CrossRef]
42. Essigmann, J.M.; Barker, L.J.; Fowler, K.W.; Francisco, M.A.; Reinhold, V.N.; Wogan, G.N. Sterigmatocystin-DNA interactions: Identification of a major adduct formed after metabolic activation in vitro. *Proc. Natl. Acad. Sci. USA* **1979**, *76*, 179–183. [CrossRef] [PubMed]
43. Essigmann, J.M.; Donahue, P.R.; Story, D.L.; Wogan, G.N.; Brunengraber, H. Use of the isolated perfused rat liver to study carcinogen-DNA adduct formation from aflatoxin B_1 and sterigmatocystin. *Cancer Res.* **1980**, *40*, 4085–4091.
44. Noda, K.; Umeda, M.; Ueno, Y. Cytotoxic and mutagenic effects of sterigmatocystin on cultured chinese hamster cells. *Carcinogenesis* **1981**, *2*, 945–949. [CrossRef] [PubMed]
45. Trienens, M.; Rohlfs, M. Experimental evolution of defense against a competitive mold confers reduced sensitivity to fungal toxins but no increased resistance in *Drosophila* larvae. *BMC Evol. Biol.* **2011**, *11*, 206. [CrossRef] [PubMed]
46. Ueno, Y.; Umemori, K.; Niimi, E.C.; Tanuma, S.I.; Nagata, S.; Sugamata, M.; Ihara, T.; Sekijima, M.; Kawai, K.I.; Ueno, I.; et al. Induction of apoptosis by T-2 toxin and other natural toxins in HL-60 human promyelotic leukemia cells. *Nat. Toxins* **1995**, *3*, 129–137. [CrossRef] [PubMed]
47. Zingales, V.; Fernández-Franzón, M.; Ruiz, M.J. Sterigmatocystin: Occurrence, toxicity and molecular mechanisms of action—A review. *Food Chem. Toxicol.* **2020**, *146*, 111802. [CrossRef] [PubMed]
48. Guidance for Industry: Action Levels for Poisonous or Deleterious Substances in Human Food and Animal Feed. Available online: https://www.fda.gov/regulatory-information/search-fda-guidance-documents/guidance-industry-action-levels-poisonous-or-deleterious-substances-human-food-and-animal-feed (accessed on 6 January 2025).

49. Commission Regulation (EC) No 1881/2006 of 19 December 2006 Setting Maximum Levels for Certain Contaminants in Foodstuffs (Text with EEA Relevance). Available online: https://www.legislation.gov.uk/eur/2006/1881 (accessed on 9 January 2025).
50. Armijo, A.L.; Thongararm, P.; Fedeles, B.I.; Yau, J.; Kay, J.E.; Corrigan, J.J.; Chancharoen, M.; Chawanthayatham, S.; Samson, L.D.; Carrasco, S.E.; et al. Molecular origins of mutational spectra produced by the environmental carcinogen *N*-nitrosodimethylamine and S_N1 chemotherapeutic agents. *Nucleic Acids Res. Cancer* **2023**, *5*, zcad015. [CrossRef] [PubMed]
51. Fedeles, B.I.; Essigmann, J.M. Chapter 25: Mutational Spectra Provide Insight into the Mechanisms Bridging DNA Damage to Genetic Disease. In *DNA Damage, DNA Repair and Disease*; Royal Society of Chemistry: London, UK, 2020; pp. 214–253.
52. Thongararm, P.; Fedeles, B.I.; Khumsubdee, S.; Armijo, A.L.; Kim, L.; Thiantanawat, A.; Promvijit, J.; Navasumrit, P.; Ruchirawat, M.; Croy, R.G.; et al. Modulation of *N*-methyl-*N*-nitrosourea mutagenesis in mouse embryo fibroblasts derived from the *gpt* delta mouse by an inhibitor of the O^6-methylguanine methyltransferase, MGMT. *Chem. Res. Toxicol.* **2020**, *33*, 625–633. [CrossRef] [PubMed]
53. Chancharoen, M.; Yang, Z.; Dalvie, E.D.; Gubina, N.; Ruchirawat, M.; Croy, R.G.; Fedeles, B.I.; Essigmann, J.M. 5-chloro-2′-deoxycytidine induces a distinctive high-resolution mutational spectrum of transition mutations in vivo. *Chem. Res. Toxicol.* **2024**, *37*, 486–496. [CrossRef]
54. Varma, S.K.; Verma, R.A.; Jha, A.K. Ecotoxicological aspects of *Aspergilli* present in the phylloplane of stored leaves of chewing tobacco (*Nicotiana tobaccum*). *Mycopathologia* **1991**, *113*, 19–23. [CrossRef]
55. Pauly, J.L.; Paszkiewicz, G. Cigarette smoke, bacteria, mold, microbial toxins, and chronic lung inflammation. *J. Oncol.* **2011**, *2011*, 819129. [CrossRef] [PubMed]
56. Croy, R.G.; Wogan, G.N. Temporal patterns of covalent DNA adducts in rat liver after single and multiple doses of aflatoxin B_1. *Cancer Res.* **1981**, *41*, 197–203. [PubMed]
57. Mao, H.; Deng, Z.; Wang, F.; Harris, T.M.; Stone, M.P. An intercalated and thermally stable FAPY adduct of aflatoxin B_1 in a DNA duplex: Structural refinement from ^{1}H NMR. *Biochemistry* **1998**, *37*, 4374–4387. [CrossRef]
58. Denissenko, M.F.; Cahill, J.; Koudriakova, T.B.; Gerber, N.; Pfeifer, G.P. Quantitation and mapping of aflatoxin B_1-induced DNA damage in genomic DNA using aflatoxin B_1-8,9-epoxide and microsomal activation systems. *Mutat. Res.* **1999**, *425*, 205–211. [CrossRef] [PubMed]
59. Wogan, G.N.; Kensler, T.W.; Groopman, J.D. Present and future directions of translational research on aflatoxin and hepatocellular carcinoma. A review. *Food Addit. Contam. Part. A Chem. Anal. Control Expo. Risk Assess.* **2012**, *29*, 249–257. [CrossRef]
60. Eaton, D.L.; Williams, D.E.; Coulombe, R.A. Species differences in the biotransformation of aflatoxin B_1: Primary determinants of relative carcinogenic potency in different animal species. *Toxins* **2025**, *17*, 30. [CrossRef] [PubMed]
61. Groopman, J.D.; Croy, R.G.; Wogan, G.N. In vitro reactions of aflatoxin B_1-adducted DNA. *Proc. Natl. Acad. Sci. USA* **1981**, *78*, 5445–5449. [CrossRef]
62. Groopman, J.D.; Donahue, P.R.; Zhu, J.Q.; Chen, J.S.; Wogan, G.N. Aflatoxin metabolism in humans: Detection of metabolites and nucleic acid adducts in urine by affinity chromatography. *Proc. Natl. Acad. Sci. USA* **1985**, *82*, 6492–6496. [CrossRef]
63. Sivakumar, V.; Thanislass, J.; Niranjali, S.; Devaraj, H. Lipid peroxidation as a possible secondary mechanism of sterigmatocystin toxicity. *Hum. Exp. Toxicol.* **2001**, *20*, 398–403. [CrossRef] [PubMed]
64. Gao, W.; Jiang, L.; Ge, L.; Chen, M.; Geng, C.; Yang, G.; Li, Q.; Ji, F.; Yan, Q.; Zou, Y.; et al. Sterigmatocystin-induced oxidative DNA damage in human liver-derived cell line through lysosomal damage. *Toxicol. In Vitro* **2015**, *29*, 1–7. [CrossRef] [PubMed]
65. Kucab, J.E.; Zou, X.; Morganella, S.; Joel, M.; Nanda, A.S.; Nagy, E.; Gomez, C.; Degasperi, A.; Harris, R.; Jackson, S.P.; et al. A compendium of mutational signatures of environmental agents. *Cell* **2019**, *177*, 821–836.e16. [CrossRef] [PubMed]
66. Jakšić, D.; Ćurtović, I.; Kifer, D.; Rašić, D.; Kopjar, N.; Micek, V.; Peraica, M.; Klarić, M.Š. Single-dose toxicity of individual and combined sterigmatocystin and 5-methoxysterigmatocistin in rat lungs. *Toxins* **2020**, *12*, 734. [CrossRef] [PubMed]
67. Wood, M.L.; Dizdaroglu, M.; Gajewski, E.; Essigmann, J.M. Mechanistic studies of ionizing radiation and oxidative mutagenesis: Genetic effects of a single 8-hydroxyguanine (7-hydro-8-oxoguanine) residue inserted at a unique site in a viral genome. *Biochemistry* **1990**, *29*, 7024–7032. [CrossRef] [PubMed]
68. Basu, A.K.; Loechler, E.L.; Leadon, S.A.; Essigmann, J.M. Genetic effects of thymine glycol: Site-specific mutagenesis and molecular modeling studies. *Proc. Natl. Acad. Sci. USA* **1989**, *86*, 7677–7681. [CrossRef]
69. Hill-Perkins, M.; Jones, M.D.; Karran, P. Site-specific mutagenesis in vivo by single methylated or deaminated purine bases. *Mutat. Res.* **1986**, *162*, 153–163. [CrossRef] [PubMed]
70. Gopalakrishnan, S.; Liu, X.; Patel, D.J. Solution structure of the covalent sterigmatocystin-DNA adduct. *Biochemistry* **1992**, *31*, 10790–10801. [CrossRef]
71. Muench, K.F.; Misra, R.P.; Humayun, M.Z. Sequence specificity in aflatoxin B_1-DNA interactions. *Proc. Natl. Acad. Sci. USA* **1983**, *80*, 6–10. [CrossRef]
72. Brown, K.L.; Bren, U.; Stone, M.P.; Guengerich, F.P. Inherent stereospecificity in the reaction of aflatoxin B_1 8,9-epoxide with deoxyguanosine and efficiency of DNA catalysis. *Chem. Res. Toxicol.* **2009**, *22*, 913–917. [CrossRef]

73. Alexandrov, L.B.; Kim, J.; Haradhvala, N.J.; Huang, M.N.; Tian Ng, A.W.; Wu, Y.; Boot, A.; Covington, K.R.; Gordenin, D.A.; Bergstrom, E.N.; et al. The repertoire of mutational signatures in human cancer. *Nature* **2020**, *578*, 94–101. [CrossRef] [PubMed]
74. Fremlin, L.J.; Piggott, A.M.; Lacey, E.; Capon, R.J. Cottoquinazoline A and cotteslosins A and B, metabolites from an Australian marine-derived strain of *Aspergillus versicolor*. *J. Nat. Prod.* **2009**, *72*, 666–670. [CrossRef]
75. Zhu, F.; Lin, Y. Three xanthones from a marine-derived mangrove endophytic fungus. *Chem. Nat. Comp.* **2007**, *43*, 132–135. [CrossRef]

toxins

MDPI

Article

Green-Engineered Montmorillonite Clays for the Adsorption, Detoxification, and Mitigation of Aflatoxin B1 Toxicity

Johnson O. Oladele [1,2], Xenophon Xenophontos [3], Gustavo M. Elizondo III [1,4], Yash Daasari [2], Meichen Wang [5], Phanourios Tamamis [3,6], Natalie M. Johnson [1,4] and Timothy D. Phillips [1,2,*]

1 Interdisciplinary Faculty of Toxicology, Texas A&M University, College Station, TX 77843, USA; oladelejohn2007@tamu.edu (J.O.O.); gelizondo@exchange.tamu.edu (G.M.E.III); nmjohnson@tamu.edu (N.M.J.)
2 Department of Veterinary Physiology and Pharmacology, College of Veterinary Medicine & Biomedical Sciences, Texas A&M University, College Station, TX 77843, USA
3 Artie McFerrin Department of Chemical Engineering, College of Engineering, Texas A&M University, College Station, TX 77843, USA; xxenop01@tamu.edu (X.X.); tamamis@tamu.edu (P.T.)
4 Department of Environmental & Occupational Health, Texas A&M University, College Station, TX 77843, USA
5 Department of Environmental Health Sciences, University of Massachusetts Amherst, Amherst, MA 01003, USA; meichenwang@umass.edu
6 Department of Materials Science and Engineering, College of Engineering, Texas A&M University, College Station, TX 77840, USA
* Correspondence: tphillips@cvm.tamu.edu

Abstract: Dietary and environmental exposure to aflatoxins via contaminated food items can pose major health challenges to both humans and animals. Studies have reported the coexistence of aflatoxins and other environmental toxins. This emphasizes the urgent need for efficient and effective mitigation strategies for aflatoxins. Previous reports from our laboratory have demonstrated the potency of the green-engineered clays (GECs) on ochratoxin and other toxic chemicals. Therefore, this study sought to investigate the binding and detoxification potential of chlorophyll (CMCH and SMCH) and chlorophyllin (CMCHin and SMCHin)-amended montmorillonite clays for aflatoxin B1 (AFB1). In addition to analyzing binding metrics including affinity, capacity, free energy, and enthalpy, the sorption mechanisms of AFB1 onto the surfaces of engineered clays were also investigated. Computational and experimental studies were performed to validate the efficacy and safety of the clays. CMCH showed the highest binding capacity (Qmax) of 0.43 mol/kg compared to the parent clays CM (0.34 mol/kg) and SM (0.32 mol/kg). Interestingly, there were no significant changes in the binding capacity of the clays at pH2 and pH6, suggesting that the clays can bind to AFB1 throughout the gastrointestinal track. In silico investigations employing molecular dynamics simulations also demonstrated that CMCH enhanced AFB1 binding as compared to parent clay and predicted hydrophobic interactions as the main mode of interaction between the AFB1 and CMCH. This was corroborated by the kinetic results which indicated that the interaction was best defined by chemosorption with favorable thermodynamics and Gibbs free energy (ΔG) being negative. In vitro experiments in Hep G2 cells showed that clay treatment mitigated AFB1-induced cytotoxicity, with the exception of 0.5% (w/v) SMCH. Finally, the in vivo results validated the protection of all the clays against AFB1-induced toxicities in Hydra vulgaris. This study showed that these clays significantly detoxified AFB1 (86% to 100%) and provided complete protection at levels as low as 0.1%, suggesting that they may be used as AFB1 binders in feed and food.

Keywords: aflatoxin; food safety; mycotoxin; enterosorbent; NovaSil; Alphasil; clay; molecular dynamics; isotherms; kinetics

Key Contribution: Green-engineered clays revealed a high binding for aflatoxin B1 as supported by in vitro adsorption, HepG2 cell models, in silico computation simulations, and the in vivo Hydra vulgaris model, thus implying that these engineered clays may facilitate AFB1 elimination and detoxification.

1. Introduction

Aspergillus fungus, especially *A. flavus*, generates a class of secondary fungal metabolites called aflatoxins, commonly referred to as mycotoxins. The discovery of aflatoxins emerged after the "Turkey X disease" outbreak in England in 1960, when more than 100,000 turkeys unexpectedly fell ill and perished over several months. The turkeys suffered liver necrosis and extensive intestinal inflammation, according to post-mortem examination. It was quickly revealed that a large number of the turkeys were given Brazilian groundnut meal, which was shown to be highly poisonous when offered to poultry in feeding trials [1]. Later, it was shown that *Aspergillus flavus* metabolites (known as aflatoxins) were the cause of these toxicities. Aflatoxin G2, aflatoxin G1, aflatoxin B2, and Aflatoxin B1 (AFB1) are the four metabolites that are produced by *A. flavus* and are members of the aflatoxin class [2]. According to the International Agency for Research on Cancer (IARC), there is a sufficient indication to categorize aflatoxins as carcinogens in humans, which was discovered after assessing published epidemiological research that showed a substantial correlation between AFB1 ingestion and the development of cancer. The most carcinogenic of the aflatoxins, AFB1, has a long history of being linked to growth retardation, immune system regulation, malnutrition, and hepatocellular carcinoma (HCC) [3].

A. flavus is widely distributed in soil and pollutes a variety of crops around the globe, including peanuts, rice, and corn. Controlling aflatoxin-related contamination is challenging because fungus can grow on food at any time before or after harvest. Furthermore, nations with high humidity and temperatures, such as Southeast Asia and Sub-Saharan Africa, tend to have higher levels of AFB contamination since these regions encourage the growth of fungi. Furthermore, a significant amount of AFB1 exposure happens during storage because many of these nations lack the capacity to preserve food in dry, temperature-controlled settings [4–6]. About 4.5 billion people in underdeveloped nations were considered to be at risk for chronic, unregulated exposure to aflatoxins in 2004 [7,8], underscoring the challenges of preventing aflatoxin contamination. The agricultural sector suffers significant losses every year as a result. Numerous researchers have calculated the annual losses resulting from crop contamination with aflatoxin in different nations. Between USD 20 million and USD 2 billion have been estimated to be lost annually in the United States [9–11]. Both Asian and African nations suffer significant losses. Thailand, Indonesia, and the Philippines were predicted to lose USD 1 billion a year if the European guidelines of aflatoxin contamination were imposed, whereas African exporters were predicted to lose USD 670 million, or 64% of their revenues [12,13]. Additionally, it has been predicted that nations may begin to see larger levels of AFB1 contamination in crops, and that new locations may begin to experience issues with AFB1 exposure as climate change influences average temperatures and annual rainfall [14,15]. Therefore, remedies to AFB1 exposure and toxicities must be developed before aflatoxins become an even more serious worldwide health and economic issue.

Research activities in the laboratory of Dr. T.D. Phillips over the past four decades have pioneered and explored various mitigation and detoxification approaches using materials that are generally recognized as safe (GRAS) to reduce the exposure and toxicities of aflatoxins, both in animals and humans [16–21]. These studies include the development of an aflatoxin enterosorbent to inhibit the adsorption of AFB1 in the gastrointestinal tract, reducing its uptake into the circulatory system and preventing its delivery to target organs, which is responsible for its major toxicity. This work has led to commercialization of aflatoxin binders worldwide, including NovaSil (a calcium montmorillonite clay) and Alphasil (a sodium montmorillonite clay). The addition of these clays to animal feeds has been shown to reduce AFB1 absorption and AFM1 levels in milk, establishing proof-of-concept and the protective ability of these clays against AFB1 toxicities in a number of experimental animals. In many animal models, NovaSil clay significantly reduced the harmful effects of aflatoxin-contaminated diets in farm animals [16,17]. A long-term trial in rodents was also conducted, in which rats were given up to 2.0% *w/w* of NovaSil for 28 weeks. According to Afriyie-Gyawu et al. [18], there were no detectable toxic effects of the clay observed throughout this investigation, suggesting that this clay would be safe to use in further work.

Following a Phase I dose titration study in human participants in Texas, selected oral doses of a placebo and low and high doses of refined NovaSil clay were administered by capsule to Ghanaians living in an area at high risk for AFB1 exposure. After three months, participants in the low- and high-dose groups showed significantly decreased serum AFB1-albumin and urine AFM1 biomarkers. Furthermore, only minor adverse effects (such as nausea, diarrhea, heartburn, and dizziness) were recorded in both placebo and treatment groups, and NovaSil was not demonstrated to significantly change the health parameters of study participants [19,20]. These findings suggested that incorporating NovaSil into the diet may be effective way to diminish AFB1 toxicity. Further clinical trials in Africa showed that NovaSil was safe and effective when administered in the diet and in flavored water [21].

There is a high possibility that aflatoxins coexist with other mycotoxins and environmental chemicals such as benzene, pesticides, and PFAS. Thus, there is a critical need for the development of sorbent materials that will bind both mycotoxins and environmental chemicals. We have recently shown that the addition of various forms of chlorophyll to NovaSil clay can result in clays with enhanced hydrophobicity and attraction for lipophilic mycotoxins like ochratoxin A and zearalenone and chemicals such as PFAS and benzene [22–25].

In this current study, we investigated the activity of green-engineered clays (GECs) to bind and mitigate mixtures of aflatoxin B1. More specifically, aflatoxin B1 binding and interactions were assessed using in vitro, in silico, in vivo, and cell line models to achieve the following: (i) evaluate the adsorption characteristics of AFB1 on the surfaces of GECs using well-established methods of isothermal analyses, (ii) assess the kinetic and thermodynamic profile of AFB1 binding to and desorption from the clays, (iii) explore the atomistic dynamics and binding modes of the binding using computational approaches based on molecular dynamics simulations, (iv) determine the protective efficiency of GECs in hepatic cells, and (v) validate the safety and efficacy of GECs in living organisms (*Hydra vulgaris*).

2. Results

2.1. Isothermal Adsorption of AFB1 on the Clays at pH2 (Gastric Condition)

The results shown in Figure 1 demonstrate the isothermal adsorption of AFB1 on both the parent montmorillonites and the GECs at pH2 and 37 °C. The isothermal plot of AFB1 on both parent montmorillonites (CM and SM) fit the Langmuir model, and the curved shapes indicate that AFB1 binding was saturable and tight on these clay surfaces. The binding capacities (Qmax) of CM and SM for AFB1 were 0.34 mol/kg and 0.32 mol/kg, respectively, while their binding affinities (Kd) were 1.89×10^4 and 2.40×10^4, respectively. The adsorption isotherm of AFB1 for GECs showed that the amendment of montmorillonites with chlorophyll and chlorophyllin improved their binding capacities. Chlorophyll increased the Qmax of CM and SM to 0.43 mol/kg and 0.38 mol/kg, respectively. Similarly, chlorophyllin enhanced the Qmax of CM (0.40 mol/kg) and SM (0.39 mol/kg). The Gibbs free energies (ΔG) of the adsorption of AFB1 onto the clay surfaces were between −19.19 kJ/mol to −20.28 kJ/mol, indicating chemosorption. A summary of all the adsorption parameters is displayed in Table 1.

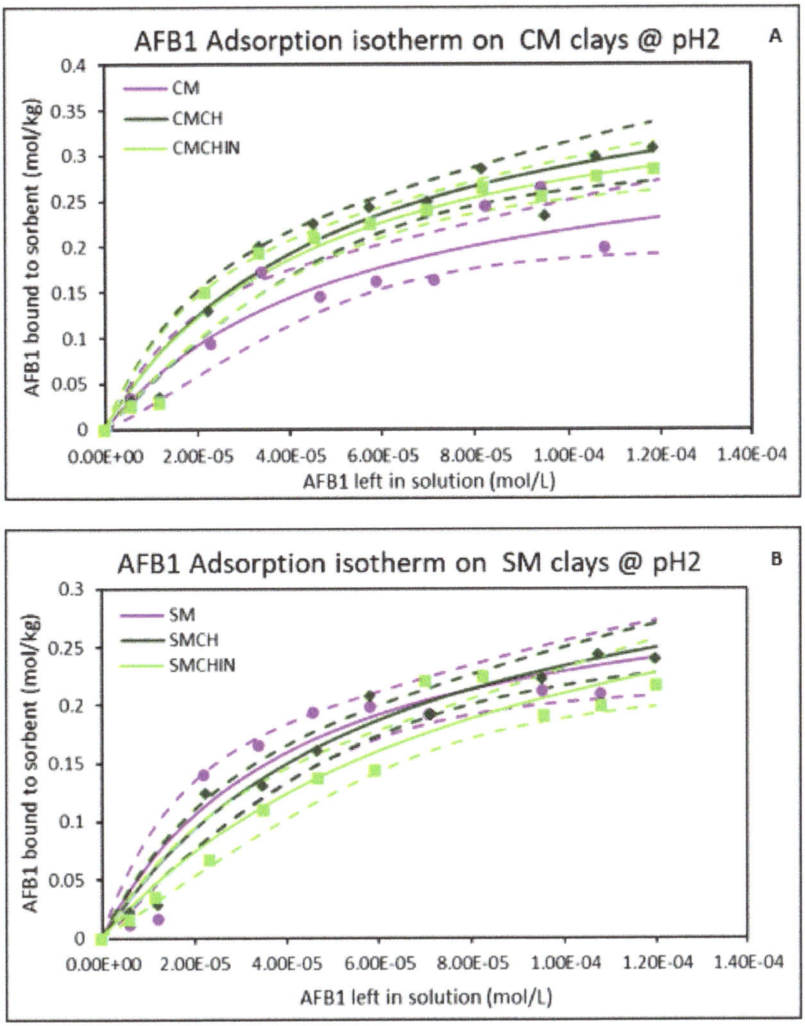

Figure 1. Adsorption isotherms of AFB1 onto binding surfaces of (**A**) CM-clays and (**B**) SM-clays at pH2. SMCHin; chlorophyllin-amended sodium montmorillonite; SMCH: chlorophyll-amended sodium montmorillonite; SM: sodium montmorillonite; CMCHin; chlorophyllin-amended calcium montmorillonite; CMCH: chlorophyll-amended calcium montmorillonite; CM: calcium montmorillonite.

Table 1. Parameters and correlation coefficients of adsorption isotherms of AFB1 on binding surfaces of the clays.

Sorbents	Adsorption Parameters @ pH2				Adsorption Parameters @ pH6			
	Q_{max}	K_d	ΔG	r^2	Q_{max}	K_d	ΔG	r^2
CM	0.34	1.89×10^4	−19.19	0.88	0.35	2.07×10^4	−19.83	0.93
CMCH	0.43	2.01×10^4	−20.28	0.95	0.41	1.86×10^4	−19.95	0.96
CMCHin	0.40	2.18×10^4	−20.07	0.96	0.36	2.09×10^4	−19.71	0.96
SM	0.32	2.40×10^4	−19.72	0.92	0.31	1.91×10^4	−19.32	0.93
SMCH	0.38	1.66×10^4	−19.60	0.97	0.33	2.68×10^4	−19.71	0.94
SMCHin	0.39	1.14×10^4	−19.33	0.94	0.38	1.63×10^4	−19.83	0.92

Q_{max}: binding capacity (mol/kg); K_d: binding affinity; ΔG: Gibbs free energy (kJ/mol); r^2: correlation coefficients. SMCHin; chlorophyllin-amended sodium montmorillonite; SMCH: chlorophyll-amended sodium montmorillonite; SM: sodium montmorillonite; CMCHin; chlorophyllin-amended calcium montmorillonite; CMCH: chlorophyll-amended calcium montmorillonite; CM: calcium montmorillonite.

2.2. Isothermal Adsorption of AFB1 on the Clays at pH6 (Intestinal Condition)

At pH6 (intestinal pH) and 37 °C, the adsorption plots of AFB1 binding on the surfaces of the parent montmorillonites (CM and SM) exhibited good fit to a Langmuir model based on correlation coefficients and a curved shape, suggesting the presence of monolayer binding and saturable active sites (Figure 2). The binding of AFB1 onto parent montmorillonites and green-engineered clays showed high binding capacities of 0.35 and 0.31 mol/kg for CM and SM, respectively. Higher binding capacities ranging from 0.33 to 0.41 mol/kg were recorded for the green-engineered clays with chlorophyll-amended clay (CMCH) having the highest capacity of 0.41 mol/kg. Furthermore, all the clays exhibited high affinities in the magnitudes of 10^4 (Table 1). Interestingly, these results showed that the change in pH did not affect the binding of AFB1 on the surfaces of the montmorillonite clays. The binding potency of these clays was enhanced following amendment with chlorophyll and chlorophyllin, with increased Qmax, as shown in Table 1. Remarkably, the chlorophyll-engineered clays exhibited higher binding capacities than the chlorophyllin clays.

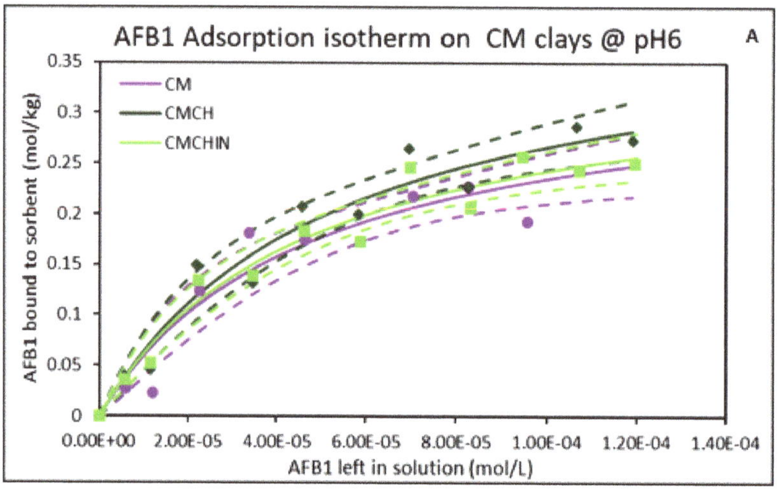

Figure 2. *Cont.*

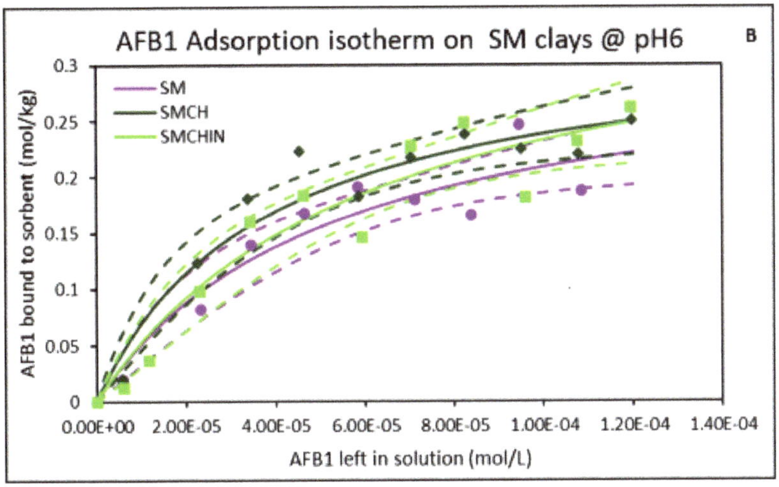

Figure 2. Adsorption isotherms of AFB1 onto binding surfaces of (**A**) CM-clays and (**B**) SM-clays at pH6. SMCHin; chlorophyllin-amended sodium montmorillonite; SMCH: chlorophyll-amended sodium montmorillonite; SM: sodium montmorillonite; CMCHin; chlorophyllin-amended calcium montmorillonite; CMCH: chlorophyll-amended calcium montmorillonite; CM: calcium montmorillonite.

2.3. Kinetics of the Binding of AFB1 on the Clays

Nonlinear pseudo-first-order, pseudo-second-order, and Elovich models were used to better understand the AFB1 adsorption kinetics on the binding surfaces of the parent and engineered clays. The adsorption of AFB1 onto the CM clays (Figure 3A) and SM clays (Figure 3B) sorbents' binding surfaces was best described by the pseudo-second-order kinetic model, according to the correlation coefficient value and the consistency between the modeled values (qe, cal) and experimental binding capacity (qe, exp). Table 2 displays the kinetic model's parameters. The greatest binding capacity (qe, exp) values are 0.08 mg/kg for CMCH, 0.07 mg/kg for SMCH and SMCHin, and 0.05 mg/kg for CM and SM.

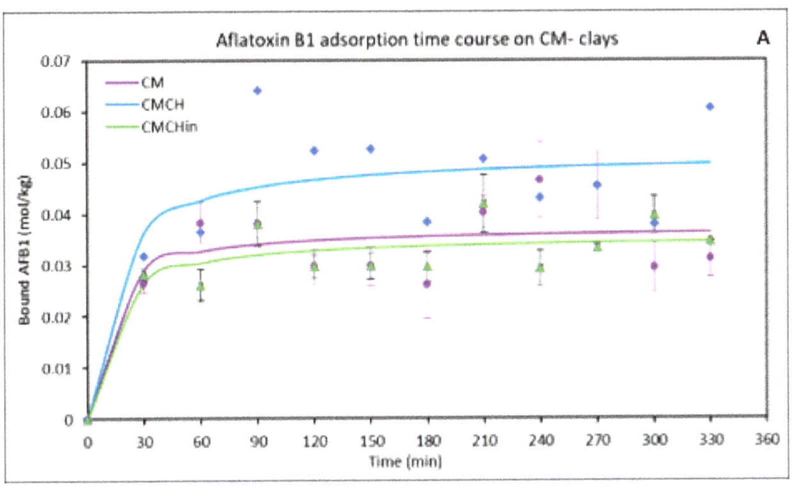

Figure 3. *Cont.*

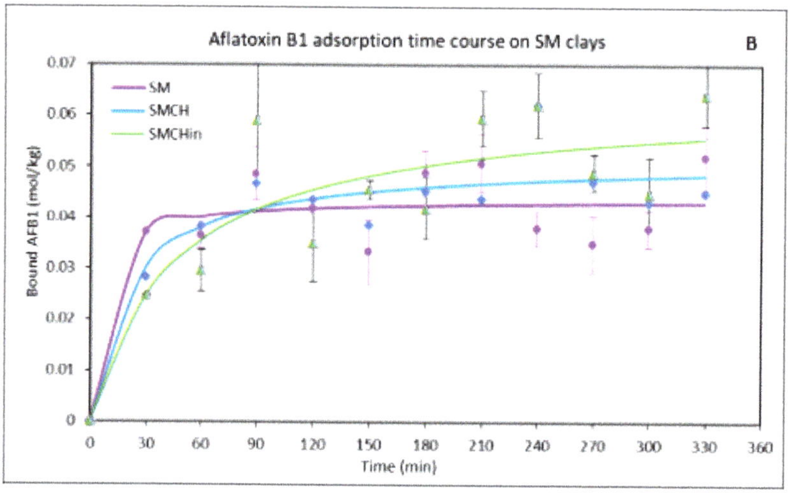

Figure 3. Effect of contact time on the adsorption of AFB1 on binding surfaces of (**A**) CM-clays and (**B**) SM-clays. SMCHin; chlorophyllin-amended sodium montmorillonite; SMCH: chlorophyll-amended sodium montmorillonite; SM: sodium montmorillonite; CMCHin; chlorophyllin-amended calcium montmorillonite; CMCH: chlorophyll-amended calcium montmorillonite; CM: calcium montmorillonite.

Table 2. Adsorption kinetic parameters for AFB1 on the clays.

Pseudo-Second Order Parameters	qe (exp $mgkg^{-1}$)	qe (cal $mgkg^{-1}$)	K_2	r^2
CM	0.05	0.04	8.32×10^0	0.85
CMCH	0.08	0.05	3.41×10^0	0.87
CMCHin	0.04	0.04	1.36×10^0	0.93
SM	0.05	0.04	3.66×10^0	0.89
SMCH	0.07	0.05	1.36×10^0	0.94
SMCHin	0.07	0.06	2.75×10^{-1}	0.84

qe (exp): binding at equilibrium in experiment; qe (cal): binding at equilibrium calculated by pseudo-second order; K_2: rate constant of the second order; r^2: correlation coefficients.

2.4. In Silico Molecular Dynamics (MD) Simulations Investigating AFB1 Binding to Surfaces of Clay (CM) and Chlorophyll-Engineered Clay (CMCH)

Figure 4 shows the average binding percentage probability of AFB1 to CMCH and CM at both pH2 and pH7 (Figure 4A,B, respectively). Both CM and CMCH showed high binding probability >70% at both pH conditions. CMCH showed a ~20% increase in the binding probability when compared to the parent clay at pH2 and a ~10% increase at pH7. The total binding capacity of AFB1 to CM and CMCH at both pH conditions is highly similar to the slightly higher probability occurring at pH7 compared to pH2 for CM and direct interactions in CMCH. This could be attributed to the slightly higher tendency of AFB1 to participate in contacts with the edges in the clay surfaces of the neutral clay compared to the acidic clay surfaces. CMCH variably contributed to AFB1's binding due to both direct-assisted and indirect-assisted interactions (Figure 4).

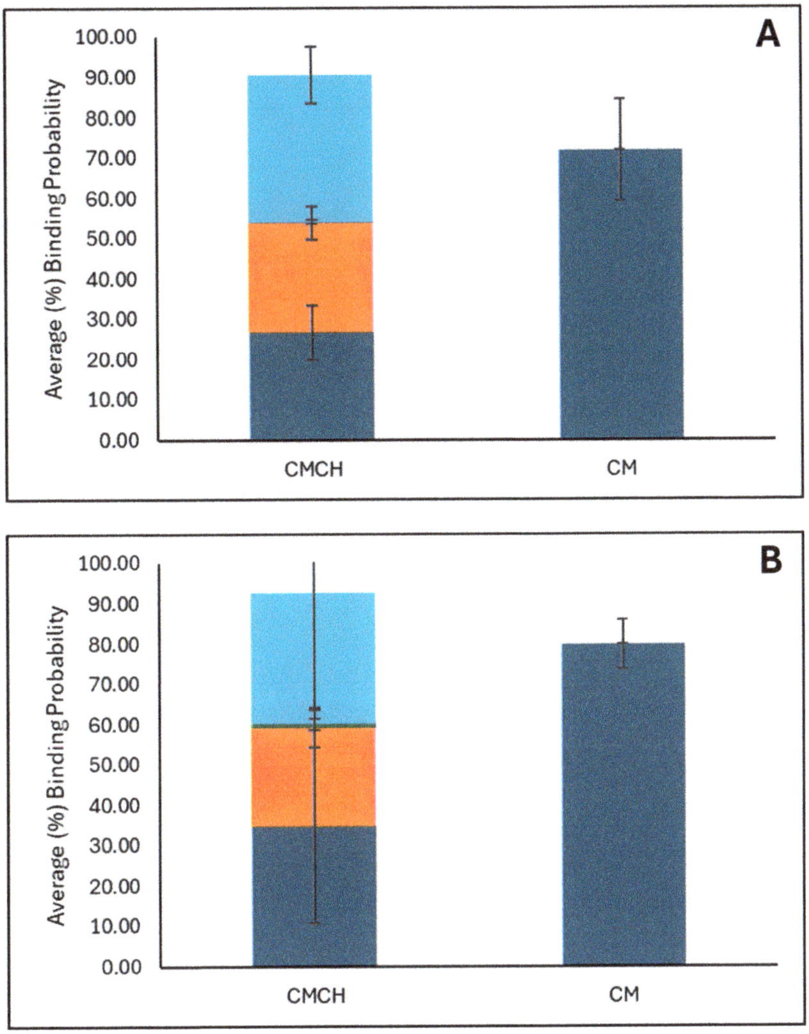

Figure 4. The panels (**A**,**B**) show the average percentage binding probability of AFB1 at pH2 and pH7, respectively, to chlorophyll-amended clay (CMCH) and parent clay (CM). Direct, direct-assisted, direct-helped, and indirect-assisted interactions are shown in dark blue, orange, green, and cyan, respectively. The average values are calculated from triplicate runs. The error bars denote the standard deviation values calculated from triplicate runs.

Figure 5 presents the percentage contribution of each chlorophyll chemical group to the interactions with AFB1 at both pH2 and pH7 (Figure 5A,B, respectively). The interaction between AFB1 and chlorophyll's chlorin ring (head) or alkyl chai (tail) is approximately equally probable at both pH conditions within the simulations.

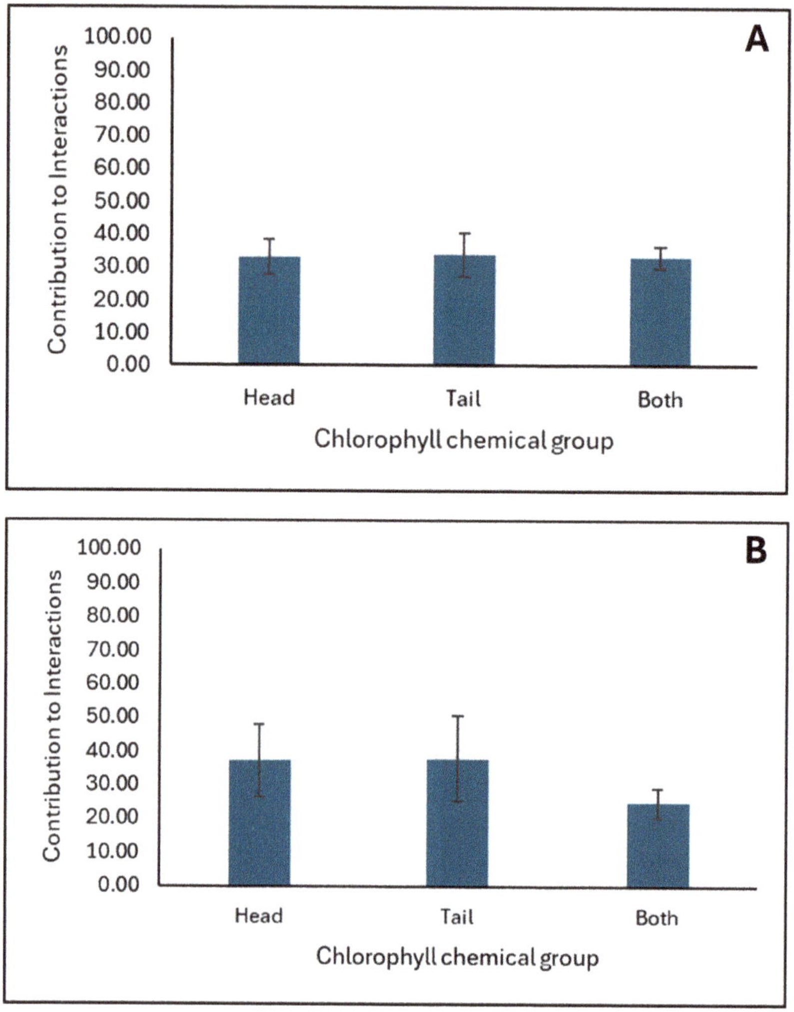

Figure 5. The panels (**A**,**B**) show the average contribution of chlorophyll's chemical groups to the interactions with AFB1 at pH2 and pH7, respectively. The average values are calculated from triplicate runs. The error bars denote standard deviation values calculated from triplicate runs.

2.5. Cytotoxicity Effect of AFB1 on Hep G2 and Protective Ability of Green-Engineered Clays

AFB1 exposure caused significantly elevated levels of LDH in Hep G2 cells, reflecting hepatic toxicity (Figure 6). Each clay-treated exposure condition did not show significantly elevated levels of LDH in spent media, with the exception of 0.5% (w/v) SMCH. Generally, there appeared to be a protective effect associated with clay treatment.

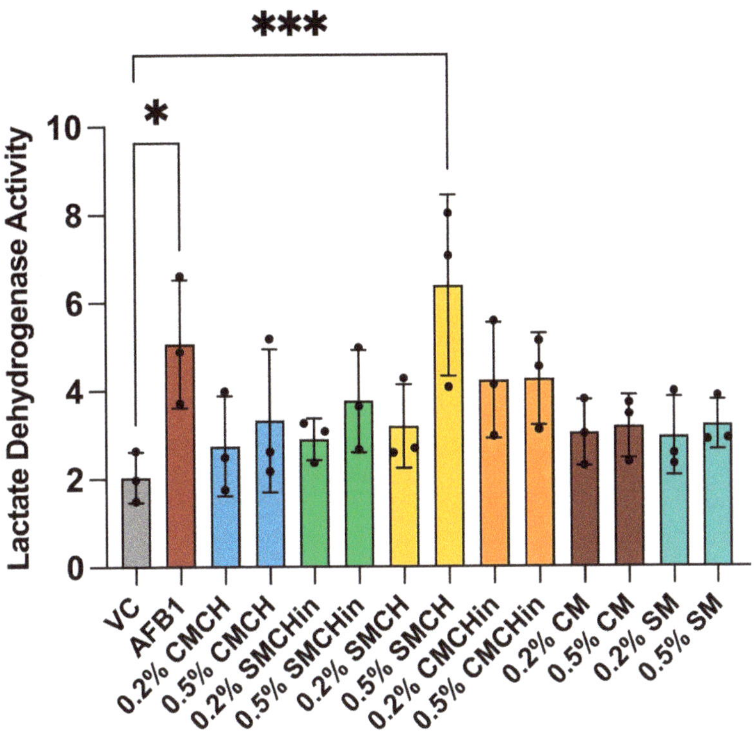

Figure 6. Cytotoxicity of aflatoxin B1 and effects of clay treatments in Hep G2 cells measured by LDH release after 24 h exposure. Relative amount of LDH released into cell culture medium was determined after 24 h exposure to either 20 ppm aflatoxin B1 or clay-treated media containing aflatoxin-1 B and compared to vehicle control. Bars are color-coded to represent vehicle control, aflatoxin B1, and six different clays, with each clay having two dose levels. Individual data points are shown as circles. Values are presented as mean ± standard deviation (SD). N = 3 for each treatment. Significant differences are indicated by (*) for $p < 0.05$ and (***) for $p < 0.001$.

2.6. *Effect of AFB1 on Hydra Vulgaris and Detoxification Efficacy of Green-Engineered Clays*

Figure 7 displays the findings of the AFB1 toxicity assessment conducted on hydra in vivo. AFB1 exposure between 10 and 200 ppm showed significant toxicity to hydra morphology. In particular, AFB1 impaired the hydra's morphology between 50 and 100 percent at different doses of 10, 20, 40, 80, 100, and 200 ppm. Notably, after 48 h of exposure, the hydra subjected to concentrations greater than 20 ppm of AFB1 completely disintegrated. Therefore, 20 ppm was used for the detoxification studies and evaluation. The hydra colony was considerably shielded against AFB1 toxicity by treatment with different doses of the montmorillonite-clay-based sorbent additives, ranging from 0.05% to 0.5% (w/v), as seen in Figure 8. In particular, protection ranged from 33% to 93% for SM-amended clays (SMCH and SMCHin) at 0.2% and 0.5% inclusion, whereas it ranged from 87% to 100% for CM-amended clays (CMCH and CMCHin). Interestingly, CMCH provided full (100%) protection at both 0.2% and 0.5% inclusion. The feeding behavior of Hydra vulgaris was significantly impaired by 20 ppm of AFB1; however, the inclusion of the clays prevented this toxicity.

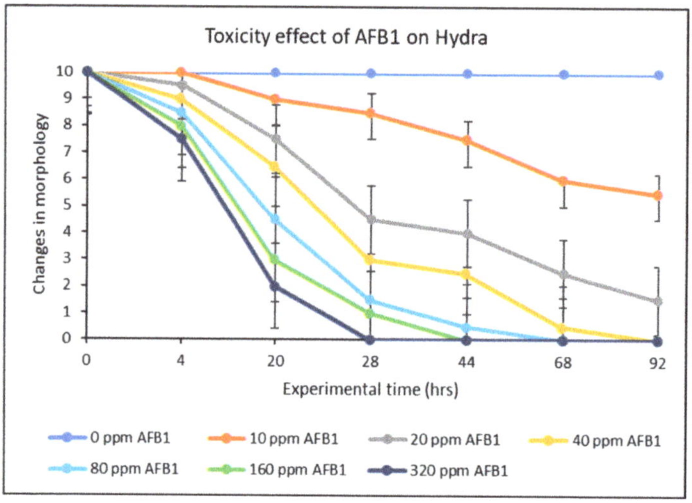

Figure 7. Toxicity effects of AFB1 exposure to hydra.

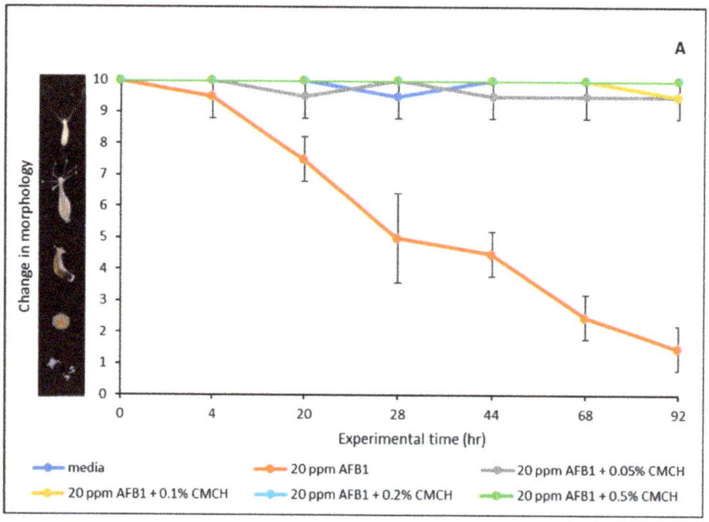

Figure 8. *Cont.*

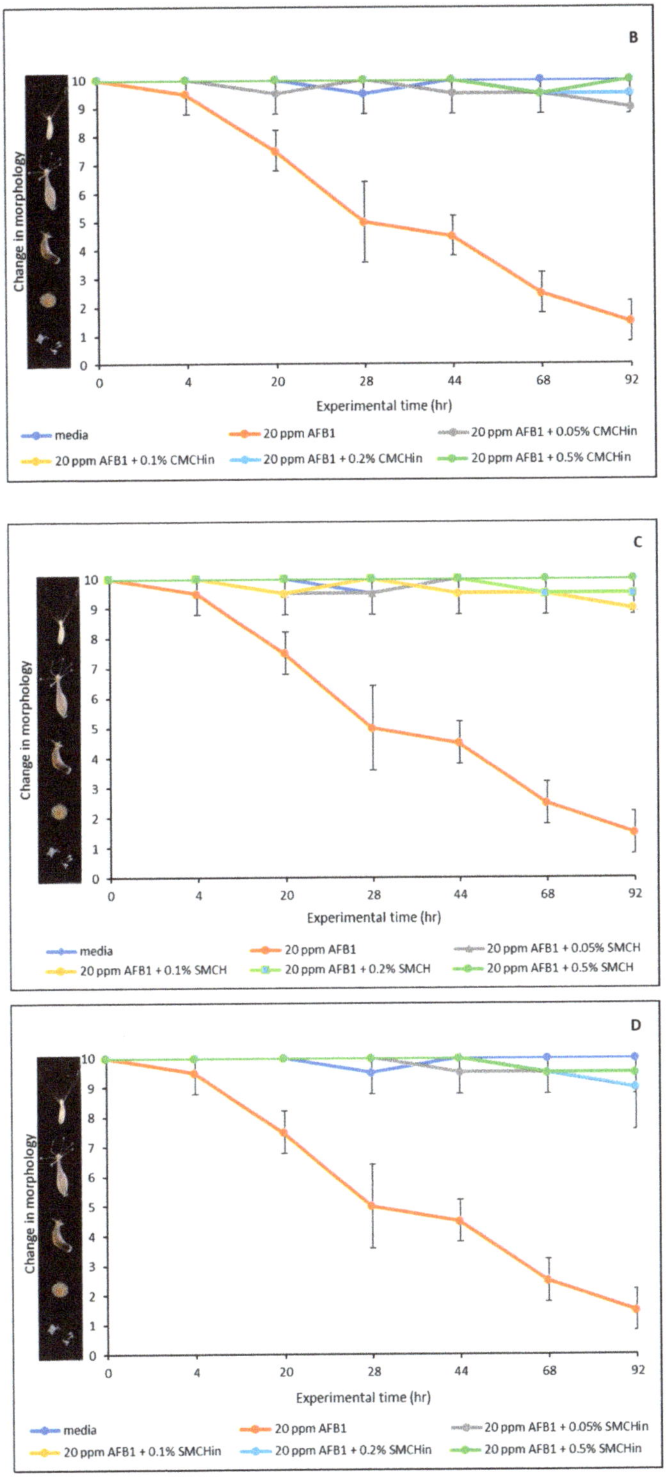

Figure 8. *Cont.*

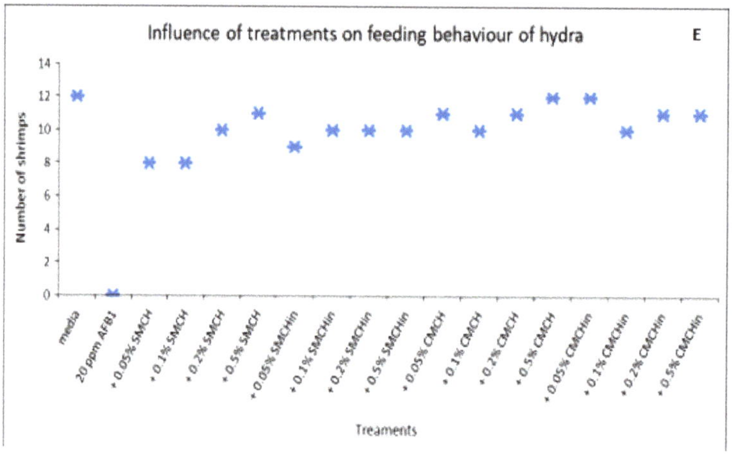

Figure 8. Protective effects of green-engineered clays on AFB1-toxicities to hydra (**A**) with chlorophyll-amended calcium montmorillonite; (**B**) with chlorophyllin-amended calcium montmorillonite; (**C**) chlorophyll-amended sodium montmorillonite; (**D**) chlorophyllin-amended sodium montmorillonite. (**E**) Influence of treatment on feeding behavior of hydra.

3. Discussion

The inclusion of selected clays to diet are novel ways to address AFB1 contamination [26–29]; they work as binding agents to reduce the bioavailability of AFB1 from the gastrointestinal tract following consumption, hence preventing AFB1's uptake by the blood and effects in the body. As shown in the results of this study, both the parent clay and GECs significantly reduced the amount of aflatoxin in the simulated gastrointestinal fluids. Previous studies in our laboratory have established the parent clay (NovaSil) as an excellent binder of aflatoxin [20,21,30–33]. Interestingly, the amendment of these clays with both chlorophyll and chlorophyllin increased the binding capacities of the clays. Interestingly, the inclusion of chlorophyll and chlorophyllin as dietary supplements in human foods and animal diets has been reported to decrease systemic absorption of aflatoxins. According to Breinholt et al. [34], the AFB1-DNA adduct in rainbow trout was reduced by 37% when chlorophyllin was added to contaminated feed, resulting in a 77% decrease in the prevalence of cancer [34]. Similarly, the addition of chlorophyllin to AFB1-contaminated diet reduced AFM1 in rat urine by 90%, AFB1-DNA adducts by 42%, and AFB1-albumin adducts by 65% [35]. Furthermore, chlorophyll also demonstrated efficacy in the same trial by lowering urinary AFM1 levels by 92%, AFB1-DNA adducts by 55%, and AFB1-albumin adducts by 51% [35]. A human study also observed that adding chlorophyllin to the diets of those living in high-risk locations for AFB1 exposure decreased AFB1-N7-guanine levels by 55% when compared to those who did not receive chlorophyllin [36].

In this study, chlorophyll-amended clays showed a higher binding capacity for aflatoxin B1 than the parent clays. Our observation is similar to animal and clinical studies that used chlorophyll and chlorophyllin compounds as preclinical interventions. When chlorophyllin and chlorophyll were added to aflatoxin B1-contaminated diets, the tumor incidence in the experimental rats decreased by 74 and 77%, respectively [35]. Also, four participants in a clinical study involving human volunteers received a single dose of 30 ng of AFB1 three times. Chlorophyll and chlorophyllin were given together with the AFB1 dose for the second and third doses. According to the findings, chlorophyll decreased urinary AFM1 levels by 41% and chlorophyllin by 28% [37].

Previous research has demonstrated that parent clays (calcium montmorillonite, CM and sodium montmorillonite, SM) are highly effective binders for AFB1 and significantly mitigate toxicity when included in aflatoxin-contaminated animal feed. It is noteworthy that these base clays are now included as aflatoxin binders in feed worldwide. Importantly, the findings from this study for GECs revealed better binding than the parent montmorillonite clays. Isothermal analyses indicated that the binding of AFB1 to these clays was high affinity and high capacity. Computational studies demonstrated that AFB1 could interact with both the ring and long alkyl tail of the chlorophyll-engineered clay, suggesting the key role of hydrophobic interactions between the two moieties. The final simulation snapshot from one of triplicate runs performed for AFB1 in complex with CM and CMCH at acidic conditions are shown in Figure 9 (Panels A and B, respectively). In CM, AFB1 depicted an overall increased tendency to aggregate by stacking in parallel and form a cluster interacting with the clays, shown in Figure 9A with a dashed circle. Individual AFB1 molecules also interacted with clay by either lying flat on its surface or with the methyl groups, shown in Figure 9A with dashed arrows (i) and (ii), respectively. In CMCH, AFB1 clusters additionally participated in primarily hydrophobic interactions with chlorophyll amendments of CMCH, both via direct-assisted and indirect-assisted interactions, as shown in Figure 9B with dashed arrows (i) and (ii), respectively.

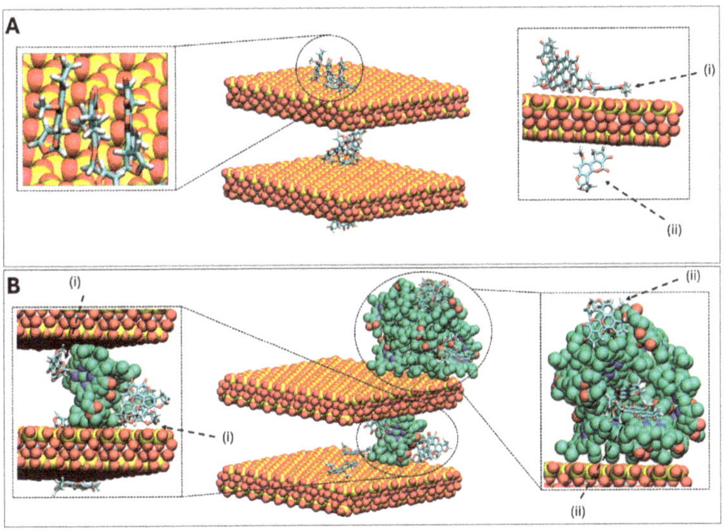

Figure 9. Panels (**A**,**B**) show the last snapshot of a particular simulation of AFB1 in complex with CM and CMCH, respectively, at pH2. The pictures in the center of the panels are zoomed-out representations while the picture on the left and the right of the panels correspond to zoomed-in representations, with different angles shown for clarity. The clay layers are shown in vdW representation, colored by atom type. The carbon atoms of chlorophyll amendments are colored in green, while the magnesium, nitrogen, and oxygen atoms are colored by atom type. The AFB1 molecules are shown in licorice representation, colored by atom type. The calcium ions that are within a distance of 3.5 Å of clay, chlorophyll, or AFB1 are shown in vdW representation, colored in tan. The hydrogen atoms of clay and chlorophyll molecules were omitted for clarity. The indicated molecules (i) and (ii) are discussed in the main text.

Furthermore, the binding ability of these GECs has been established with hazardous lipophilic environmental substances such as benzene, toluene, and xylene, and lipophilic mycotoxins such as ochratoxin A [23–25]. This highlights the added benefits of these clays in real-world scenarios containing mixtures of these and other toxic chemicals. AFB1 treatment significantly elevated the levels of LDH in spent media after 24 h exposure; however, AFB1-induced cytotoxicity was mitigated in hepatic cells after treatment with GECs, with the exception to this being clay 0.5% (*w*/*v*) SMCH. The next steps would be to repeat the exposures and assess a time point up to 72 h with media collection each 24 h to assess LDH activity in spent media. Also, the inclusion of clay treatments alone to assess the cytotoxicity of the clay types on liver cells would also be beneficial.

The safety and protective capacities of GECs were determined utilizing the hydra assay. As shown in the studies, all the clays at inclusion rates ranging from 0.05 to 0.5% (*w*/*v*) provided significant protection to hydra against AFB1 toxicity. The in vivo protection supports the in vitro isothermal findings. The >99% protection offered by these clays suggests that clay amendments with chlorophyll and chlorophyllin are safe and provide excellent protection against AFB1 in adult hydra.

4. Conclusions

This study evaluated the capacity of GECs to adsorb and detoxify aflatoxin B1. In vitro, in silico, and in vivo techniques were used to evaluate the binding properties of these green organoclays. At the physiological pH of the gastrointestinal tract, in vitro isothermal analyses revealed that GECs had significantly higher adsorption capacities, affinities, and free energy levels of sorption for aflatoxin B1 versus the parent clays. The results suggested that chemosorption was the mechanism by which aflatoxin B1 was bound to the GECs. The sorption and detoxification of aflatoxin B1 was confirmed by the notable protection against aflatoxin B1 toxicity. The combined in vitro and in silico findings provided a distinct perspective on the aflatoxin B1-binding processes on the surfaces of the clays. The in vivo investigations confirmed the effectiveness and efficacy of the clays. Taken together, the findings of this study suggested that these clays may be used for the mitigation of aflatoxin B1 toxicities during acute outbreaks of aflatoxicosis and may reduce unintentional exposures to people and animals from contaminated food and feed. Moreover, these chlorophyll-amended clays have been shown to sequester and neutralize environmental chemicals such as benzene, toluene, ochratoxin A, and other hazardous substances, which will enhance their impact on health.

5. Materials and Methods

5.1. Reagents and Chemicals

AFB1 was acquired from Sigma Aldrich, located in Saint Louis, MO, USA. Aldrich Chemical Co. (Milwaukee, WI, USA) supplied the sulfuric acid (H_2SO_4, 95–98%) and chlorophyllin. The source of the chlorophyll was Santa Cruz Biotechnology, located in Dallas, TX, USA. Acetonitrile, for high-pressure liquid chromatography (HPLC) quality and pH buffers (4.0, 7.0, and 10.0), was obtained from VWR (Atlanta, GA, USA). Human hepatocellular carcinoma (Hep G2) cells were obtained from ATCC, (Manassas, VA, USA) with product number HB-8065. The Elga^{TM} automatic filtration system (Woodridge, IL, USA) was utilized to produce ultrapure deionized water (18.2 MΩ), which was used in the experiments. The Source Clay Minerals Repository at the University of Missouri–Columbia provided sodium montmorillonite (SM), which has a cation exchange capacity of 75 cmol kg^{-1}. Engelhard Corp. (Cleveland, OH, USA) provided the calcium montmorillonite (CM), which has a cation exchange capacity of 97 cmol kg^{-1}, an exterior surface area of about 70 m^2 g^{-1}, and an average total surface area of up to 850 m^2 g^{-1} [38]. Both clays are represented by the general formula $(Na,Ca)_{0.3}(Al,Mg)_2Si_4O_{10}(OH)_2{\cdot}nH_2O$. In addition to mesopores of around 5 nm in diameter, the samples also contained some mica, quartz, sanidine, and calcite as impurities [30].

5.2. Synthesis and Amendment of GECs

Previously established methods from our laboratory [22,24] were used to amend the parent clays (CM and SM). Briefly, at 150% cation exchange capacity, the SM and CM clays were modified with water-soluble chlorophyllin to yield hydrophilic SMCHin and CMCHin, respectively, and with water-insoluble chlorophyll to develop organoclays, SMCH and CMCH, respectively. To help oversaturate exchangeable sites with chlorophyllin or chlorophyll, SM or CM at 5% w/w in pH 4.2 water were swiftly agitated with chlorophyll or chlorophyllin for 24 h. Following a 20 min centrifugation at 3000× g, the suspensions were rinsed with distilled water. Following three iterations of the washing procedure, each sample was dried in a desiccator before being ground up and run through a 150 μm sieve. The stability of chlorophyll in clay interlayers and the full characterization of these clays including light sensitivity, lipophilicity, expansibility in water, particle size, zeta potential, scanning electron microscopy (JSM-7500F, JEOL, Peabody, MA, USA), X-ray powder diffraction (Bruker D8 Endeavour, Bruker, Karlsruke, Germany), and Fourier-transform infrared spectroscopy (IRPrestige-21, Shimadzu, Japan) has been previously established in our laboratories [22,25]. The physicochemical characteristics such as pH, moisture content, coefficient of expansibility in water, hydrophobicity, bulk density, and pHpzc have also been reported [24].

5.3. Sorption Isotherms at Physiological pHs (pH2 and 6)

To replicate gastric acid and intestinal neutral pH conditions, adsorption isotherms were performed at pH2 and 6 following the procedure of Oladele et al. [23]. Briefly, pure crystals of AFB1 were dissolved in acetonitrile to make its stock solution. A UV-visible spectrophotometer was used to scan and read the absorbance at 362 nm after a calculated amount of the stock solution was injected into distilled water with a pH of 2 or 6 to prepare an 8 ppm AFB1 solution. In order to prevent AFB1 precipitation in the solutions, the maximum AFB1 concentration was fixed at 8 ppm, which is significantly below the solubility range of 11–33 ppm. Next, a gradient of increasing concentrations of AFB1 solution (ranging from 0.4 ppm to 8 ppm) was applied to 100 μg of sorbents. To prepare the concentration gradient of AFB1 solutions, polypropylene centrifuge tubes were filled with a determined volume of 8 ppm solution. A corresponding volume of distilled water (5 mL) followed by 50 μL of a 2 mg/mL clay solution were injected to accomplish the 100 μg sorbent inclusion. The suspension was thoroughly mixed using an autopipette throughout the transfer to the sorbent/toxin mixture. Three tubes containing 8 ppm AFB1 solution, distilled water, and 100 μg sorbent in distilled water served as the three controls. An electric shaker was used to shake the test and control groups for two hours at 37 °C and 1000 rpm. After that, all samples were centrifuged for 20 min at 2000× g in order to separate the clay/AFB1 complex from the solution. Samples and controls were tested for AFB1 absorption in the supernatant using a UV-visible spectrophotometer.

5.4. Adsorption Kinetics

The ability of green clays to bind AFB1 over a 6 h exposure time was assessed in this study using adsorption kinetic models. A 100 ug aliquot of each GEC was combined with 8 ppm of AFB1 in pH2 water at 37 °C. After agitating the mixture at 800 rpm, the residual AFB1 concentration was measured using a UV-visible spectrophotometer at 30 min intervals to examine the adsorption kinetics. To analyze the adsorption dynamics, the study looked at pseudo-second-order, pseudo-first-order, and Elovich models [39,40].

5.5. Data Calculations and Curve Fitting

Using Beer's law, the concentration of AFB1 remaining in solution (c) was determined using the UV-visible absorption data. The concentration difference between the test and control groups was used to compute the quantity adsorbed for each data point. More precisely, the quantity of AFB1 bound by sorbents (in mol/kg) was represented on the y-axis. It was computed by dividing the mass of the contained clays by the difference between the moles of free AFB1 in the test solution and control groups.

$$\text{Beer's law: absorbance} = eLC \tag{1}$$

where e is the molar extinction coefficient (e for AFB1 = 21,865 cm^{-1} mol^{-1}), and L is the path length of the cell holder = 1 cm, dependent on the cuvette.

Table-curve 2D V. 5.01 (Systat Software, Inc., Palo Alto, CA, USA) and the R programming language were employed to examine the adsorption data and ascertain specific parameters. The R code was used to calculate the adsorption data, and maximum likelihood estimation was used to confirm that the data conformed to well-known and accepted models. Confidence intervals and standard errors were calculated using the information matrix approach [41,42].

Adsorption isotherms based on the mean of the observed data points and the 95% confidence intervals from triplicate studies were displayed using the Langmuir model. The Langmuir model illustrates the adsorption of a monolayer on a surface with uniform adsorption energies and a finite number of identical sites. In an ideal Langmuir scenario, adsorption sites with the same energy level suggest a homogenous surface with the least amount of interaction between the adsorbed species.

$$\text{Langmuir model } q = Q_{max}\frac{K_d C_w}{1 + K_d C_w} \tag{2}$$

where C_w = equilibrium concentration of AFB1 (mol L^{-1}), K_d = Langmuir distribution constant, Q_{max} = maximum binding capacity (mol kg^{-1}), and q = the amount of AFB1 adsorbed (mol kg^{-1}).

To determine Ke° from K_d, the following equation was used:

$$Ke^\circ = \frac{K_d[\text{adsorbate}]^o}{\gamma} \tag{3}$$

where Ke° is the thermodynamic equilibrium constant, $[adsorbate]^\circ$ is the standard concentration of the adsorbate = 1 mol L^{-1}, and γ is the coefficient of activity.

The enthalpy (ΔH) and free energy (ΔG°) were determined by using the Gibbs free energy equation together with the adsorption parameters and van't Hoff equation as given below:

$$\Delta G = \Delta G^\circ + RTInKe^\circ \tag{4}$$

$$\Delta H = \frac{-RIn(\frac{K_{d2}}{K_{d1}})}{(\frac{1}{T_2}) - (\frac{1}{T_1})} \tag{5}$$

where T (absolute temperature) = 273 + t (°C) and R (gas constant) = 8.314 J mol^{-1} K^{-1}. When ΔG° is positive, the adsorption process is not favored and cannot be significant ($Ke^\circ < 1$). However, if the value is negative, it is an indication that the adsorption process is enhanced thermodynamically and is proceeding forward ($Ke^\circ > 1$). ΔG will be zero for an adsorption system in equilibrium.

The expression for the nonlinear pseudo-first-order rate equation is displayed as follows:

$$q_t = q_e \times [1 - \exp(-K_1 \times t)] \quad (6)$$

where q_e and q_t denote the amounts in mg/kg of AFB1 adsorbed onto the binding surfaces of various sorbents at equilibrium and time t (min). The rate constant of the first order is K_1 (min^{-1}).

The expression for the nonlinear pseudo-second-order rate equation is as follows:

$$q_t = \frac{K_2 \times {q_e}^2 \times t}{1 + q_e \times K_2 \times t} \quad (7)$$

where q_e and q_t denote the amounts in mg/kg of AFB1 adsorbed onto the binding surfaces of various sorbents at equilibrium and time t (min). The rate constant of the second order is K_2 (mg kg^{-1} min^{-1}).

The expression for the Elovich equation is as follows:

$$q_t = 1/b \ln ab + 1/b \ln t \quad (8)$$

This study involves calculating the initial adsorption rate represented by the symbol a (in mg/kg min) and the parameter b, which are related to the amount of surface covered and the activation energy involved in chemisorption (in mg kg^{-1}). The kinetic parameters of nonlinear models were determined by a trial-and-error method of computational operations. By minimizing the squared deviation and the coefficient of determination between the observed experimental data and the expected values during computer simulations, the parameters were determined.

5.6. In Silico Studies of AFB1 onto the Binding Surfaces of Chlorophyll-Amended Clay

We used MD simulations to investigate the binding of aflatoxin B1 (AFB1) to chlorophyll-amended clay (CMCH), as well as to parent (unamended) clay (CM) at acidic and neutral conditions. The AFB1 model structure was taken from PubChem (ID: 186907), chlorophyll was taken from PDB (molecule entry CLA) [43,44], while two layers of montmorillonite clay in acidic conditions were constructed, in accordance with our previous study [24], using CHARMM-GUI [45–48]. A separation distance of 21 Å was used between the clay layers, while the Na^+ were removed and Ca^{2+} were introduced in random positions within the box. The edges of the clay layers were modified as in our previous studies [22,24] to simulate the clay model in neutral conditions. Topology and parameters for clay were taken from INTERFACE FF [49] in conjunction with CHARMM-GUI [45–48] for AFB1 from CGenFF [50], while for chlorophyll, a combination of CGenFF [50] and parameters from Guerra et al. [51] were used, as in our previous studies [22,24]. The input files for the preparation and simulation setup, used to (a) amend the clay with chlorophyll, and subsequently (b) test the binding of AFB1 to CMCH and CM, were initially generated by CHARMM-GUI [45–48], and were partially modified by us. The preparation of systems in both (a) and (b) was performed using CHARMM [46] and a 100 Å^3 cubic water box. In (a), acidic clay conditions were used, with CM being centered and 12 copies of chlorophyll randomly being placed. The final simulation structure from (a) was used as an initial structure to prepare setup of (b), at which 12 copies of AFB1 randomly being placed away from, and without clashing with, clay or chlorophyll molecules. In (b), triplicate runs were performed, with clay represented independently at both acidic and neutral conditions. The simulations for both (a) and (b) were performed using OpenMM [52]. An equilibration (NVT) was performed at 300 K for 200 ps before the production (NPT) at 300 K and 1 atm (isotropic barostat) for 100 ns for (a) and 200 ns for (b), and in all cases magnesium/aluminum atoms of clay were constrained, analogously to our previous studies [22,24]. Upon completion of the simulations described in (b), analysis was performed with in-house programs to calculate the binding percentage probabilities of AFB1 to CM and CMCH and to understand and provide insight into the mechanisms of binding. This was conducted by decomposing chlorophyll into two chemical groups, the chlorin ring (referred to as "head") and the alkyl chain (referred to as "tail"). The binding percentage probability was calculated by counting the total number of instances that an AFB1 molecule was in contact with the parent and amended clays, and it was normalized by the total number of AFB1 molecules in the simulations and the total number of snapshots analyzed. Subsequently, the average binding percentage probability was calculated from the triplicate runs for each system. Two entities were considered to be in contact, and thus interact with each other, when the distance between any pair of their atoms (including H) was $\leq$3.5 Å. Also, interactions between AFB1 and CM or CMCH were decomposed into direct, direct-assisted, and indirect-assisted interactions in accordance with our studies [22,24].

5.7. Cell Culture and Treatment

Human hepatocellular carcinoma (Hep G2) cells were cultured in Dulbecco's Modified Eagle Medium (DMEM) supplemented with 10% fetal bovine serum (FBS), 1% non-essential amino acids, and 1% antibiotic-antimycotic. Cells were maintained on a collagen-coated surface (PureCol® collagen at a concentration of 50 µg/mL) at 37 °C in a 5% CO_2 atmosphere and subcultured once they reached 70–80% confluency. For the experiments, cells were seeded on collagen-coated 12-well plates at a density of 2×10^5 cells per well and allowed to adhere overnight, or for 12 to 24 h. The cells were then exposed to various treatments consisting of vehicle control, aflatoxin B1 suspended in media, and clay-treated media containing aflatoxin B1. The vehicle control consisted of basal DMEM. Aflatoxin B1 was dissolved in acetonitrile and added to basal media to achieve a final concentration of 20 ppm. An aliquot of the aflatoxin B1 suspension was reserved to serve as the aflatoxin B1 treatment condition. For clay treatment, parent clays (CM and SM) and the GECs (CMCH, CMHCIN, SMCHIN, and SMCH) were tested each at a 0.2% (w/v) and 0.5% (w/v) inclusion rate in 2 mL of 20 ppm AFB1. The mixture was shaken on an electric shaker for two hours at 37 °C and 1000 rpm after which they were centrifuged for 20 min at 2000× g. The aliquots of the supernatants were reserved to serve as clay-treated exposure conditions. All samples were sterile filtered using a 0.22 µm syringe filter to reduce the possibility of contamination. Complete media were aspirated from each well of the seeded 12-well plates and 1 mL of each exposure condition was overlayed onto the cells and allowed to incubate for 24 h. After a 24 h exposure period, the spent media were collected and stored at −80 °C until further analysis. The exposure experiment was repeated three times on three separate occasions for a total of three biological replicates per treatment group. Each biological replicate consisted of separate cultures of cells treated with the respective conditions.

5.7.1. Cytotoxicity Assessment

Cytotoxicity was assessed using the Lactate Dehydrogenase (LDH) Assay Kit (Colorimetric) (Cat. No. ab102526, Abcam, Inc., Cambridge, MA, USA) according to protocol Version 15a using the spent media from each exposure experiment.

5.7.2. Statistical Analysis

Data were analyzed using GraphPad Prism (Version 10.3.0). Statistical significance between treatments was assessed by one-way ANOVA comparing the mean of each condition with the mean of the vehicle control followed by Dunnett's post hoc test for multiple comparisons. A p-value of <0.05 was considered statistically significant. Data are presented in Figure 6 as mean ± standard deviation (SD) of the three biological replicates.

5.8. Hydra Vulgaris In Vivo Assay

Hydra vulgaris is a recognized in vivo model for examining the toxicity of mycotoxins [23,24,53,54]. Environmental Canada in Montreal supplied the Hydra vulgaris organisms used in this study, which were bred at a consistent temperature of 18 °C in hydra medium that contained 4 mg/L EDTA, 115 mg/L N-tris[hydroxymethyl]methyl-2-aminoethanesulfonic acid (TES), and 147 mg/L $CaCl_2$ in 18.2 MΩ water that was adjusted to pH 6.9–7.0. Using an established hydra classification scoring system ranging from 0 to 10, hydra morphology serves as a biomarker for estimating the toxicity of chemicals under a dissecting microscope. This system assigns a score of 0 to a hydra that are thought to be dead or dissolved, and a score of 10 to those that are healthy and have long tentacles. Hydra were treated at different AFB1 concentrations ranging from 10 to 320 ppm for 92 h in order to investigate the toxicity profile of AFB1. The detoxification effects of the GECs were evaluated by treating 20 ppm of AFB1 with inclusions from 0.05% (w/v) to 0.5% (w/v) of the parent and the amended clays in hydra media following exposure to the hydra colony for 92 h. Two hydra colonies each in 2 mL of testing media at 18 °C made up each of the experimental groups.

Each experiment conducted in this study, including the negative and blank controls, was carried out at least three times. A post hoc Tukey test was used after a one-way ANOVA was used to determine the data's statistical significance. Scores from toxicity and detoxification evaluations of hydra, as well as important metrics like Kd and Qmax obtained from adsorption isotherms, were examined for standard deviation and p-values. The results were deemed significant at $p < 0.05$.

Author Contributions: J.O.O.: Methodology, formal analysis, investigation, data curation, visualization, and writing—original draft. X.X.: Visualization, formal analysis, software development, and writing—original draft. G.M.E.III: formal analysis, investigation, and writing—original draft. Y.D.: Investigation, data curation. M.W.: Investigation, and writing—review and editing. P.T.: Software, funding acquisition, and writing—review and editing. N.M.J.: resources, funding acquisition, and writing—review and editing. T.D.P.: Conceptualization, supervision, funding acquisition, and writing—review and editing. All authors have read and agreed to the published version of the manuscript.

Funding: This work was supported by funding through NIEHS P42 ES027704 and USDA Hatch 6215.

Institutional Review Board Statement: Not applicable.

Informed Consent Statement: Not applicable.

Data Availability Statement: The raw data supporting the conclusions of this article will be made available by the authors on request.

Acknowledgments: All MD simulations and additional computational studies were performed using computational resources at the High-Performance Research Computing Facility, the College of Engineering, and the Artie McFerrin Department of Chemical Engineering at Texas A&M University. Xenophon Xenophontos and Phanourios Tamamis acknowledge discussions with members of Tamamis lab.

Conflicts of Interest: The authors declare no conflicts of interest.

References

1. Blount, W.P. Turkey "X" Disease. *J. Brit. Turkey Fed.* **1961**, *9*, 52–54.
2. Asao, T.; Büchi, G.; Abdel-Kader, M.M.; Chang, S.B.; Wick, E.L.; Wogan, G.N. Aflatoxins B and G. *J. Am. Chem. Soc.* **1963**, *85*, 1706–1707. [CrossRef]

3. IARC. Aflatoxins. In *IARC Monographs on the Evaluation of Carcinogenic Risks to Humans*; International Agency for Research on Cancer: Lyon, France, 2012.
4. Scudamore, K.A.; Livesey, C.T. Occurrence and Significance of Mycotoxins in Forage Crops and Silage: A Review. *J. Sci. Food Agric.* **1998**, *77*, 1–17. [CrossRef]
5. Klich, M.A. Aspergillus flavus: The Major Producer of Aflatoxin. *Mol. Plant Pathol.* **2007**, *8*, 713–722. [CrossRef] [PubMed]
6. Liu, Y.; Wu, F. Global Burden of Aflatoxin-Induced Hepatocellular Carcinoma: A Risk Assessment. *Environ. Health Perspect.* **2010**, *118*, 818–824. [CrossRef] [PubMed]
7. Shepherd, G.S. Aflatoxin and Food Safety: Recent African Perspectives. *Toxin Rev.* **2003**, *22*, 267–286. [CrossRef]
8. Williams, J.H.; Phillips, T.D.; Jolly, P.E.; Stiles, J.K.; Jolly, C.M.; Aggarwal, D. Human Aflatoxicosis in Developing Countries: A Review of Toxicology, Exposure, Potential Health Consequences, and Interventions. *Am. J. Clin. Nutr.* **2004**, *80*, 1106–1122. [CrossRef]
9. Robens, J.; Cardwell, K. The Costs of Mycotoxin Management to the USA: Management of Aflatoxins in the United States. *J. Toxicol. Toxin Rev.* **2003**, *22*, 139–152. [CrossRef]
10. Wu, F.; Liu, Y.; Bhatnagar, D. Cost-Effectiveness of Aflatoxin Control Methods: Economic Incentives. *Toxin Rev.* **2008**, *27*, 203–225. [CrossRef]
11. Mitchell, N.J.; Bowers, E.; Hurburgh, C.; Wu, F. Potential Economic Losses to the USA Corn Industry from Aflatoxin Contamination. *Food Addit. Contam. Part A Chem. Anal. Control Expo. Risk Assess.* **2016**, *33*, 540–550. [CrossRef]
12. Lubulwa, A.S.; Davis, J. Estimating the Social Costs of the Impacts of Fungi and Aflatoxins in Maize and Peanuts. In Proceedings of the 6th International Working Conference on Stored-Product Protection, Canberra, Australia, 17–23 April 1994; pp. 1017–1042.
13. Otsuki, T.; Wilson, J.S.; Sewadeh, M. Saving Two in a Billion: Quantifying the Trade Effect of European Food Safety Standards on African Exports. *Food Policy* **2001**, *26*, 495–514. [CrossRef]
14. Battilani, P.; Toscano, P.; Van der Fels-Klerx, H.J.; Moretti, A.; Camardo Leggieri, M.; Brera, C.; Rortais, A.; Goumperis, T.; Robinson, T. Aflatoxin B1 Contamination in Maize in Europe Increases Due to Climate Change. *Sci. Rep.* **2016**, *6*, 24328. [CrossRef]
15. Wu, F.; Bhatnagar, D.; Bui-Klimke, T.; Carbone, I.; Hellmich, R.; Munkvold, G.; Paul, P.; Payne, G.; Takle, E. Climate Change Impacts on Mycotoxin Risks in US Maize. *World Mycotoxin J.* **2011**, *4*, 79–93. [CrossRef]
16. Phillips, T.D.; Afriyie-Gyawu, E.; Williams, J.; Huebner, H.; Ankrah, N.A.; Ofori-Adjei, D.; Jolly, P.; Johnson, N.; Taylor, J.; Marroquin-Cardona, A.; et al. Reducing Human Exposure to Aflatoxin through the Use of Clay: A Review. *Food Addit. Contam. Part A Chem. Anal. Control Expo. Risk Assess.* **2008**, *25*, 134–145.
17. Phillips, T.D.; Kubena, L.F.; Harvey, R.B.; Taylor, D.R.; Heidelbaugh, N.D. Hydrated Sodium Calcium Aluminosilicate: A High Affinity Sorbent for Aflatoxin. *Poult. Sci.* **1988**, *67*, 243–247. [CrossRef] [PubMed]
18. Afriyie-Gyawu, E.; Mackie, J.; Dash, B.; Wiles, M.; Taylor, J.; Huebner, H.; Tang, L.; Guan, H.; Wang, J.S.; Phillips, T.D. Chronic Toxicological Evaluation of Dietary NovaSil Clay in Sprague-Dawley Rats. *Food Addit. Contam.* **2005**, *22*, 259–269. [CrossRef] [PubMed]
19. Afriyie-Gyawu, E.; Ankrah, N.; Huebner, H.J.; Ofosuhene, M.; Kumi, J.; Johnson, N.M.; Tang, L.; Xu, L.; Jolly, P.E.; Ellis, W.O.; et al. NovaSil Clay Intervention in Ghanaians at High Risk for Aflatoxicosis. I. Study Design and Clinical Outcomes. *Food Addit. Contam.* **2007**, *25*, 76–87. [CrossRef]
20. Wang, P.; Afriyie-Gyawu, E.; Tang, Y.; Johnson, N.M.; Xu, L.; Tang, L.; Huebner, H.J.; Ankrah, N.A.; Ofori-Adjei, D.; Ellis, W.; et al. NovaSil Clay Intervention in Ghanaians at High Risk for Aflatoxicosis: II. Reduction in Biomarkers of Aflatoxin Exposure in Blood and Urine. *Food Addit. Contam. Part A Chem. Anal. Control Expo. Risk Assess.* **2008**, *25*, 622–634. [CrossRef]
21. Phillips, T.D.; Wang, M.; Elmore, S.E.; Hearon, S.; Wang, J. NovaSil Clay for the Protection of Humans and Animals from Aflatoxins and Other Contaminants. *Clays Clay Miner.* **2019**, *67*, 99–110. [CrossRef]
22. Rivenbark, K.J.; Wang, M.; Lilly, K.; Tamamis, P.; Phillips, T.D. Development and characterization of chlorophyll-amended montmorillonite clays for the adsorption and detoxification of benzene. *Water Res.* **2022**, *221*, 118788. [CrossRef]
23. Oladele, J.O.; Wang, M.; Rivenbark, K.J.; Phillips, T.D. Application and efficacy of beidellite clay for the adsorption and detoxification of deoxynivalenol (vomitoxin). *Emerg. Contam.* **2024**, *10*, 100390. [CrossRef]
24. Oladele, J.O.; Wang, M.; Xenophontos, X.; Kendall, L.; Tamamis, P.; Phillips, T.D. Chlorophyll-amended organoclays for the detoxification of ochratoxin A. *Toxins* **2024**, *16*, 479. [CrossRef] [PubMed]
25. Wang, M.; Phillips, T.D. Green-engineered barrier creams with montmorillonite-chlorophyll clays as adsorbents for benzene, toluene, and xylene. *Separations* **2023**, *10*, 237. [CrossRef]
26. Jaynes, W.F.; Zartman, R.E. Aflatoxin Toxicity Reduction in Feed by Enhanced Binding to Surface-Modified Clay Additives. *Toxins* **2011**, *3*, 551–565. [CrossRef]
27. Gouda, G.A.; Khattab, H.M.; Abdel-Wahhab, M.A.; Abo El-Nor, S.A.; El-Sayed, H.M.; Kholif, S.M. Clay Minerals as Sorbents for Mycotoxins in Lactating Goat's Diets: Intake, Digestibility, Blood Chemistry, Ruminal Fermentation, Milk Yield and Composition, and Milk Aflatoxin M1 Content. *Small Rumin. Res.* **2019**, *175*, 15–22. [CrossRef]

28. Hassan, A.A.; Salma, H.; Hafsa, A.; Elghandour, M.M.M.Y.; Reddy, P.R.K.; Monroy, J.C.; Salem, A.Z.M. Dietary Supplementation with Sodium Bentonite and Coumarin Alleviates the Toxicity of Aflatoxin B1 in Rabbits. *Toxicon* **2019**, *171*, 35–42. [CrossRef]
29. Adegbeye, M.J.; Reddy, P.R.K.; Chilaka, C.A.; Balogun, O.B.; Elghandour, M.M.M.Y.; Rivas-Caceres, R.R.; Salem, A.Z.M. Mycotoxin Toxicity and Residue in Animal Products: Prevalence, Consumer Exposure, and Reduction Strategies—A Review. *Toxicon* **2020**, *177*, 96–108. [CrossRef] [PubMed]
30. Marroquin-Cardona, A.; Deng, Y.; Garcia-Mazcorro, J.; Johnson, N.M.; Mitchell, N.; Tang, L.; Robinson, A., II; Taylor, J.; Wang, J.-S.; Phillips, T.D. Characterization and Safety of Uniform Particle Size NovaSil Clay as a Potential Aflatoxin Enterosorbent. *Appl. Clay Sci.* **2011**, *54*, 248–257. [CrossRef]
31. Wang, J.-S.; Luo, H.; Billam, M.; Wang, Z.; Guan, H.; Tang, L.; Goldston, T.; Afriyie-Gyawu, E.; Lovett, C.; Griswold, J.; et al. Short-Term Safety Evaluation of Processed Calcium Montmorillonite Clay (NovaSil) in Humans. *Food Addit. Contam.* **2005**, *22*, 270–279. [CrossRef] [PubMed]
32. Zychowski, K.E.; Pohlenz, C.; Mays, T.; Romoser, A.; Hume, M.; Buentello, A.; Gatlin, D.M., III; Phillips, T.D. Effects of Dietary NovaSil on Aflatoxin B1-Exposed Nile Tilapia (Oreochromis niloticus). *Aquaculture* **2013**, *376–379*, 117–123. [CrossRef]
33. Zychowski, K.E.; Rodrigues Hoffmann, A.; Ly, H.J.; Pohlenz, C.; Buentello, A.; Romoser, A.; Gatlin, D.M.; Phillips, T.D. The Effect of Aflatoxin-B1 on Red Drum (Sciaenops ocellatus) and Assessment of Dietary Supplementation of NovaSil for the Prevention of Aflatoxicosis. *Toxins* **2013**, *5*, 1555–1573. [CrossRef]
34. Breinholt, V.; Hendricks, J.; Pereira, C.; Arbogast, D.; Bailey, G. Dietary Chlorophyllin Is a Potent Inhibitor of Aflatoxin B1 Hepatocarcinogenesis in Rainbow Trout. *Cancer Res.* **1995**, *55*, 57–62.
35. Simonich, M.T.; Egner, P.A.; Roebuck, B.D.; Orner, G.A.; Jubert, C.; Pereira, C.; Groopman, J.D.; Kensler, T.W.; Dashwood, R.H.; Williams, D.E.; et al. Natural Chlorophyll Inhibits Aflatoxin B1-Induced Multi-Organ Carcinogenesis in the Rat. *Carcinogenesis* **2007**, *28*, 1294–1302. [CrossRef] [PubMed]
36. Egner, P.A.; Wang, J.B.; Zhu, Y.R.; Zhang, B.C.; Wu, Y.; Zhang, Q.N.; Qian, G.S.; Kuang, S.Y.; Gange, S.J.; Jacobson, L.P.; et al. Chlorophyllin Intervention Reduces Aflatoxin-DNA Adducts in Individuals at High Risk for Liver Cancer. *Proc. Natl. Acad. Sci. USA* **2001**, *98*, 14601–14606. [CrossRef] [PubMed]
37. Jubert, C.; Mata, J.; Bench, G.; Dashwood, R.; Pereira, C.; Tracewell, W.; Turteltaub, K.; Williams, D.; Bailey, G. Effects of Chlorophyll and Chlorophyllin on Low-Dose Aflatoxin B1 Pharmacokinetics in Human Volunteers. *Cancer Prev. Res.* **2009**, *2*, 1015–1022. [CrossRef]
38. Grant, P.G.; Phillips, T.D. Isothermal adsorption of aflatoxin B1 on HSCAS clay. *J. Agric. Food Chem.* **1998**, *46*, 599–605. [CrossRef]
39. Tran, H.N.; You, S.J.; Hosseini-Bandegharaei, A.; Chao, H.P. Mistakes and Inconsistencies Regarding Adsorption of Contaminants from Aqueous Solutions: A Critical Review. *Water Res.* **2017**, *120*, 88–116. [CrossRef]
40. Yuvaraja, G.; Prasad, C.; Vijaya, Y.; Subbaiah, M.V. Application of ZnO Nanorods as an Adsorbent Material for the Removal of As(III) from Aqueous Solution: Kinetics, Isotherms, and Thermodynamic Studies. *Int. J. Integr. Care* **2018**, *9*, 17–25. [CrossRef]
41. Yan, F.; Chu, Y.Y.; Zhang, K.; Zhang, F.F.; Bhandari, N.; Ruan, G.D.; Dai, Z.Y.; Liu, Y.; Zhang, Z.; Kan, A.T. Determination of adsorption isotherm parameters with correlated errors by measurement error models. *Chem. Eng. J.* **2015**, *281*, 921–930. [CrossRef]
42. Gong, J. Rshiny. 2020. Available online: https://jgong9.shinyapps.io/chemistry_app/ (accessed on 30 September 2023).
43. Berman, H.M.; Westbrook, J.; Feng, Z.; Gilliland, G.; Bhat, T.N.; Weissig, H.; Shindyalov, I.N.; Bourne, P.E. The protein data bank. *Nucleic Acids Res.* **2000**, *28*, 235–242. [CrossRef]
44. PDB. 2022 Chlorophyll A CLA. Available online: https://www.rcsb.org/ligand/CLA (accessed on 6 March 2025).
45. Jo, S.; Kim, T.; Iyer, V.G.; Im, W. CHARMM-GUI: A Web-based Graphical User Interface for CHARMM. *J. Comput. Chem.* **2008**, *29*, 1859–1865. [CrossRef] [PubMed]
46. Brooks, B.R.; Brooks, C.L., III; MacKerell, A.D., Jr.; Nilsson, L.; Petrella, R.J.; Roux, B.; Won, Y.; Archontis, G.; Bartels, C.; Boresch, S.; et al. CHARMM: The biomolecular simulation program. *J. Comput. Chem.* **2009**, *30*, 1545–1614. [CrossRef] [PubMed]
47. Lee, J.; Cheng, X.; Swails, J.M.; Yeom, M.S.; Eastman, P.K.; Lemkul, J.A.; Wei, S.; Buckner, J.; Jeong, J.C.; Qi, Y.; et al. CHARMM-GUI Input Generator for NAMD, GROMACS, AMBER, OpenMM, and CHARMM/OpenMM Simulations Using the CHARMM36 Additive Force Field. *J. Chem. Theory Comput.* **2016**, *12*, 405–413. [CrossRef] [PubMed]
48. Choi, Y.K.; Kern, N.R.; Kim, S.; Kanhaiya, K.; Afshar, Y.; Jeon, S.H.; Jo, S.; Brooks, B.R.; Lee, J.; Tadmor, E.B.; et al. CHARMM-GUI Nanomaterial Modeler for Modeling and Simulation of Nanomaterial Systems. *J. Chem. Theory Comput.* **2022**, *18*, 479–493. [CrossRef] [PubMed] [PubMed Central]
49. Heinz, H.; Lin, T.J.; Mishra, R.K.; Emami, F.S. Thermodynamically consistent force fields for the assembly of inorganic, organic, and biological nanostructures: The INTERFACE force field. *Langmuir* **2013**, *29*, 1754–1765. [CrossRef]
50. Vanommeslaeghe, K.; MacKerell, A.D., Jr. Automation of the CHARMM General Force Field (CGenFF) I: Bond perception and atom typing. *J. Chem. Inf. Model.* **2012**, *52*, 3144–3154. [CrossRef]
51. Guerra, F.; Adam, S.; Bondar, A.N. Revised force-field parameters for chlorophyll-a, pheophytin-a and plastoquinone-9. *J. Mol. Graph. Model.* **2015**, *58*, 30–39. [CrossRef]

52. Eastman, P.; Swails, J.; Chodera, J.D.; McGibbon, R.T.; Zhao, Y.; Beauchamp, K.A.; Wang, L.P.; Simmonett, A.C.; Harrigan, M.P.; Stern, C.D.; et al. OpenMM 7: Rapid development of high performance algorithms for molecular dynamics. *PLoS Comput. Biol.* **2017**, *13*, e1005659. [CrossRef]
53. Eagles, E.J.; Benstead, R.; MacDonald, S.; Handy, R.D.; Hutchinson, T.H. Environmental Risks to Freshwater Organisms from the Mycotoxins Deoxynivalenol and Zearalenone Using Species Sensitivity Distributions. *Chemosphere* **2021**, *267*, 129279. [CrossRef]
54. Marchesano, V.; Ambrosone, A.; Bartelmess, J.; Strisciante, F.; Tino, A.; Echegoyen, L.; Tortiglione, C.; Giordani, S. Impact of Carbon Nano-Onions on Hydra vulgaris as a Model Organism for Nanoecotoxicology. *Nanomaterials* **2015**, *5*, 1331–1350. [CrossRef]

toxins

MDPI

Obituary

Thomas W. Kensler (1948–2025): A Legend in Antioxidant Response Pathways and Aflatoxin Carcinogenesis Research

David L. Eaton [1,*] and John D. Groopman [2]

1 Department of Environmental and Occupational Health Sciences, School of Public Health, University of Washington, Seattle, WA 98105, USA
2 Department of Environmental Health & Engineering, Bloomberg School of Public Health, The Johns Hopkins University, Baltimore, MD 21205, USA
* Correspondence: deaton@uw.edu

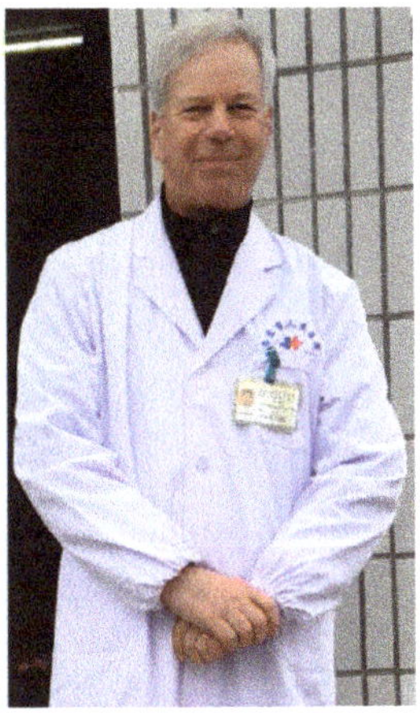

It is with great sadness that we must include in this Special Volume of *Toxins* a memorial to our close friend and colleague, Dr. Thomas W. Kensler, who passed away from a hiking accident on Mt. Blanc, France, on 11 July 2025, at the age of 76. Dr. Kensler was born in New York City in 1948, the son of Charles J. Kensler and Elizabeth B. K. Williams. He grew up in Lexington, Massachusetts. After earning his AB in biology from Hamilton College, he then received his PhD in toxicological sciences from the Massachusetts Institute of Technology in 1976, in the laboratory of Dr. Gerald Wogan. He then completed postdoctoral training at the McArdle Laboratory for Cancer Research at the University of Wisconsin and at the National Cancer Institute in cancer therapeutics before joining the faculty of the Johns Hopkins Bloomberg School of Public Health in 1980. Tom spent 30 years at Hopkins before he and his wife, Dr. Nancy Davidson, moved to the University of Pittsburgh in 2010 (he maintained his appointment and collaborations with his colleagues at Hopkins Bloomberg School of Public Health). In 2017, he and Dr. Davidson moved to Seattle where Nancy was appointed as President and Executive Director of the Seattle Cancer Care Alliance and Senior Vice President at Fred Hutchinson Cancer Center and Tom continued his research in the Public Health Sciences Division for 7 more years, retiring in 2024. Dr. Kensler was a giant in several related areas in toxicology, including the toxicology of aflatoxins, on which this Special Issue of *Toxins* is focused. Over his nearly 50 years of research, Dr. Kensler published nearly 500 research papers, book chapters and reviews, of which 400 were published in peer-reviewed journals.

https://doi.org/10.3390/toxins17100517

His research has been cited by others over 45,000 times, giving him an "H-Index" of 109, which is remarkable (Figure 1) One online source states that "for top-tier professionals, H-indices greater than 40 are generally considered excellent, and 60 or higher may be considered remarkable or exceptional". Tom mentioned to one of us many years ago, "My goal is to have an H-factor higher than my age when I die." He more than met that goal! This is itself an incredible testament to the scientific impact that Dr. Kensler has had in toxicology and more specifically cancer prevention research.

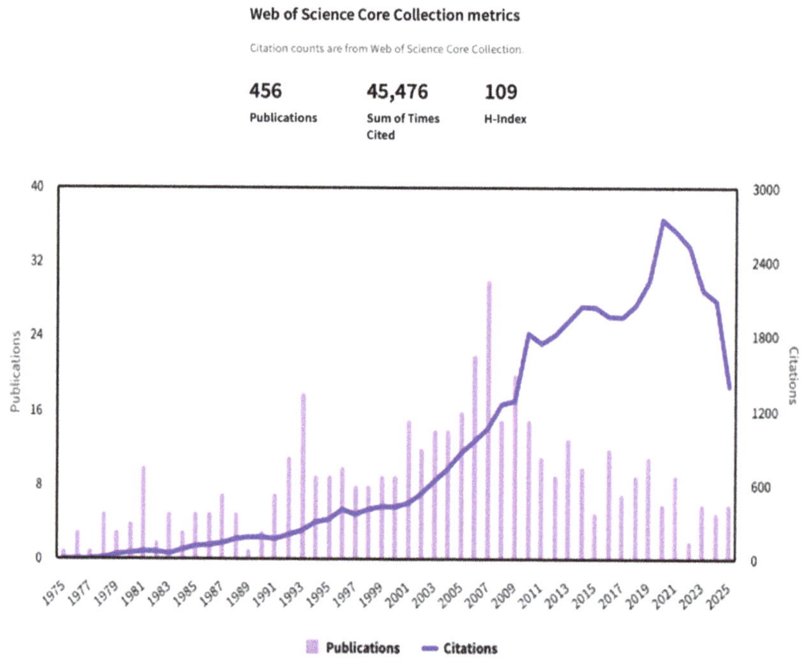

Figure 1. Web of Science Publications and Citations of Dr. Thomas Kensler 1975–2025.

Tom was a major contributor to the field of cancer chemoprevention, with much of his work focused on novel approaches to dietary modulation of aflatoxin biotransformation [1–6]. His contributions in the area focused on prevention of dietary aflatoxin-induced liver cancer, yet only 25% of his research publications were related to aflatoxins. He made significant contributions in the broader (albeit related) area of 'redox biology', with a focus on understanding how certain vegetable components in the diet can modify gene expression of antioxidant pathways that help protect against oxidative stress [7–9]. His research was both fundamental (e.g., at the molecular level) and directly applicable to 'real-world' cancer prevention. His elegant studies on the Keap1-Nrf2 antioxidant pathway and its modification by dithiolthiones (including sulforaphane found in broccoli and other cruciferous vegetables) led the way for direct human intervention studies in populations at increased risk for certain cancers [10–17].

Despite the molecular details of much of his research, he never lost sight of the bigger picture and was an outstanding collaborator with many clinicians interested in research that saves lives. For example, in 2016, he was first author on a review titled "Transforming Cancer Prevention through Precision Medicine and Immune-oncology" [18]. The 11 co-authors (including his wife, Nancy) were leading cancer prevention researchers from 12 of the most prestigious cancer research and treatment centers in the United States. In this article, the authors note "Just as precision medicine and immune-oncology are revolutionizing cancer therapy, these approaches are transforming cancer prevention. Here, we set out a brief agenda for the immediate future of cancer prevention research (including a "Pre-Cancer Genome Atlas" or "PCGA"), which will involve the inter-related fields of precision medicine and immunoprevention—pivotal elements of a broader domain of personalized public health."

Tom's contributions to cancer prevention research were widely recognized by his colleagues and by major professional organizations. For example, in 2007, he was honored by the American Association for Cancer Research and the American Cancer Society through with the annual "Award for Research Excellence in Cancer Epidemiology and Prevention". Two years later in 2009, the Society of Toxicology recognized Tom with one of their highest awards, the Translational Impact Award. His research had a global impact and was greatly appreciated in China. In 2011, he received a National Friendship Award in Beijing, People's Republic of China, which is the highest award for foreign civilians, and was made an honorary Professor at the Nantong Tumor Institute, Nantong, China, in 2015.

In addition to his remarkable contributions to cancer prevention research, Tom was an outstanding mentor and educator. Over his 40+ years in academia, he served as mentor/advisor for 28 doctoral students, 16 postdoctoral fellows, and 8 master's degree students. He also served on over 120 other graduate student committees, alongside conducting viva voce exams and performing other mentoring roles. But his mentorship and influence on other scientists extend well beyond the hundreds of graduate students and postdocs he directly mentored. For example, Dr. Donna Zhang, a full Professor in Pharmacology and Toxicology at the University of Arizona, was quoted in Tom's obituary in the Baltimore Sun: "His quiet brilliance, deep integrity, and unwavering generosity shaped not only the field of redox biology, but also my own journey in science." We know that this perspective is shared by all who have known and worked with Tom over the years. As a testament to Tom's passion to be a 'good mentor, one of our colleagues shared this story: "I recall being with him at Hopkins as a visiting scientist. I attended a student seminar being presented by one of his students. Tom was really grilling the students to a point that it was difficult to see why he was being so critical. Patricia Egner [Tom's senior lab tech] explained afterwards that Tom wanted his students to go out into the world, be respected from the first sentence they shared, be accurate with their sharing, and think about the bigger issues. It was better that life was uncomfortable for them in a safe environment (the seminar) than when they were out in the real world."

He will be greatly missed as a dear friend and colleague, but we find solace that his tremendous work in the field will continue to inspire new research and save lives, and that—as tragic as his accident was—he left us doing something he loved.

Tom is survived by his wife of 43 years, Nancy E. Davidson, son Kevin H. Kensler, daughter Caroline B. Kensler and son-in-law Nikolas F. Iubel, brother-in-law and sister-in-law David L. Davidson and Kathy Reigstad, nephews David M. Davidson and Keith L. Davidson, and stepsisters Aimée Margolis and Nadia Margolis.

Contributions in Dr. Kensler's memory can be made to the American Association for Cancer Research at www.aacr.org (accessed on 15 October 2025).

Funding: This research received no external funding.

Acknowledgments: We would like to express our deep gratitude to Nancy Davidson for her 50+ years of devotion to Kensler's personal and professional development and to all of Tom's trainees, who provided him with the motivation to continue his research.

Conflicts of Interest: The authors declare no conflicts of interest.

References

1. Chen, J.G.; Zhu, Y.R.; Qian, G.S.; Wang, J.B.; Lu, J.H.; Kensler, T.W.; Jacobson, L.P.; Munoz, A.; Groopman, J.D. Fifty Years of Aflatoxin Research in Qidong, China: A Celebration of Team Science to Improve Public Health. *Toxins* **2025**, *17*, 79. [CrossRef] [PubMed]
2. Davis, C.P.; Fest, S.; Cushing-Haugen, K.; Kensler, T.W.; Chavarro, J.E.; Harris, H.R. Dietary patterns and age at menarche in a prospective study of girls in the USA. *Hum. Reprod.* **2025**, *40*, 1087–1093. [CrossRef] [PubMed]
3. Egner, P.A.; Munoz, A.; Kensler, T.W. Chemoprevention with chlorophyllin in individuals exposed to dietary aflatoxin. *Mutat. Res.* **2003**, *523–524*, 209–216. [CrossRef] [PubMed]
4. Fahey, J.W.; Kensler, T.W. Role of dietary supplements/nutraceuticals in chemoprevention through induction of cytoprotective enzymes. *Chem. Res. Toxicol.* **2007**, *20*, 572–576. [CrossRef] [PubMed]
5. Guyton, K.Z.; Kensler, T.W. Prevention of liver cancer. *Curr. Oncol. Rep.* **2002**, *4*, 464–470. [CrossRef] [PubMed]
6. Kensler, T.W.; Eaton, D.L. 65 Years on-Aflatoxin Biomarkers Blossoming: Whither Next? *Toxins* **2024**, *16*, 496. [CrossRef] [PubMed]
7. Agyeman, A.S.; Chaerkady, R.; Shaw, P.G.; Davidson, N.E.; Visvanathan, K.; Pandey, A.; Kensler, T.W. Transcriptomic and proteomic profiling of KEAP1 disrupted and sulforaphane-treated human breast epithelial cells reveals common expression profiles. *Breast Cancer Res. Treat.* **2012**, *132*, 175–187. [CrossRef] [PubMed]
8. Kensler, T.W.; Egner, P.A.; Dolan, P.M.; Groopman, J.D.; Roebuck, B.D. Mechanism of protection against aflatoxin tumorigenicity in rats fed 5-(2-pyrazinyl)-4-methyl-1,2-dithiol-3-thione (oltipraz) and related 1,2-dithiol-3-thiones and 1,2-dithiol-3-ones. *Cancer Res.* **1987**, *47*, 4271–4277. [PubMed]
9. Laso, N.; Mas, S.; Lafuente, M.J.; Llobet, J.M.; Molina, R.; Ballesta, A.; Kensler, T.W.; Lafuente, A. Induction of NAD(P)H quinone oxidoreductase by vegetables widely consumed in Catalonia, Spain. *Nutr. Cancer* **2005**, *52*, 49–58. [CrossRef] [PubMed]
10. Camoirano, A.; Bagnasco, M.; Bennicelli, C.; Cartiglia, C.; Wang, J.B.; Zhang, B.C.; Zhu, Y.R.; Qian, G.S.; Egner, P.A.; Jacobson, L.P.; et al. Oltipraz chemoprevention trial in Qidong, People's Republic of China: Results of urine genotoxicity assays as related to smoking habits. *Cancer Epidemiol. Biomark. Prev.* **2001**, *10*, 775–783.
11. Chen, J.; Zhu, J.; Wang, G.; Groopman, J.D.; Kensler, T.W. Qidong: A crucible for studies on liver cancer etiology and prevention. *Cancer Biol. Med.* **2019**, *16*, 24–37. [CrossRef] [PubMed]
12. Chen, J.G.; Kensler, T.W.; Zhu, J.; Zhu, Y.R.; Wang, J.B.; Lu, J.H.; Munoz, A.; Groopman, J.D. Profound primary prevention of liver cancer following a natural experiment in China: A 50-year perspective and public health implications. *Int. J. Cancer* **2025**, *156*, 756–763. [CrossRef] [PubMed]
13. Groopman, J.D.; Wogan, G.N.; Roebuck, B.D.; Kensler, T.W. Molecular biomarkers for aflatoxins and their application to human cancer prevention. *Cancer Res.* **1994**, *54*, 1907s–1911s. [PubMed]
14. Kensler, T.W.; Egner, P.A.; Agyeman, A.S.; Visvanathan, K.; Groopman, J.D.; Chen, J.G.; Chen, T.Y.; Fahey, J.W.; Talalay, P. Keap1-nrf2 signaling: A target for cancer prevention by sulforaphane. *Top. Curr. Chem.* **2013**, *329*, 163–177. [CrossRef] [PubMed]
15. Kensler, T.W.; Egner, P.A.; Wang, J.B.; Zhu, Y.R.; Zhang, B.C.; Lu, P.X.; Chen, J.G.; Qian, G.S.; Kuang, S.Y.; Jackson, P.E.; et al. Chemoprevention of hepatocellular carcinoma in aflatoxin endemic areas. *Gastroenterology* **2004**, *127*, S310–S318. [CrossRef] [PubMed]
16. Kensler, T.W.; Roebuck, B.D.; Wogan, G.N.; Groopman, J.D. Aflatoxin: A 50-year odyssey of mechanistic and translational toxicology. *Toxicol. Sci.* **2011**, *120* (Suppl. S1), S28–S48. [CrossRef] [PubMed]
17. Yates, M.S.; Kensler, T.W. Keap1 eye on the target: Chemoprevention of liver cancer. *Acta Pharmacol. Sin.* **2007**, *28*, 1331–1342. [CrossRef] [PubMed]
18. Kensler, T.W.; Spira, A.; Garber, J.E.; Szabo, E.; Lee, J.J.; Dong, Z.; Dannenberg, A.J.; Hait, W.N.; Blackburn, E.; Davidson, N.E.; et al. Transforming Cancer Prevention through Precision Medicine and Immune-oncology. *Cancer Prev. Res.* **2016**, *9*, 2–10. [CrossRef] [PubMed]

toxins

MDPI

Article

AI and Biotechnology to Combat Aflatoxins: Future Directions for Modern Technologies in Reducing Aflatoxin Risk

Charitha J. Gamlath [1] and Felicia Wu [1,2,*]

1 Department of Food Science and Human Nutrition, Michigan State University, East Lansing, MI 48824, USA; pahalaga@msu.edu
2 Department of Agricultural, Food, and Resource Economics, Michigan State University, East Lansing, MI 48824, USA
* Correspondence: fwu@msu.edu

Abstract: Although a decades-old problem in food safety, aflatoxin has largely resisted human control methods. This situation could be mitigated using new technologies that could provide better control all along the food supply chain, for crops frequently infected with the causative fungi *Aspergillus flavus* and *A. parasiticus*, which produce aflatoxin. Generative artificial intelligence (AI) and modern biotechnology could offer, and have offered, a suite of potential solutions to reducing both fungal infection and aflatoxin contamination of foods. In this paper, we describe these technologies, as well as means by which they may be utilized to reduce aflatoxin risk along the food supply chain. We discuss how regulatory frameworks worldwide may be restrictive for biotechnologies in certain parts of the world, but are relatively less stringent for AI at present. To the extent that these technologies can be harnessed and deployed safely to combat the problem of aflatoxins, we encourage research and development in these areas to improve the precision, accuracy, and speed by which to deal with this food safety risk.

Keywords: AI; artificial intelligence; biotechnology; aflatoxins; control strategies

Key Contribution: This article reviews recent AI and biotechnology applications for aflatoxin control from farm to fork and proposes a conceptual scenario to illustrate where these technologies can be incorporated into the corn food supply chain.

1. Introduction

This article describes the potential applications of a convergence of technologies, artificial intelligence (AI) and biotechnologies, to reduce aflatoxin contamination in food and feed. Artificial intelligence (AI) has existed as a branch of computer science and an application in technology for decades. But in recent years, AI has garnered greater attention across multiple fields because more advanced forms have become much more accessible to the general public for the first time. Moreover, one does not need to know the details of how AI works to be able to use it across many domains. AI tools such as ChatGPT-5 or Gemini (Google AI) allow users to do many things: gather summary information on any topic they seek, do both rudimentary and complex calculations, write programming code or poems, create images, rewrite documents in particular styles, formats, and languages, detect patterns in data and images, design spaces, help with household and work tasks, and much more.

On a larger scale, AI is being used in industries and governmental and non-governmental organizations, in diverse ways. One of the ways that the use of AI could be enhanced in agriculture, food, and public health is in conjunction with emerging biotechnologies that help to curb risks associated with climate change, economic shocks, and geopolitical instability. Unlike AI, biotechnology has been used in agriculture since the 1980s, for multiple purposes: to prevent the freezing of citrus fruits (ice-minus: genetically engineered bacteria), to confer viral or insect pest resistance or herbicide tolerance in crops, to biofortify grains with micronutrients, to enhance growth rates of salmon, and to produce textiles from crops. One paper describes how biotechnology can be used to reduce mycotoxins in corn, either by reducing fungal infection or by degrading the toxins [1]. Combined with AI, biotechnologies could become more selective and informed in mitigating aflatoxin risk.

In this paper, we explore how AI and modern biotechnologies can be harnessed to advance aflatoxin-related research, detection, and mitigation strategies from farm to fork. We begin by providing an overview of aflatoxins, AI, and contemporary biotechnological tools. Subsequently, we synthesize the existing literature to highlight potential applications and their benefits for aflatoxin control and the promotion of human health. Finally, we propose a conceptual scenario to illustrate how AI and biotechnology can be incorporated into the entire food supply chain to manage aflatoxin contamination, using corn—one of the most susceptible crops—as a case study. This work offers a unique perspective on leveraging AI and modern biotechnological innovations for comprehensive aflatoxin management, aiming to inform future research, identify existing knowledge gaps, and accelerate the effective integration of emerging technologies in this field.

2. Background: Aflatoxins

Aflatoxins are toxic and carcinogenic secondary metabolites of the fungi *Aspergillus flavus* and *A. parasiticus*. As these fungi infect the food and feed crops such as corn, peanuts, tree nuts, cottonseed, and sunflower seeds grown in tropical and subtropical climates, aflatoxin is frequently a contaminant of these foods. Aflatoxins were first discovered in 1960 in a gruesome manner: when over 100,000 turkey poults died in the United Kingdom as a result of eating moldy peanut meal [2]. Since then, the exposure of aflatoxins was extensively investigated and subsequently recognized to cause liver toxicity and cancer (hepatocellular carcinoma) in multiple animal species. In 1993, the International Agency for Research on Cancer (IARC) classified "naturally occurring mixtures of aflatoxins" as a Group 1 carcinogen [3]. Further, aflatoxins are particularly carcinogenic in individuals exposed to high levels of both aflatoxins and hepatitis B virus (HBV). Exposure to both agents increases lifetime liver cancer risk multiplicatively when compared with the risk imposed by just one agent [4–6].

Out of the four common aflatoxins (B1, B2, G1, and G2), aflatoxin B1 (AFB1) is of the greatest concern worldwide, due to its toxicity, carcinogenicity, and prevalence in staple foods and feeds worldwide [7]. When ingested, AFB1 is metabolized in the liver by the P450 enzyme system into the carcinogenic intermediate, aflatoxin B1-8,9-epoxide (AFBO). This compound exists in two isomeric forms: endo-8,9-epoxide and exo-8,9-epoxide. Due to its highly electrophilic nature, AFBO readily reacts with biological amines in proteins and nucleic acids. When interacting with DNA, AFBO forms a covalent bond at the N7 position of guanine, producing the adduct AFB1-N7-guanine. The AFBO exo isomer exhibits a much greater affinity for guanine residues than the endo isomer and is therefore regarded as the primary carcinogenic metabolite [8]. The resulting DNA damage can initiate the development of hepatocellular carcinoma (liver cancer), or, at high exposure levels, cause acute liver failure leading to aflatoxicosis [9]. Increasing evidence also suggest that AFB1 can induce oxidative stress in cell function [10]. Globally, 5–28% of all liver cancer cases can be attributed to aflatoxin exposure, exceeding over 100,000 new aflatoxin-induced liver cancer cases per year. The majority of these cases occur in sub-Saharan Africa, Southeast Asia, and China, where both HBV infection rates and aflatoxin contamination in food remain high and poorly controlled [11]. To minimize dietary exposure to AFB1, regulatory limits have been established globally to ensure that contamination levels in food and feed remain sufficiently low. Regulatory limits for AFB1 in maize and peanuts—two of the most frequently contaminated food commodities, set by various nations and regulatory authorities are available in Wu et al. (2013) [12].

While farm-to-fork strategies currently exist to reduce aflatoxin in food, or its harmful effects in the body [13], oftentimes these strategies can be difficult to implement in real time, in the populations of interest. For example, biocontrol—atoxigenic strains of *Aspergillus* applied to crop soils to competitively exclude toxigenic strains on crops—can only be applied at the start of the growing season, before a farmer knows whether aflatoxin would even be a problem in that season. If later in the summer, the farmer detects high aflatoxin risk in the crops, it is too late then to apply biocontrol [14]. Similarly: many dietary chemopreventive strategies, such as incorporation of *Brassica* or *Allium* vegetables to the diet to reduce the risk of aflatoxin epoxide-mediated DNA damage [15], are not always feasible, as they are not readily available in sufficient amounts in the diets of populations where aflatoxin-contaminated maize and peanut consumption is high; and public awareness of these dietary chemopreventive agents is low.

The combined use of AI and modern biotechnologies could enhance the utility of these existing aflatoxin control strategies, as well as provide new strategies. These technologies are described below.

3. Background: AI

The term artificial intelligence (AI) refers to a suite of tools that simulates human intelligence and ability to perform tasks by means of machines; principally computer systems, robotics, and digital equipment [16,17]. Specifically, generative AI refers to AI that creates new material by processing large amounts of existing data. How can it do this? *Machine learning* (ML) is one of the key themes of AI. It involves the development of algorithms or models, sometimes called large language models or LLM, that are trained from ideally copious amounts of data to identify patterns or make predictions [18]. It is by machine learning that AI tools such as ChatGPT and Google Gemini can provide answers to the questions that users ask on virtually any topic: solving mathematical problems, helping to write essays and letters, coding, providing interior decorating or grocery shopping tips, or even imitating a therapist. This paper will not delve into the ethical and moral hazards associated with AI use, but will focus very specifically on possible applications in aflatoxin reduction.

Several statistical and mathematical methods are used when developing such algorithms. Some of the commonly used ML algorithms used in Aflatoxin control are described below:

Artificial neural networks (ANN) are a computational method that mimics the biological neural functions of the human brain. ANN consists of layers that are interdependent of each other. Each layer consists of processing nodes or "neurons," linked by weighted connections that transfers outputs from one nodes input to another [19]. When the weighted sum of inputs exceeds a predefined threshold value of a node, it passes the signal to neighboring nodes via a function known as the transfer function [20]. Neural networks have many applications such as pattern recognition, prediction, and classifications, and are employed in the detection of fungal growth by image processing and for identifying complex metabolic pathways that lead to toxin-induced cellular alteration using molecular descriptors [19,21,22].

Principal component analysis (PCA) is a dimension reduction method that has commonly been used in research long before the advent of generative AI. PCA is useful when analyzing highly correlated data with a large number of variables, with multiple observations associated with each variable. PCA identifies key categories (referred to as principal components) that represent the original data with minimal loss of information. It projects the data into a new-lower dimensional subspace and reduces storage space, collinearity and noise in data [19,23]. A potential application of PCA during aflatoxin control is coupling it with spectral images to screen signals and identify signals that are specific to aflatoxins [24].

Support vector machines (SVM) are algorithms that distinguish between two classes by finding the hyperplane that maximizes the gap between the closest data points of opposite classes. The number of features in the input data dictates if the hyperplane is a line in a 2-D space or a plane in a n-dimensional space. Since multiple hyperplanes may demarcate two classes of data, maximizing the gap between points allows the algorithm to find the best boundary between classes [25]. SVM has diverse applications in disease detection, crop quality classification and yield prediction during agricultural activities.

Decision trees are classification or regression algorithms with a tree-like architecture that progressively organize a dataset into smaller homogeneous clusters known as subpopulations. Decision tree algorithms consist of internal nodes that represent a different pairwise comparison of a selected feature. A branch consists of several such nodes and represents the outcome of the comparison [26]. A *random forest* forms when multiple decision trees connect to each other to achieve a single outcome [19]. Random forests are used for crop classification and detection of mycotoxin contamination levels in crops using image analysis [27].

Deep learning is a specific type of an ANN with complex multilayers that consists of a large number of functions that allow data representation in a hierarchical manner. Deep learning has added advantages of automatic data extraction from raw data, with characteristics from higher levels of the hierarchy being formed by the components of lower levels. Compared to other approaches, deep learning can solve complex problems quickly and effectively due to the complex models used [28]. Similar to PCA, deep learning can be coupled with spectral approaches to detect aflatoxins in crops; however, with better performance [29].

All of these AI methods are useful in solving agricultural and food problems; from robotic harvesting machines operated from a distance, to supply chain solutions in optimal food distribution across multiple sites. Additionally, other technologies can help to ensure food productivity and safety. Many of these fall under modern biotechnologies, discussed next.

4. Background: Biotechnology

Biotechnology has its roots in understanding the properties of DNA, genes, and how these can be engineered by humans for specific purposes. The discovery of recombinant DNA and its possibilities in the 1970s has led to breakthroughs in medicine, engineering, and all of the life sciences [30]. Agricultural biotechnology had its first application in 1987 in "Ice-minus": a genetic variant of the bacterium *Pseudomonas syringae* to spray onto crops to prevent frost damage [31]. Although this product was field-tested, it was never commercialized. Larger agbiotech applications were commercialized and deployed in US agriculture in the mid-1990s: transgenic corn, cotton, potato, and soybean that were modified to produce insecticides (Bacillus thuringiensis (Bt) treated crops), tolerate herbicides (Roundup Ready or Liberty Link crops), or both. To date, a vast majority of the field corn and soybeans produced in the US are biotech varieties. More biotech crops have been developed and commercialized that are not simply transgenic, but gene-edited or genetically modified using RNA-interference methods. Some biotech methods used in agriculture are described below.

Transgenic crops, often called genetically modified organisms (GMOs) in the public dialogue, contain genes introduced from foreign (non-host) species using genetic engineering techniques such as gene guns (older method) or *Agrobacterium tumefaciens* to allow gene introgression. These foreign genes confer desired attributes in the host plant such as pest protection, herbicide tolerance, viral resistance, and enhanced nutritional content. As described above, transgenic crops are the earliest biotech crops commercialized worldwide, with the introduction of insect-protected Bt crops and herbicide-tolerant crops in the 1990s in the US and other countries worldwide. Transgenic Bt corn, for example, contains genes from a soil bacterium *Bacillus thuringiensis* (hence Bt) that produce delta-endotoxins, selectively toxic to certain insect pests. Transgenic crops can aid aflatoxin control in several ways. The lower levels of insect pest damage mean fewer entry wounds on kernels that fungi can then easily infect. Additionally, transgenic crops can be developed to express synthetic peptides and enzymes that can retard fungal growth. These are explained in detail in Section 9.

Another type of biotechnology more recently employed in agriculture that can fight against fungal infections is *RNA interference (RNAi)*. RNAi refers to a bioengineering process that allows the host organism (e.g., a corn plant) to interact with another species (e.g., an insect pest or a fungal pathogen) to interfere with particular processes in that species as a protective mechanism to the host. In contrast to Bt corn, which produces proteins that are toxic to insects, RNAi corn silences specific genes in potential pests or pathogens that attack it. In 2017, the US Environmental Protection Agency (EPA) approved a variety of RNAi corn that controls for corn rootworm, to be commercialized in the US (https://www.epa.gov/pesticide-registration/epa-registers-innovative-tool-control-corn-rootworm (accessed on 7 September 2025)). Now, RNAi corn hybrids are being developed that can also control aflatoxin by silencing particular *A. flavus* genes in the aflatoxin biosynthetic pathway [32].

Clustered regularly interspaced short palindromic repeats (CRISPR) is an adaptive immune system in bacteria that employs small guide RNAs (crRNAs) to interfere with invading nucleic acids. CRISPR-Cas (also known as CRISPR associated) systems consist of a genomic locus that holds together short repetitive elements (repeats) separated by unique sequences (spacers), which are originally produced in mobile genetic elements (MGEs) such as bacteriophages, transposons, or plasmids. In nature, CRISPR-Cas system acts in a sequence-specific way to recognize and cleave foreign DNA or RNA [33]. In the presence of an invading MGE, a distinct sequence of the MGE is incorporated into the CRISPR array, leading to the formation of a new spacer. The new spacer incorporated CRISPR array is then transcribed into long precursor crRNA and further processed into mature RNA that remembers the invader's DNA. Finally, the crRNA forms a complex with a Cas nuclease (an enzyme), that ultimately identifies and cleaves the invading DNA with the complementary sequence [33,34]. CRISPR has potential applications in mycotoxin control in food where a guide crRNA could be designed and delivered along with Cas nuclease to cleave genes in fungi responsible for mycotoxin production. In addition to DNA cleavage, different Cas enzymes have different functions that can be utilized for diagnostic purposes. For instance, after recognizing and cleaving a specific target, Cas12a, Cas13, and Cas14 exhibit collateral, nonspecific cleavage activities against single-stranded DNA (ssDNA) or single-stranded RNA (ssRNA). Therefore, by incorporating a ssRNA or ssDNA reporter molecule that can be cleaved by such Cas enzymes resulting in a fluorescent signal, to the CRISPR system, a bio sensor could be designed to generate a signal when a target genetic material is present [35]. Transcriptomics and proteomics can complement CRISPR applications by identifying regulatory targets and resistance traits of plants for reducing the risk of fungal infection and subsequent aflatoxin production.

The remainder of this paper describes how AI and biotechnology can be used to improve aflatoxin detection and control, from seed production to understanding of its toxicology. Figure 1 summarizes how AI could improve methods of aflatoxin control from farm to fork, and beyond to human health.

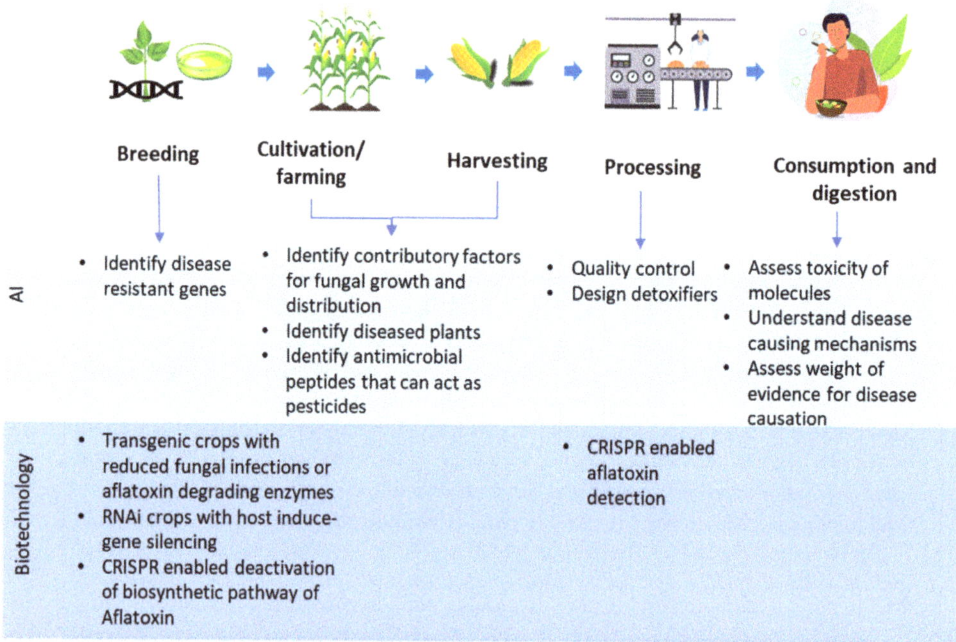

Figure 1. Potential areas of aflatoxin control that AI and biotechnology can enhance.

5. AI Applications in Plant Breeding: Conventional or Biotechnological

Today, AI models trained on DNA sequences can generate new sequences encoding potentially novel biological functions. Separately, large language models (LLM) trained on the scientific literature can guide novices in pursuing sophisticated biological work. For example, LLMs can be trained on using the scientific literature about which genes in plants confer resistance to fungal infection and subsequent aflatoxin production. Even more practically, AI can be used in the laboratory to evaluate different crop plant strains with different genetic sequences for *A. flavus* infection, and subsequent aflatoxin contamination, to determine which genes or gene clusters might offer better protection without compromising yield. These genes can then be inserted using conventional breeding or transgenic methods to arrive at crops that are high-yielding and also have lower aflatoxin levels.

Gene expression in plants is affected by environmental stressors, which can be classified into abiotic and biotic stress. Fungal infections are a form of biotic stress that can activate genes responsible for stress responses in the plant. Machine learning has been successfully utilized to identify disease resistance genes specifically under fungal infections in plants including rice [36], sugarcane [37], oilseed rape, and coffee [38]. These studies mainly use genome wide SNP and genotype by sequencing datasets to carry out genomic predictions using different model architectures varying from decision tree, Best Linear

Unbiased Prediction (BLUP) models, Recurrent Neural networks to Deep Learning. When these techniques are used, the prediction power of the genomic regions that are responsible for fungal disease resistance was found to be higher compared to traditional methods such as Genome Wide Association Studies (GWAS) [37,39]. Similar approaches can be taken to predict genes responsible for fungal resistance, which then can be used to reduce fungal infections in plants.

6. AI Applications in the Field to Detect and Mitigate Aflatoxins

The occurrence of aflatoxins in crops at harvest is impacted by climate and biogeochemical characteristics of the soil that in turn impact both crops and fungi. For instance, soil characteristics such as carbonate content, saturated hydraulic conductivity, pH, bulk density, and texture, influence soil microbial communities, and determine which species of fungi might dominate in a given soil environment [40,41]. Other factors such as fungal dispersion and growth mechanisms also play a role in the occurrence of aflatoxins in crops in a specific soil. Machine learning models can be used to identify the correlation between multiple weather, soil and fungal characteristics, and aflatoxin occurrence to identify risk factors that lead to aflatoxin occurrence in crops [41]. Such knowledge could help develop agricultural practices and mitigation strategies that eliminate or control the identified risk factors.

In a study conducted in corn fields of Illinois, Castano-Duque et al. (2023) [41] employed a gradient boosting machine (GBM) learning models and a neural network (NN) machine learning model to identify the key geospatial and climate properties that correlate with aflatoxin occurrence in corn. GBM identified temperature and precipitation prior to sowing, as significant influential factors contributing to high aflatoxin contamination. The Aflatoxin-GBM model showed that a higher aflatoxin risk index (ARI) in January, March, July, and November, reflecting faster fungal growth and dispersion rates, led to higher aflatoxin contamination in the southern regions of Illinois. Higher values of corn-specific normalized difference vegetation index (NDVI) in July, reflecting denser corn vegetation, led to lower aflatoxin contamination in Central and Southern Illinois. A similar relationship was also observed by Castano-Duque et al. (2022) [42] by using GBM and Bayesian network (BN) modeling.

Computer vision and pattern recognition are AI methods by which we can train models to recognize images corresponding to aflatoxin risk in the field. Right now, very little can help a farmer other than marketing strategies and filing a crop insurance claim [43], if they detect aflatoxin problems in the field; because by the time aflatoxin problems present themselves in the field, it is too late to apply biocontrol or to plant a different hybrid, or even apply good agricultural practices. Currently existing fungicides, which are effective against Fusaria, do not work against Aspergilli. While this is yet to be applied in the field, it could potentially give farmers a head-start on understanding the need for testing, reporting to the US Department of Agriculture, and filing an insurance claim. This will help in funneling potentially contaminated grain to uses that may not require as stringent an aflatoxin standard (e.g., certain types of animal feeds and industrial uses).

Apart from growth conditions and fungal dispersion dynamics that determine the extent of fungal growth in crops, cropping system variables such as sowing and harvesting time and type of tillage determine the extent of contamination that ensues. Using a Deep Neural Network (DNN) approach, Camardo Leggieri et al. (2021) [44] combined both meteorological and cropping system information collected from the fields of Northern Italy to predict the occurrence of aflatoxins in corn with better accuracy compared to traditional linear regression models.

AI could be utilized to identify the antimicrobial activity of peptides, which could potentially be used as a fungicide during cultivation and food processing. Antimicrobial peptides have become more popular in recent decades as an alternative to antibiotics due to their ability to overcome the resistance mechanisms developed by disease pathogens and their ability to generate multiple physiological outcomes by targeting different intracellular components. In particular, their strong DNA binding affinity and the ability to penetrate cell membranes have been identified as key factors for achieving enhanced therapeutic efficacy. Traditional chemoinformatic approaches used to identify antimicrobial activity are less applicable when screening multiple molecules, as exploring large databases becomes a highly tedious and time-consuming task. Instead, trained deep learning models can rapidly screen millions of molecules at once, identifying the most promising candidates within minutes [45]. Although not directly applied to identify the antifungal activity against Aspergilli, recently a deep learning model called AMPs-Net successfully identified four antimicrobial peptides derived from *E. coli*'s fragmented genome. Out of the four identified peptides, three were tested in vitro and all demonstrated antimicrobial activity [45]. Further, detailed peptide—membrane/ligand interactions of such identified molecules could be elucidated using molecular dynamic simulations to predict their biological activity and pharmacological relevance [45,46].

7. AI Applications in Food Processing to Reduce Aflatoxins

A key approach to reducing the carry-over of aflatoxins during food processing is sorting the harvest to remove seeds and grains infested with *Aspergillus* species, prior to further processing. Fungal infections generally lead to alterations in the color and appearance of nuts, seeds, and grains, enabling their detection through image processing techniques coupled with AI. In a study conducted with peanuts, Ziyaee et al. (2021) [21] employed three different machine learning tools: ANN, SVM, and adaptive neuro-fuzzy inference system (ANFIS) to detect the presence of *Aspergillus flavus* in images of peanuts seeds taken using LED, UV, and fluorescent lights. The results showed that the combination of LED light in a white background with ANN had 99.7% accuracy in detecting fungal growth on peanuts after 72 h from infection. Similarly, UV lights and a black background with ANFIS achieved 99.9% accuracy in detecting fungal growth after 48 h of infection.

In a similar study, Manhando et al. (2021) [47] employed an error-correcting output code (ECOC)-based SVM trained on features extracted using a pre-trained Deep Convolutional Neural Network (DCNN), to detect *Aspergillus flavus* growth in peanuts using images taken by optical coherence tomography. Their model was successful in identifying fungal growth with a promising accuracy on both the training and testing datasets.

In addition to direct imaging of the infested sample, color changes that take place in colorimetric sensor arrays as a result of mold growth, can also be coupled with AI to detect *Aspergillus* presence in peanuts. For instance, Zhu et al. (2022) [48] used the color changes resulting from the reaction between moldy peanut powder and a colorimetric sensor, to train a support vector regression (SVR) quantitative analysis model that detects AFB1 in peanuts with strong specificity.

Spectral approaches such as fluorescence spectroscopy, and hyperspectral imaging have shown promising results in detecting aflatoxins in food products, due to the fluorescence characteristics of aflatoxins under ultraviolet light [24,49]. However, the multitude of chemical compounds in food matrices can produce autofluorescence, contributing to artifacts in results. Therefore, these approaches require optimization of data acquisition conditions and utilization of suitable chemometric models to analyze results. Machine learning algorithms such as deep neural networks, random forest, SVM, and PCA are previously used alongside spectral approaches to detect aflatoxins in almonds [24], peanuts [27,29,49,50], and figs [51]. Deep learning approaches have shown better performance compared to traditional models such as neural network, random forest and SVM, when detecting aflatoxin contamination using spectral images [29].

In addition to AI-aided detection of aflatoxin for quality control of materials, machine learning could potentially be used to design composite mycotoxin detoxifiers (MDT). MDTs are food or feed additives that form bulky-non absorbable complexes with mycotoxins in the gastrointestinal tract, thereby reducing the absorbability and the bio availability of the toxin. They can also reduce the toxicity of the chemical by promoting their degradation into non-toxic metabolites by the use of bio-transforming agents such as bacteria and enzymes [52]. Development of MDTs on a large scale requires the integration of seemingly conflicting research and development strategies such as computational screening of a large number of materials for their performance and compatibility, high-throughput synthesis and characterization of the material and testing using living animals.

Alternatively, machine learning models can incorporate data obtained from material characterization, mycotoxin assessment and in vitro absorption experiments to identify suitable MDTs for a single or an array of mycotoxins. Using this approach Lo Dico et al. (2022) [52] searched the material space for possible material formulations with high removal capacity of several food toxins including AFB1, while gaining insight into their modes of action. They observed optimum detoxifying performance in a clay composite material consisting of epiolite, montmorillonite, and activated carbon. This builds upon the body of work conducted by Phillips et al. (2019) [53] over decades, on clays that can bind aflatoxin in the intestinal tracts of livestock and humans to allow excretion rather than systemic absorption.

8. AI Applications in Understanding Toxicology of Aflatoxins: Whether and How It Affects Child Growth Impairment, Immune System Dysfunction, and Other Diseases and Conditions

It has been known for over 60 years that aflatoxin causes liver cancer, but all the other health effects that have been associated with aflatoxin exposure have a lower weight of evidence, due to a combination of fewer years of research and yet-undetermined mechanisms of toxicity (and thereby unclear associations). Reviewing all the existing literature to evaluate the weight of evidence linking aflatoxin exposure to different health outcomes is a formidable task.

To this end, LLM that effectively and efficiently extracts crucial information from publications on aflatoxin-related health risks, may enable rapid assessment of the weight of evidence linking aflatoxin exposure to the health endpoints in question (e.g., immunological effects, neurological effects, growth stunting). Although LLMs have not yet been used in assessing aflatoxin's health effects, attempts are currently underway to fine-tune existing Generative Pre-trained Transformer (GPT) models to extract data for chemical risk assessment [54]. While currently available GPT models are increasingly used for general text search and data extraction, model performance decreases as the task becomes more complex and specific. In a case study conducted on bisphenol A (BPA), a GPT3-model (*Curie* base model) was refined using language tokens of 78 publications to answer an array structured questions on the toxicity of the chemical. The fine-tuned model demonstrated markedly better performance than the currently available LLM model used for comparison in the study, suggesting that proper prompt engineering is essential for successful use of LLMs [54].

Complex metabolic pathways that lead to toxin-induced cellular alterations could potentially be modeled using machine learning. One such pathway by which mycotoxins cause cellular damage is lipid peroxidation. For example, in Galvez-Llompart et al.

(2023) [22], a machine learning quantitative structure–activity relationship (QSAR) model was employed to predict the lipid peroxidation activity of an array of mycotoxins. QSAR models use molecular descriptors, that is, numerical representations of a molecule's chemical structure that can capture features such as atom type, shape, and connectivity to predict its ability to induce lipid oxidation. Using an ANN and a linear discriminant analysis approach, the study was able to classify the lipid peroxidation activity of 70 mycotoxins with 88% accuracy.

9. Biotechnology Applications in Plant Breeding to Reduce Aflatoxin Occurrence

Transgenic crop technology has enabled the development of crop lines that are resistant to fungal growth, and more recently by directly targeting invading fungi. For instance, Bt corn, which was first developed to confer insect pest control, has significantly less insect damage on its kernels. As kernel wounds allow fungal spores to invade, reduction in insect damage results in reduced mycotoxin occurrence in corn kernels. One of the first commercial applications of transgenic crop technology was the development of Bt corn that contains transgenes from the soil bacterium *Bacillus thuringiensis* that enable the production of crystal proteins, toxic to certain insect pests that reduce corn yield [55]. As kernel wounds caused by insect damage allow fungal spores to invade, reduction in insect damage results in reduced mycotoxin occurrence in corn kernels. Shortly after Bt corn was first commercialized in the US, it was found to have lower *Fusarium verticillioides* infection because of lower insect pest damage, and thereby lower contamination of the mycotoxin fumonisin [56], which has been implicated in neural tube defects and esophageal cancer [57]. More recently, in a study of corn growers' insurance claims, Bt corn planting was also found to result in lower aflatoxin levels [58]. Newer Bt corn varieties that contain insecticidal proteins in particular, provide significantly improved resistance to the insects such as corn earworm (*Helicoverpa zea*) and fall armyworm (*Spodoptera frugiperda*) that make corn susceptible to aflatoxin accumulation [59]. A recent meta-analysis of the impact of genetically engineered corn suggested that genetically engineered maize results in a 28.8–36.5% reduction in mycotoxin levels [60].

More recent advancements in transgenic corn have been successful in going beyond insect pest control to impart antifungal activity, thereby directly reducing mycotoxin levels in the crop. In particular, transgenic corn expressing the synthetic peptide AGM182 has successfully reduced fungal growth in seeds resulting in a 79–98% reduction in aflatoxin levels [61]. Similarly, transgenic corn transformed using a gene from *Lablab purpureus* beans have successfully expressed α-amylase inhibitor-like protein (AILP) that effectively inhibits α-amylase activity in *A. flavus*, resulting in a 35–72% reduction in *A. flavus* growth [62]. In addition to expressing proteins that can inhibit enzymes necessary for fungal growth, transgenic corn could be developed to express enzymes that chemically degrade aflatoxins present in corn kernels. A recent example is the development of three transgenic maize lines that were modified to express an aflatoxin-degrading enzyme isolated from the edible Honey mushroom *Armillariella tabescens* [63].

Another approach to developing transgenic crops that may inhibit fungal infections is the use of RNA interference (RNAi) in corn. To control aflatoxin occurrence, RNAi corn could enable host-induced gene silencing (HIGS) where the corn plant silences genes in the well-defined aflatoxin biosynthesis pathway of *Aspargillus* [64], allowing the fungi to colonize the corn kernel without producing the toxin [1]. In this approach, the corn plant is modified to produce double-stranded RNA (dsRNA) molecules that correspond to essential genes in the fungal aflatoxin biosynthetic pathway, such as *aflR*, *aflS*, and *omtA*. When *Aspergillus* infects the corn kernel, these dsRNAs are absorbed by the fungus and processed into small interfering RNAs (siRNAs), which guide the degradation of complementary fungal RNAs. This silences the targeted genes, disrupting the expression of enzymes and regulatory proteins necessary for aflatoxin biosynthesis [65].

Maize plants modified with a kernel-specific RNAi gene cassette targeting the *aflC* gene, which encodes an enzyme in the *Aspergillus* aflatoxin biosynthetic pathway, have been successful in stopping aflatoxin occurrence in kernels after pathogen infection [65]. Under similar conditions, transgenic corn with the modified aflC gene did not produce detectable levels of aflatoxin, whereas the non-transgenic control kernels produced toxin levels reaching thousand parts per billion. However, no differences were observed between transcripts from developing aflatoxin-free transgenic kernels and those from non-transgenic kernels [65]. Similarly, a corn variety modified to express an RNAi construct targeting the *A. flavus* alpha-amylase gene *amy1*, has been successful in reducing *amy1* gene expression thereby reducing fungal colonization and aflatoxin accumulation in kernels [66]. Development of a maize variety incorporated with an RNAi vector containing a portion of the *A. flavus* Alkaline protease (alk) gene has resulted in an 87% reduction in both *A. flavus* growth and aflatoxin accumulation under laboratory conditions [32]. In field conditions, corn incorporated with an RNAi vector containing a portion of the *aflM* gene that targets versicolorin dehydrogenase, a key enzyme involved in the aflatoxin biosynthetic pathway, reduced aflatoxin presence in kernels by up to 60% compared to the non-transgenic samples when planted in the field and allowed to self-pollinated by hand [67].

As opposed to transgenic crops, which are produced by artificially inserting an exogenous DNA stretch into a plant genome, usually from a foreign species to achieve a desired trait, CRISPR can achieve desired attributes by precisely editing the host's DNA itself. While CRISPR has not been used directly for aflatoxin reduction in crops, recent advances in this technology may prove useful to reduce aflatoxins in crops. For instance, a CRISPR/Cas system was successfully used to delete large genomic fragments in polykaryotic fungi that blocked the production of the mycotoxin citrinin, produced by the fungus species *Monascus purpureus*, which contaminates Monascus Red food pigment [68]. In vitro reconstituted CRISPR-Cas9 has successfully been used to induce targeted gene deletions in *Penicillium polonicum*, that disabled production of verrucosidin, a mycotoxin commonly found in food such as fresh and cured meat, nuts, and some fruits [69].

These examples demonstrate the potential of using CRISPR technology to lower the risk of aflatoxin contamination in corn by targeting and disrupting the biosynthetic pathways responsible for toxins formation, or by modifying host traits that make corn susceptible to fungal infection. These traits may involve genes related to heat tolerance, drought resistance, and defense against insect pests. Although such characteristics are often controlled by multiple genes, advances in multiplex CRISPR and other gene editing tools may soon enable effective modifications to achieve desired phenotypic traits [1].

Machine learning and genomic prediction models could potentially be coupled with biotechnology to assist researchers in identifying genomic regions associated with aflatoxin resistance in crops. By analyzing large datasets of genetic markers and phenotypic traits, these models detect patterns and estimate the contribution of specific loci to resistance. The identified genomic regions can then be cross-referenced with GWAS or functional annotations to pinpoint candidate genes for further modification or incorporation into resistance breeding programs.

10. Biotechnology Applications to Enhance Aflatoxin Detection in Food and Feed

CRISPR is increasingly used to develop biosensors that detect aflatoxins in food. Since aflatoxins are small, non-nucleic acid molecules, CRISPR cannot detect them directly.

However, biosensors may be developed via indirect strategies that convert aflatoxins into a specific DNA-based signal identifiable by CRISPR technology.

One indirect strategy is using an aptamer—activator complex; a composite molecule made by coupling an aptamer (a synthetic DNA or RNA molecule with a specific 3D structure that binds to a target analyte) to an activator protein. In the presence of aflatoxin, the aptamer binds to it, while the activator triggers the activation of the CRISPR-Cas system. Depending on the design, the CRISPR-Cas system performs its diagnostic function, which is typically the collateral cleavage of a reporter molecule (generally a fluorescently labeled ssDNA or ssRNA), which generate a signal upon cleavage. This approach was successfully used by Zhu and Zhao (2024) [70] who developed a dual functional DNA probe by linking an AFB1 aptamer with Cas12a activator. They prepared the diagnostic probe by linking the AFB1 aptamer—A32 and the acDNA of Cas12a (activator) via a poly-thymine (poly-T) space sequence (A32-acDNA). A reporter system was separately prepared as a solution containing a ribonucleoprotein complex (RNP) and fluorescently labeled T10 reporter. For detection, a sample containing AFB1 should be mixed with the probe to facilitate the preferential binding between the probe and AFB1. Then the binding solution is applied on a microplate coated with bovine serum albumin (BSA)-AFB1 conjugates, where free unbound probes are captured on the microplate by the high binding affinity between A32 aptamers and AFB1 conjugates on the microplate. The microplate containing the attached probes is then incubated in the reporter solution, where acDNA region interacts with RNP complex, leading to the cleavage of the fluorescently labeled reporters and the production of fluorescence signal. With the increase in AFB1 in the tested sample, more A32-acDNA probes binds to the free AFB1, reducing the quantities captured by BSA-AFB1 on the microplate. This results in a concentration dependent reduction in the fluorescent signal when immersed in the reporter solution, facilitating AFB1 quantification [70].

Another, novel fluorescence biosensor was constructed with CRISPR/Cas12 by intergrading MXenes-Ti_3C_2Tx, a novel two-dimensional metal carbide with a surface rich in –OH, –F, and –O groups, which can easily interact with biomolecules in the CRISPR/Cas12 system. The biosensor had a detection range from 0.001 to 80 ng mL^{-1}, with a detection limit of 0.92 pg mL^{-1}, and the ability to detect within 80 min. It demonstrated excellent detection performance in real peanut samples [71]. Similarly, a multimodal sensor with detection limits of 0.85, 0.79, and 1.65 pg mL^{-1} was constructed by a CRISPR/Cas12a system consisting of tetramethylbenzidine as a colorimetric agent for visual detection of AFB1 [72].

Nano particle technology often is coupled with CRISPR-Cas systems to enhance the sensitivity of the biosensors. In a recent study, activator strands were introduced to initiate the *trans*-cleavage of CRISPR/Cas12a for cutting the nanoparticles-tagged-magnetic beads, which were transduced to nanoparticle count signals measurable by single-particle mode inductively coupled plasma mass spectrometry (Sp-ICPMS) [73]. In another study [74], a surface-enhanced Ramen Spectroscopy (SERS) platform was developed by combining CRISPR/Cas12 and nano particle technology. SERS is increasingly used for diagnostics purposes; however, the beacon molecules used for SERS detection often overlap with the signal of biological samples, disturbing the target signal. In an attempt to resolve this problem, Zhang et al. (2023) [74] synthesized a sensor consisting of nano particles embedded with the dye molecule, Prussian blue, which is released and gives a signal in the Ramen silent region, enabling interference free detection when coupled with the CRISPR/Cas 12 system. Visual detection of AFB1 was accomplished by Chen et al. (2023) [75] who used multiple isothermal amplifications coupled with CRISPR/Cas14a. This technique utilized composite nanoprobes comprising magnetic nanoparticles and gold nanoparticles. AFB1 was efficiently identified through an aptamer competition process where the activation of CRISPR/Cas14a in the presence of AFB1 triggers the cleavage of composite nano probes and nano particle release, resulting in significant changes in both color and colorimetric signal.

11. Case Study in AI and Biotechnology to Reduce Aflatoxin from Farm to Fork

The previous discussion demonstrates how one or a number of combined potential strategies could be deployed—with a consideration for cost—to reduce aflatoxin risk at different points in the food supply chain. Below is a hypothetical scenario of how a suite of AI- and biotechnology-informed strategies, could be applied to corn, a key crop frequently contaminated with aflatoxin worldwide.

First, the development of corn varieties that are more resistant to *A. flavus* infection and subsequent aflatoxin production without compromising yield may benefit from high-throughput screening of genes and gene clusters not just in existing corn varieties, but in other species that provide these desired qualities. These may aid in breeding—through either conventional or transgenic methods—corn varieties that are better able to resist aflatoxin while still providing high yields. To date, it has been a challenge to find fungal-resistant varieties of crops that do not also suffer from compromised yield. AI may aid crop breeders in finding the right gene or combination of genes across multiple existing landraces (traditional varieties) and hybrids of corn that have both acceptable yield performance and a greater ability to resist *A. flavus* infection and subsequent aflatoxin production.

Additionally, biotech corn varieties, such as described above, can resist insect damage that predisposes the corn to fungal infection (transgenic Bt corn) or in the future, can degrade aflatoxin in the kernels to reduce human and animal exposures.

Machine learning may be applied to historical data of both climatic conditions (daily temperatures, relative humidity, precipitation, and soil moistures) and real-time images of corn throughout growth stages, to identify and be trained on conditions that result in high aflatoxin risk. For example, there might be a visual cue that human eyes have missed or cannot easily discern in a large corn field (discoloration, spotting, etc.), which indicates that an aflatoxin problem may occur; (i.e., detected by computer vision and pattern recognition enabled by machine learning, that is not evident to the human eye). Then new biotechnological methods of developing peptides that are specifically antifungal to *Aspergillus* could be applied to the corn (unlike biocontrol, it could be applied early in fungal infection and not at the very start of the growing season).

In postharvest conditions, AI combined with biotechnology could be used to reduce aflatoxin risk. Currently, when harvested corn is taken to a grain elevator, aflatoxin measurements are frequently inaccurate. Aflatoxin can concentrate in a very small segment of an entire consignment: in one or a few kernels, or in a "hot spot" in a bin [76]. This is the main source of sampling error: what has traditionally made sampling for aflatoxin analysis difficult. If the elevator operator happens to take an analytical sample that either has a much higher or lower aflatoxin concentration than the rest of the lot on average, it is an inaccurate measure of the actual aflatoxin in that bin. One method of dealing with this currently is for the farmer to request an appeal sample if the analytical sample showed excessively high aflatoxin levels for market purposes [77]; but overall, this practice biases analyses to lower aflatoxin levels than that may exist. A combination of AI and biotechnology, through computer vision and heat maps for aflatoxin detection, could allow farmers to find the hot spots of aflatoxin in their bins; allowing the them to remove or separate the contaminated portion for destruction or for sale in a market that allows higher aflatoxin levels (e.g., ethanol or other industrial production).

If, despite all control efforts, aflatoxin nonetheless finds its way into human diets, more solutions may be possible using biotechnologies to reduce risks to human health. As described earlier, certain compounds in *Brassica* and *Allium* vegetables are bio-transformed in human digestion to induce Phase 2 enzymes that help detoxify aflatoxin. Conceivably, these compounds or their metabolites (sulforaphane, allicin) could be engineered into corn so that the corn could produce these compounds as well. Then even if aflatoxin is present, its harmful effects could be partially ameliorated in the diet, if *Brassica* and *Allium* vegetables are not easily available.

12. Discussion

It is an exciting time for new technologies, particularly as they converge and become more available and accessible to diverse stakeholder groups, including the general public. There is no reason that these new technologies could not be used in agriculture to solve global, millennia-old societal problems, including those surrounding foodborne mycotoxins. In particular, aflatoxin—the most widely recognized mycotoxin because of its toxicity, carcinogenicity, and prevalence in foods worldwide—has continued to cause economic, and human and animal health risks in some of the most vulnerable parts of the world. While a number of control strategies have been developed, the implementation and success of these has varied widely worldwide.

Now AI and biotechnology have both matured to a level that allows not just companies, but the general public, to access them to a higher degree than ever before. In this paper, we have described how these technologies can be used from farm to fork to reduce aflatoxin risk, to a degree that is likely to substantially reduce it so that human and animal health can be protected from its serious effects. In particular, what these technologies offer is a level of precision and accuracy in relatively quick time that previously would have taken an extremely long time, and large amounts of resources, to achieve. The benefit is that solutions emerging from these technologies could be deployed anywhere in the world.

Nonetheless, barring a few field trials [41,44] that have utilized AI to identify geospatial, climatic, and cropping system variables contributing to aflatoxin occurrence, most AI technologies currently under investigation have yet to be implemented on a large scale in real-world settings. Even the studies reviewed in this work are largely concentrated in developed countries such as those in Europe and the United States. Research efforts in developing regions—including Asia, Africa, and Latin America, where aflatoxin prevalence is particularly high—remain scarce. Significant progress is still needed in customizing and training LLMs which is still at the preliminary stage of being used in toxicology, to extract and analyze data from the existing literature to predict metabolic pathways through which aflatoxins induce cellular damage, assess toxicity, and perform automated risk analyses to identify diseases associated with aflatoxin exposure.

One of the primary challenges limiting AI application in aflatoxin control is the need for extensive, high-quality, and well-labeled datasets to train reliable models. Acquiring such datasets requires substantial human expertise and financial resources, both of which are often limited in developing nations. AI for aflatoxin detection may falter in the field due to poor cross-region transfer (different climates, cultivars, storage, and *Aspergillus* species) and sensor drift or inconsistent calibration that distorts the results. Additionally, the high initial investment required to deploy AI-based technologies such as computer vision systems and spectrometric approaches in agricultural fields serves as a deterrent for many traditional farmers.

Similarly, biotechnology-based tools such as CRISPR-enabled biosensors remain at the bench-scale stage and involve several labor-intensive steps before results can be obtained.

Considerable research is still required to scale up these technologies and develop user-friendly, in situ devices suitable for diverse farming and food processing environments.

Beyond scaling challenges, we identify two short-term research directions that could advance the integration of AI and biotechnology for aflatoxin control. The first is a quantitative comparison of the accuracy, reproducibility of computer vision and machine learning–assisted detection approaches against conventional detection techniques such as ELISA and liquid chromatography–tandem mass spectrometry (LC-MS/MS). Such a study coupled with a cost benefit analysis would assess the feasibility of employing these technologies on a large scale. The second is a quantitative feasibility assessment of the proposed case study of integrating of AI and biotechnology across the corn supply chain, using data from both the existing literature and future field trials.

These potential solutions and directions described above, however, are highly dependent on nations' and communities' acceptance of AI and biotechnologies. Over the last decade, several nations that have had recorded problems of aflatoxin have commercialized transgenic Bt corn that can help to reduce this problem, such as Kenya (https://www.isaaa.org/gmapprovaldatabase/ (accessed on 7 September 2025)). But notably, Bt corn has already been commercialized in other nations for nearly 30 years. It is likely that any further biotech crop application approvals would take considerably longer. By contrast, AI regulation at a national level has been relatively lacking worldwide. Despite legitimate ethical and moral considerations, which regulators and the industry are actively managing, AI and biotechnology present a timely avenue to mitigate aflatoxin contamination and associated public-health risks. We encourage further research in these areas to combat the millennia-old problem of aflatoxin, to ensure a safer food supply worldwide.

Author Contributions: Conceptualization, F.W.; investigation, F.W. and C.J.G.; resources, F.W.; writing—original draft preparation, F.W. and C.J.G.; writing—review and editing, F.W.; visualization, C.J.G.; supervision, F.W. All authors have read and agreed to the published version of the manuscript.

Funding: This research received no external funding.

Data Availability Statement: The original contributions presented in this study are included in the article. Further inquiries can be directed to the corresponding author.

Conflicts of Interest: The authors declare no conflicts of interest.

References

1. Wu, F. Mycotoxin risks are lower in biotech corn. *Curr. Opin. Biotechnol.* **2022**, *78*, 102792. [CrossRef] [PubMed]
2. Kensler, T.W.; Roebuck, B.D.; Wogan, G.N.; Groopman, J.D. Aflatoxin: A 50-Year Odyssey of Mechanistic and Translational Toxicology. *Toxicol. Sci.* **2011**, *120*, S28–S48. [CrossRef] [PubMed]
3. IARC. International Agency for Research on Cancer (IARC)—Monographs on the Evaluation of Carcinogenic Risks to Humans: Some Naturally Occurring Substances: Food Items and Constituents, Heterocyclic Aromatic Amines and Myco-toxins.No 50, IARC, Lyon, France: 1993. Available online: https://publications.iarc.who.int/Book-And-Report-Series/Iarc-Monographs-On-The-Identification-Of-Carcinogenic-Hazards-To-Humans/Some-Naturally-Occurring-Substances-Food-Items-And-Constituents-Heterocyclic-Aromatic-Amines-And-Mycotoxins-1993 (accessed on 7 September 2025).
4. Qian, G.S.; Ross, R.K.; Yu, M.C.; Yuan, J.M.; Gao, Y.T.; Henderson, B.E.; Wogan, G.N.; Groopman, J.D. A follow-up study of urinary markers of aflatoxin exposure and liver cancer risk in Shanghai, People's Republic of China. *Cancer Epidemiol. Biomark. Prev.* **1994**, *3*, 3–10.
5. JECFA (Joint FAO/WHO Expert Committee on Food Additives). Safety evaluation of certain food additives and con-taminants, WHO Food Additives Series 40, Aflatoxins. In Proceedings of the The Forty-Ninth Meeting of the Joint FAO/WHO Expert Committee on Food Additives, Rome, Italy, 17–26 June 1997; World Health Organization: Geneva, Switzerland, 1998.
6. Liu, Y.; Chang, C.-C.H.; Marsh, G.M.; Wu, F. Population attributable risk of aflatoxin-related liver cancer: Systematic review and meta-analysis. *Eur. J. Cancer* **2012**, *48*, 2125–2136. [CrossRef]
7. Do, J.H.; Choi, D.-K. Aflatoxins: Detection, toxicity, and biosynthesis. *Biotechnol. Bioprocess Eng.* **2007**, *12*, 585–593. [CrossRef]

8. Rushing, B.R.; Selim, M.I. Aflatoxin B1: A review on metabolism, toxicity, occurrence in food, occupational exposure, and detoxification methods. *Food Chem. Toxicol.* **2019**, *124*, 81–100. [CrossRef] [PubMed]
9. Groopman, J.D.; Johnson, D.; Kensler, T.W. Aflatoxin and hepatitis B virus biomarkers: A paradigm for complex environmental exposures and cancer risk. *Cancer Biomarkers* **2005**, *1*, 5–14. [CrossRef]
10. Benkerroum, N. Chronic and Acute Toxicities of Aflatoxins: Mechanisms of Action. *Int. J. Environ. Res. Public Heal.* **2020**, *17*, 423. [CrossRef]
11. Liu, Y.; Wu, F. Global Burden of Aflatoxin-Induced Hepatocellular Carcinoma: A Risk Assessment. *Environ. Heal. Perspect.* **2010**, *118*, 818–824. [CrossRef]
12. Wu, F.; Stacy, S.L.; Kensler, T.W. Global Risk Assessment of Aflatoxins in Maize and Peanuts: Are Regulatory Standards Adequately Protective? *Toxicol. Sci.* **2013**, *135*, 251–259. [CrossRef]
13. Khlangwiset, P.; Wu, F. Costs and efficacy of public health interventions to reduce aflatoxin-induced human disease. *Food Addit. Contam. Part A* **2010**, *27*, 998–1014. [CrossRef]
14. Wu, F.; Khlangwiset, P. Evaluating the technical feasibility of aflatoxin risk reduction strategies in Africa. *Food Addit. Contam. Part A* **2010**, *27*, 658–686. [CrossRef]
15. Kensler, T.W.; Chen, J.-G.; Egner, P.A.; Fahey, J.W.; Jacobson, L.P.; Stephenson, K.K.; Ye, L.; Coady, J.L.; Wang, J.-B.; Wu, Y.; et al. Effects of Glucosinolate-Rich Broccoli Sprouts on Urinary Levels of Aflatoxin-DNA Adducts and Phenanthrene Tetraols in a Randomized Clinical Trial in He Zuo Township, Qidong, People's Republic of China. *Cancer Epidemiol. Biomark. Prev.* **2005**, *14*, 2605–2613. [CrossRef]
16. Ben Ayed, R.; Hanana, M. Artificial Intelligence to Improve the Food and Agriculture Sector. *J. Food Qual.* **2021**, *2021*, 1–7. [CrossRef]
17. Patel, G.S.; Rai, A.; Das, N.N.; Singh, R. *Smart Agriculture: Emerging Pedagogies of Deep Learning, Machine Learning and Internet of Things*; CRC Press: Boca Raton, FL, USA, 2021.
18. Singhal, R.; Izquierdo, P.; Ranaweera, T.; Abá, K.S.; Brown, B.N.; Lehti-Shiu, M.D.; Shiu, S.-H. Using supervised machine-learning approaches to understand abiotic stress tolerance and design resilient crops. *Philos. Trans. R. Soc. B: Biol. Sci.* **2025**, *380*, 20240252. [CrossRef]
19. Esmaeily, R.; Razavi, M.A.; Razavi, S.H. A step forward in food science, technology and industry using artificial intelligence. *Trends Food Sci. Technol.* **2023**, *143*, 104286. [CrossRef]
20. Zou, J.; Han, Y.; So, S.-S. Overview of artificial neural networks. In *Artificial Neural Networks: Methods Applications*; Springer: Berlin/Heidelberg, Germany, 2009; pp. 14–22.
21. Ziyaee, P.; Ahmadi, V.F.; Bazyar, P.; Cavallo, E. Comparison of Different Image Processing Methods for Segregation of Peanut (*Arachis hypogaea* L.) Seeds Infected by Aflatoxin-Producing Fungi. *Agronomy* **2021**, *11*, 873. [CrossRef]
22. Galvez-Llompart, M.; Zanni, R.; Manyes, L.; Meca, G. Elucidating the mechanism of action of mycotoxins through machine learning-driven QSAR models: Focus on lipid peroxidation. *Food Chem. Toxicol.* **2023**, *182*, 114120. [CrossRef] [PubMed]
23. Ferath, K.; Adeliya, L. Chapter 12—Principal component analysis. In *Machine Learning*; Mechelli, A., Vieira, S., Eds.; Academic Press: Cambridge, MA, USA, 2020.
24. Bertani, F.R.; Mencattini, A.; Gambacorta, L.; De Ninno, A.; Businaro, L.; Solfrizzo, M.; Gerardino, A.; Martinelli, E. Aflatoxins detection in almonds via fluorescence imaging and deep neural network approach. *J. Food Compos. Anal.* **2023**, *125*, 105850. [CrossRef]
25. IBM. (2023). What Are Support Vector Machines (SVMs)? Available online: https://www.ibm.com/think/topics/support-vector-machine (accessed on 7 September 2025).
26. Liakos, K.G.; Busato, P.; Moshou, D.; Pearson, S.; Bochtis, D. Machine learning in agriculture: A review. *Sensors* **2018**, *18*, 2674. [CrossRef]
27. Kabir, M.A.; Lee, I.; Mishra, G.; Panda, B.K.; Singh, C.B.; Lee, S.-H. Classification of Aflatoxin B1 Contamination Level Using Hyperspectral Images with Random Forest and QDA. In Proceedings of the 2024 IEEE/ACIS 9th International Conference on Big Data, Cloud Computing, and Data Science (BCD), Kitakyushu, Japan, 16–18 July 2024.
28. Kamilaris, A.; Prenafeta-Boldú, F.X. Deep learning in agriculture: A survey. *Comput. Electron. Agric.* **2018**, *147*, 70–90. [CrossRef]
29. Han, Z.; Gao, J. Pixel-level aflatoxin detecting based on deep learning and hyperspectral imaging. *Comput. Electron. Agric.* **2019**, *164*, 104888. [CrossRef]
30. Berg, P. Meetings that changed the world: Asilomar 1975: DNA modification secured. *Nature* **2008**, *455*, 290–291. [CrossRef] [PubMed]
31. Chemla, Y.; Sweeney, C.J.; Wozniak, C.A.; Voigt, C.A. Design and regulation of engineered bacteria for environmental release. *Nat. Microbiol.* **2025**, *10*, 281–300. [CrossRef]
32. Omolehin, O.; Raruang, Y.; Hu, D.; Han, Z.-Q.; Wei, Q.; Wang, K.; Rajasekaran, K.; Cary, J.W.; Chen, Z.-Y. Resistance to Aflatoxin Accumulation in Maize Mediated by Host-Induced Silencing of the *Aspergillus flavus* Alkaline Protease (*alk*) Gene. *J. Fungi* **2021**, *7*, 904. [CrossRef]

33. Hille, F.; Charpentier, E. CRISPR-Cas: Biology, mechanisms and relevance. *Philos. Trans. R. Soc. B: Biol. Sci.* **2016**, *371*, 20150496. [CrossRef] [PubMed]
34. Jiang, F.; Doudna, J.A. CRISPR–Cas9 structures and mechanisms. *Annu. Rev. Biophys.* **2017**, *46*, 505–529. [CrossRef]
35. Aman, R.; Mahas, A.; Mahfouz, M. Nucleic Acid Detection Using CRISPR/Cas Biosensing Technologies. *ACS Synth. Biol.* **2020**, *9*, 1226–1233. [CrossRef] [PubMed]
36. Liu, Q.; Zuo, S.-M.; Peng, S.; Zhang, H.; Peng, Y.; Li, W.; Xiong, Y.; Lin, R.; Feng, Z.; Li, H.; et al. Development of Machine Learning Methods for Accurate Prediction of Plant Disease Resistance. *Engineering* **2024**, *40*, 100–110. [CrossRef]
37. Aono, A.H.; Costa, E.A.; Rody, H.V.S.; Nagai, J.S.; Pimenta, R.J.G.; Mancini, M.C.; dos Santos, F.R.C.; Pinto, L.R.; Landell, M.G.d.A.; de Souza, A.P.; et al. Machine learning approaches reveal genomic regions associated with sugarcane brown rust resistance. *Sci. Rep.* **2020**, *10*, 1–16. [CrossRef]
38. de Sousa, I.C.; Nascimento, M.; Silva, G.N.; Nascimento, A.C.C.; Cruz, C.D.; e Silva, F.F.; de Almeida, D.P.; Pestana, K.N.; Azevedo, C.F.; Zambolim, L.; et al. Genomic prediction of leaf rust resistance to Arabica coffee using machine learning algorithms. *Sci. Agricola* **2021**, *78*, e20200021. [CrossRef]
39. Wang, X.-Y.; Ren, C.-X.; Fan, Q.-W.; Xu, Y.-P.; Wang, L.-W.; Mao, Z.-L.; Cai, X.-Z. Integrated Assays of Genome-Wide Association Study, Multi-Omics Co-Localization, and Machine Learning Associated Calcium Signaling Genes with Oilseed Rape Resistance to *Sclerotinia sclerotiorum*. *Int. J. Mol. Sci.* **2024**, *25*, 6932. [CrossRef]
40. Brady, N.C.; Weil, R.R.; Weil, R.R. *The Nature and Properties of Soils*; Prentice Hall: Upper Saddle River, NJ, USA, 2008; Volume 13.
41. Castano-Duque, L.; Winzeler, E.; Blackstock, J.M.; Liu, C.; Vergopolan, N.; Focker, M.; Barnett, K.; Owens, P.R.; van der Fels-Klerx, H.J.; Vaughan, M.M.; et al. Dynamic geospatial modeling of mycotoxin contamination of corn in Illinois: Unveiling critical factors and predictive insights with machine learning. *Front. Microbiol.* **2023**, *14*, 1283127. [CrossRef]
42. Wu, F.; Miller, J.D.; Casman, E.A. The economic impact of Bt corn resulting from mycotoxin reduction. *J Toxicol: Toxin Rev.* **2004**, *23*, 397–424. [CrossRef]
43. Yu, J.; Hennessy, D.A.; Tack, J.; Wu, F. The impact of climate change on aflatoxin contamination in US corn. *Environ. Res. Lett.* **2022**, *17*, 054017. [CrossRef]
44. Leggieri, M.C.; Mazzoni, M.; Battilani, P. Machine Learning for Predicting Mycotoxin Occurrence in Maize. *Front. Microbiol.* **2021**, *12*, 661132. [CrossRef]
45. Puentes, P.R.; Henao, M.C.; Cifuentes, J.; Muñoz-Camargo, C.; Reyes, L.H.; Cruz, J.C.; Arbeláez, P. Rational Discovery of Antimicrobial Peptides by Means of Artificial Intelligence. *Membranes* **2022**, *12*, 708. [CrossRef]
46. Puentes, P.R.; Rueda-Gensini, L.; Valderrama, N.; Hernández, I.; González, C.; Daza, L.; Muñoz-Camargo, C.; Cruz, J.C.; Arbeláez, P. Predicting target–ligand interactions with graph convolutional networks for interpretable pharmaceutical discovery. *Sci. Rep.* **2022**, *12*, 1–17. [CrossRef] [PubMed]
47. Manhando, E.; Zhou, Y.; Wang, F. Early Detection of Mold-Contaminated Peanuts Using Machine Learning and Deep Features Based on Optical Coherence Tomography. *Agriengineering* **2021**, *3*, 703–715. [CrossRef]
48. Zhu, C.; Deng, J.; Jiang, H. Parameter Optimization of Support Vector Machine to Improve the Predictive Performance for Determination of Aflatoxin B_1 in Peanuts by Olfactory Visualization Technique. *Molecules* **2022**, *27*, 6730. [CrossRef] [PubMed]
49. Zhongzhi, H.; Limiao, D. Aflatoxin contaminated degree detection by hyperspectral data using band index. *Food Chem. Toxicol.* **2020**, *137*, 111159. [CrossRef]
50. Jiang, J.; Qiao, X.; He, R. Use of Near-Infrared hyperspectral images to identify moldy peanuts. *J. Food Eng.* **2016**, *169*, 284–290. [CrossRef]
51. Cruz-Carrasco, C.; Díaz-Álvarez, J.; Chávez de la O, F.; Sánchez-Venegas, A.; Villegas Cortez, J. Detection of *Aspergillus flavus* in Figs by Means of Hyperspectral Images and Deep Learning Algorithms. *Agriengineering* **2024**, *6*, 3969–3988. [CrossRef]
52. Dico, G.L.; Croubels, S.; Carcelén, V.; Haranczyk, M. Machine learning-aided design of composite mycotoxin detoxifier material for animal feed. *Sci. Rep.* **2022**, *12*, 4838. [CrossRef]
53. Phillips, T.D.; Wang, M.; Elmore, S.E.; Hearon, S.; Wang, J.-S. NovaSil Clay for the Protection of Humans and Animals from Aflatoxins and Other Contaminants. *Clays Clay Miner.* **2019**, *67*, 99–110. [CrossRef] [PubMed]
54. Sonnenburg, A.; van der Lugt, B.; Rehn, J.; Wittkowski, P.; Bech, K.; Padberg, F.; Eleftheriadou, D.; Dobrikov, T.; Bouwmeester, H.; Mereu, C.; et al. Artificial intelligence-based data extraction for next generation risk assessment: Is fine-tuning of a large language model worth the effort? *Toxicology* **2024**, *508*, 153933. [CrossRef] [PubMed]
55. Wu, F. Mycotoxin Reduction in Bt Corn: Potential Economic, Health, and Regulatory Impacts. *Transgenic Res.* **2006**, *15*, 277–289. [CrossRef] [PubMed]
56. Munkvold, G.P.; Hellmich, R.L.; Rice, L.G. Comparison of Fumonisin Concentrations in Kernels of Transgenic Bt Maize Hybrids and Nontransgenic Hybrids. *Plant Dis.* **1999**, *83*, 130–138. [CrossRef]
57. Chen, C.; Riley, R.T.; Wu, F. Dietary Fumonisin and Growth Impairment in Children and Animals: A Review. *Compr. Rev. Food Sci. Food Saf.* **2018**, *17*, 1448–1464. [CrossRef]

58. Yu, J.; Hennessy, D.A.; Wu, F. The Impact of Bt Corn on Aflatoxin-Related Insurance Claims in the United States. *Sci. Rep.* **2020**, *10*, 1–10. [CrossRef]
59. Pruter, L.S.; Brewer, M.J.; A Weaver, M.; Murray, S.C.; Isakeit, T.S.; Bernal, J.S. Association of Insect-Derived Ear Injury with Yield and Aflatoxin of Maize Hybrids Varying in Bt Transgenes. *Environ. Èntomol.* **2019**, *48*, 1401–1411. [CrossRef]
60. Pellegrino, E.; Bedini, S.; Nuti, M.; Ercoli, L. Impact of genetically engineered maize on agronomic, environmental and toxicological traits: A meta-analysis of 21 years of field data. *Sci. Rep.* **2018**, *8*, 3113. [PubMed]
61. Rajasekaran, K.; Sayler, R.J.; Sickler, C.M.; Majumdar, R.; Jaynes, J.M.; Cary, J.W. Control of Aspergillus flavus growth and aflatoxin production in transgenic maize kernels expressing a tachyplesin-derived synthetic peptide, AGM182. *Plant Sci.* **2018**, *270*, 150–156. [CrossRef] [PubMed]
62. Rajasekaran, K.; Sayler, R.J.; Majumdar, R.; Sickler, C.M.; Cary, J.W. Inhibition of Aspergillus flavus growth and aflatoxin production in transgenic maize expressing the α-amylase inhibitor from *Lablab purpureus* L. *J. Vis. Exp.* **2019**, *144*, e59169.
63. Schmidt, M.A.; Mao, Y.; Opoku, J.; Mehl, H.L. Enzymatic degradation is an effective means to reduce aflatoxin contamination in maize. *BMC Biotechnol.* **2021**, *21*, 70. [CrossRef]
64. Bhatnagar, D.; Ehrlich, K.C.; Cleveland, T.E. Molecular genetic analysis and regulation of aflatoxin biosynthesis. *Appl. Microbiol. Biotechnol.* **2003**, *61*, 83–93. [CrossRef]
65. Thakare, D.; Zhang, J.; Wing, R.A.; Cotty, P.J.; Schmidt, M.A. Aflatoxin-free transgenic maize using host-induced gene silencing. *Sci. Adv.* **2017**, *3*, e1602382. [CrossRef]
66. Gilbert, M.K.; Majumdar, R.; Rajasekaran, K.; Chen, Z.-Y.; Wei, Q.; Sickler, C.M.; Lebar, M.D.; Cary, J.W.; Frame, B.R.; Wang, K. RNA interference-based silencing of the alpha-amylase (amy1) gene in Aspergillus flavus decreases fungal growth and aflatoxin production in maize kernels. *Planta* **2018**, *247*, 1465–1473. [CrossRef]
67. Raruang, Y.; Omolehin, O.; Hu, D.; Wei, Q.; Han, Z.-Q.; Rajasekaran, K.; Cary, J.W.; Wang, K.; Chen, Z.-Y. Host Induced Gene Silencing Targeting Aspergillus flavus aflM Reduced Aflatoxin Contamination in Transgenic Maize Under Field Conditions. *Front. Microbiol.* **2020**, *11*, 754. [CrossRef]
68. Liu, W.; An, C.; Shu, X.; Meng, X.; Yao, Y.; Zhang, J.; Chen, F.; Xiang, H.; Yang, S.; Gao, X.; et al. A Dual-Plasmid CRISPR/Cas System for Mycotoxin Elimination in Polykaryotic Industrial Fungi. *ACS Synth. Biol.* **2020**, *9*, 2087–2095. [CrossRef]
69. Valente, S.; Piombo, E.; Schroeckh, V.; Meloni, G.R.; Heinekamp, T.; Brakhage, A.A.; Spadaro, D. CRISPR-Cas9-Based Discovery of the Verrucosidin Biosynthesis Gene Cluster in Penicillium polonicum. *Front. Microbiol.* **2021**, *12*, 660871. [CrossRef]
70. Zhu, F.; Zhao, Q. Competitive aptamer assay for aflatoxin B1 detection using CRISPR/Cas12a as a signal amplifier. *Microchem. J.* **2024**, *207*, 112054. [CrossRef]
71. Wu, Z.; Sun, D.-W.; Pu, H.; Wei, Q. A novel fluorescence biosensor based on CRISPR/Cas12a integrated MXenes for detecting Aflatoxin B1. *Talanta* **2022**, *252*, 123773. [CrossRef]
72. Wu, Z.; Sun, D.-W.; Pu, H. CRISPR/Cas12a and G-quadruplex DNAzyme-driven multimodal biosensor for visual detection of Aflatoxin B1. *Spectrochim. Acta Part A: Mol. Biomol. Spectrosc.* **2023**, *302*, 123121. [CrossRef] [PubMed]
73. Zhang, C.; Zhao, X.; Huang, Z.; Li, Z.; Hu, J.; Liu, R.; Lv, Y. Highly sensitive detection of aflatoxin B1 byCRISPR/Cas12a-assisted single nanoparticle counting. *Food Chem.* **2024**, *443*, 138557. [CrossRef]
74. Zhang, J.; Jiang, L.; Li, H.; Yuan, R.; Yang, X. Construction of a SERS platform for sensitive detection of aflatoxin B1 based on CRISPR strategy. *Food Chem.* **2023**, *415*, 135768. [CrossRef] [PubMed]
75. Chen, J.; Ren, B.; Wang, Z.; Wang, Q.; Bi, J.; Sun, X. Multiple Isothermal Amplification Coupled with CRISPR–Cas14a for the Naked-eye and Colorimetric Detection of Aflatoxin B1. *ACS Appl. Mater. Interfaces* **2023**, *15*, 55423–55432. [CrossRef]
76. Whitaker, T.B.; Johansson, A.S. Sampling Uncertainties for the Detection of Chemical Agents in Complex Food Matrices. *J. Food Prot.* **2005**, *68*, 1306–1313. [CrossRef]
77. Wu, F. A tale of two commodities: How EU mycotoxin regulations have affected u.s. tree nut industries. *World Mycotoxin J.* **2008**, *1*, 95–102. [CrossRef]

toxins MDPI

Review

Fifty Years and Counting: Searching for the "Silver Bullet" or the "Silver Shotgun" to Mitigate Preharvest Aflatoxin Contamination

Baozhu Guo [1,*], Idrice Carther Kue Foka [2], Dongliang Wu [1,3], Josh P. Clevenger [4], Rong Di [2,*] and Jake C. Fountain [5,*]

1 Crop Genetics and Breeding Research Unit, USDA-Agricultural Research Service, Tifton, GA 31793, USA
2 Department of Plant Biology, Rutgers, The State University of New Jersey, New Brunswick, NJ 08901, USA; ik351@sebs.rutgers.edu
3 Department of Plant Pathology, University of Georgia, Tifton, GA 31793, USA; dongliang.wu@uga.edu
4 HudsonAlpha Institute for Biotechnology, Huntsville, AL 35806, USA; jclevenger@hudsonalpha.org
5 Department of Plant Pathology, University of Georgia, Griffin, GA 30223, USA
* Correspondence: baozhu.guo@usda.gov (B.G.); rongdi@sebs.rutgers.edu (R.D.); jfount1@uga.edu (J.C.F.)

Abstract: The year 2025 marks two significant milestones for aflatoxin research: 65 years since aflatoxin was first identified in 1960, and 50 years of focused research on preharvest aflatoxin contamination since it was first recognized in 1975. Studies in the 1970s revealed that *A. flavus* could infect crops like maize and produce aflatoxin in the field before harvest and made it possible to investigate the potential genetic resistance in crops to mitigate the issues. Tremendous efforts have been made to learn about the process and regulation of aflatoxin production along with interactions between *A. flavus* and host plants as influenced by environmental factors. This has allowed for the breeding of more resistant crops and investigations into the underlying genetic and genomic components of resistance mechanisms in crops like maize and peanut. However, despite decades of studies, many questions remain. One established "dogma" is that drought stress, especially when combined with high temperatures, is the single greatest contributing factor to preharvest aflatoxin contamination and is a perennial risk faced throughout the major agricultural production regions of the world. Although there are many reviews summarizing the decades' long wealth of information about *A. flavus*, aflatoxin biosynthesis, management and host plant resistance, there are few reports that put the spotlight on why aflatoxin contamination is exacerbated by drought stress, which places plants under severe physiological stress and weakens immune systems. Therefore, here we will focus on three major areas of research in maize: the "living embryo" theory and host resistance mechanisms, the "Key Largo hypothesis" and the causes of drought-exacerbated aflatoxin contamination, and recent advancements in CRISPR-based genome editing for enhancing drought tolerance and increasing plant immune responses. This will highlight key breakthroughs and future prospects for the continuing development of superior crop germplasm and cultivars and for mitigating aflatoxin contamination in food and feed supply chains.

Keywords: preharvest aflatoxin contamination; "living embryo" theory; "Key Largo" theory; host resistance; drought stress; oxidative stress; reactive oxygen species; ROS; CRISPRa; tissue culture; enhanced immunity; food safety

Key Contribution: This review summarized (i) the "living embryo" theory and host resistance mechanisms in resistant maize germplasm GT-MAS:gk, (ii) the "Key Largo" hypotheses and the causes of drought-exacerbated aflatoxin contamination, and (iii) emerging CRISPR-based strategies for enhancing plant immunity, drought tolerance, and aflatoxin resistance.

1. Introduction

Aspergillus flavus is a ubiquitous saprophytic and opportunistic fungal pathogen infecting, colonizing, and producing aflatoxin in agricultural commodities worldwide [1]. *A. flavus* was described as early as 1809, but the initial discovery of aflatoxin stemmed from the "Turkey X disease" outbreak in England in 1960 [2,3], which was a new, highly fatal disease that struck flocks of young turkeys in England. The disease was characterized by exceptionally high mortality in infected flocks. The cause of the disease remained a mystery for a while, leading to the designation "Turkey X disease". The subsequent identification of the toxin produced by *A. flavus* sparked a new era of aflatoxin research, one of the most potent natural carcinogens ever discovered and causing a range of health issues, including liver damage, immune suppression, and stunted growth in children [4].

Aflatoxin contamination was treated as a post-harvest storage problem until Anderson et al. (1975) reported an extensive 3-year field survey, covering all the corn-producing areas of the United States and sampling from 6 weeks prior to harvest through harvest, and supported pre-harvest aflatoxin contamination occurring by the late milk stage, and the highest rates of incidence were in the warmer and humid growing regions like southern states [5,6]. This 1975 milestone shifted mitigation strategies to intervene before harvest and made it possible to investigate crop-plant genetic resistance and to develop crops that could resist fungal infection and aflatoxin production in the field before harvest. Scully et al. (2008) reported a long-term survey, starting shortly after 1975, covering 45 Georgia counties to monitor the regional severity of aflatoxin contamination in corn before harvest for 28 years [7]. The findings were alarming, with an average of 97 ppb through the 28-year survey, well above the 20 ppb FDA limit [7]. The realization of the urgency and the unique nature of the aflatoxin problem and the need for novel technologies to ameliorate the impact of food safety became a focal point of discussion at the first U.S. Aflatoxin Elimination Workshop held in New Orleans, LA, in 1988. This workshop was held annually as an international forum to assemble scientists and representatives of the different commodities (corn, peanut, tree nuts, and cotton) and industries in a unique cooperative effort to develop aflatoxin control strategies through research and development [8,9]. Since the 1970s, with the dramatically shifted paradigm of managing *A. flavus* and aflatoxin contamination from passive post-harvest prevention to active breeding of resistant crops to fungal infection, research efforts have been focusing on determining the source of host plant resistance to prevent *A. flavus* colonization and subsequent aflatoxin production before harvest [7]. These efforts have employed numerous techniques and approaches, including modern plant breeding and genomic tools such as proteomic, transcriptomic, and biochemical analyses to discover the underlying mechanism of host plant resistance and the interaction between the host crops and the fungus [10]. To date, these efforts have revealed that resistance is quantitatively inherited with a strong genotype-by-environment component [11,12].

In the United States, the Southeastern Regional Aflatoxin Trial (SERAT) was formed under the umbrella of the U.S. Aflatoxin Elimination Workshop in 2003, and its mission is to test and identify public germplasms, inbreds, and hybrids with the most consistent resistance to aflatoxin accumulation and to evaluate their essential agronomic traits in different environments [8,9]. SERAT has been testing 30 to 40 public breeding hybrids for agronomics and aflatoxin accumulation each year since 2003 [13]. The SERAT trials demonstrated that a large portion of aflatoxin susceptibility is genetic (22%; for yield this was 19%) and heritable across very diverse but relevant environments [13,14].

Nonetheless, at this time, there is no "Silver Bullet" having been found for solving the aflatoxin contamination problem in crops before and after harvest, and the "Silver Shotgun" of all available strategies must be applied simultaneously at all stages in the supply chain to ensure a healthy crop, free of aflatoxins [12,15,16]. The most explored method for mitigating aflatoxin contamination is developing and using preharvest host resistance, because *A. flavus* infects and produces aflatoxins in susceptible crops prior to harvest. Another factor, the well-established "dogma", is that drought stress plays a crucial and multi-faceted role in both promoting and suppressing host immune responses against various abiotic and biotic stresses, resulting in exacerbated aflatoxin accumulation [17,18]. It is a complex interaction with a high degree of environmentally induced variability, with abiotic and biotic stress strongly influencing resistance or susceptibility. As early as in 1993, Brown et al. (1993) reported a "living embryo" hypothesis and suggested that a living embryo's metabolic activity in corn is crucial for maintaining the resistance and reducing aflatoxin contamination, as the resistance is lost in "non-living" damaged embryos [19]. Understanding how the viable embryo mediates resistance to aflatoxin accumulation may provide opportunities to modify corn genotypes to support lower levels of contamination, and the "living embryo" theory offers the basis for studies of the resistance mechanism of corn plants [20] in contrast to the newly reported "Key Largo" hypothesis related to investigating the potential role of reactive oxygen species (ROS) in host-drought-*A. flavus* interactions [18,21]. The success in the advancement of genome-editing, like genome-wide knockout and activation as powerful platforms, will play significant roles in research mitigating strategies of aflatoxin contamination. Therefore, this review will focus on three areas of research in maize: the "living embryo" theory and the associated host resistance mechanisms, the "Key Largo" theory and the causes of aflatoxin contamination exacerbated by drought stress, and lastly, leveraging advancements in CRISPR (clustered regularly interspaced short palindromic repeats)-based genome editing, particularly the integration of CRISPR with tissue culture techniques for enhancing drought tolerance and reducing aflatoxin contamination, highlighting key breakthroughs, challenges, and future prospects.

Because of safety concerns of the toxicological content in food and feed, it is an urgent need to search the mitigation strategies to reduce the level or eliminate the contamination in food chain. Aflatoxin B_1 is classified by the International Agency for Research on Cancer (IARC) as a Group 1 human carcinogen and is strongly associated with hepatocellular carcinoma and other adverse health outcomes [22,23]. Consequently, mitigation success must be defined by the ability to meet the maximum residue limits (MRLs) such as the U.S. FDA limit of 20 ppb for food and feed and more stricter European Union limits of 2–4 ppb for human consumption [24], and Codex Alimentarius guidelines for contaminants in food and feed [25]. Therefore, this review puts the spotlight on why aflatoxin contamination is exacerbated by drought stress and the causes of drought-exacerbated aflatoxin contamination to safeguard food and feed supply chains.

2. The "Living Embryo" Theory and Maize Host Resistance Mechanisms, a Case Study of GT-MAS:gk

Broad genetic variation regarding host resistance to aflatoxin accumulation exists across both maize and peanut germplasm. In maize, kernel infection assays and multi-environment trials of diverse inbred lines demonstrate substantial natural resistance, though none exhibit full immunity. Since Zuber et al. (1978) proved resistance to aflatoxin accumulation is a heritable trait in maize [26], many resistant breeding lines have been developed and released. Among the reported resistant germplasm, a maize germplasm GT-MAS:gk was developed and released as resistant to aflatoxin accumulation in Georgia [19,20]. However, Guo et al. (2001) demonstrated the resistance in GT-MAS:gk was still segregating [27], and inbreeding selection was made and tested in the field. Later three inbred lines, GT601, GT602, and GT603 [28,29], were released for public use.

In 1993, Brown et al. first tested GT-MAS:gk and proposed the "living embryo" theory that metabolic activity within the living corn embryo produces compounds that are key to the corn kernel's resistance to aflatoxin contamination [19], which laid the groundwork for study of causal genes, proteins, and metabolites [30]. This theory is supported by evidence that resistance diminishes when the embryo is killed, wounded, or removed, as reported by Guo (1995), who investigated the mechanisms of resistance to aflatoxin accumulation by *A. flavus* in maize genotype GT-MAS:gk [31].

Guo et al. (1995) first reported that genotype differences in aflatoxin B_1 accumulation were demonstrated between GT-MAS:gk and thirteen maize hybrids [20]. Most commercial hybrids supported high levels of aflatoxin production, with no differences in aflatoxin levels between intact and wounded kernels of these genotypes. In addition, aflatoxin levels were higher in wounded than in intact kernels. GT-MAS:gk not only supported the lowest levels of aflatoxin production in intact kernels, but aflatoxin levels in endosperm-wounded kernels were also significantly lower in GT-MAS:gk than in wounded kernels of all other tested lines. Furthermore, treatment with KOH to remove cutin from intact kernels prior to inoculation with *A. flavus* caused a substantial increase in aflatoxin accumulation in GT-MAS:gk, whereas only marginal increases were seen in the susceptible hybrid Pioneer 3154. Similarly, removing wax from the surface of GT-MAS:gk kernels greatly increased their susceptibility to aflatoxin accumulation. Interestingly, when wax removal was combined with treatment with KOH or purified cutinase, aflatoxin levels in kernels were equal to those in wounded control kernels in both genotypes. These results indicated that wax and cutin layers of maize kernel pericarps play a critical role in resistance to aflatoxin accumulation in GT-MAS:gk. In addition, detailed studies of corn kernel wax and fungal cutinase production by *A. flavus* [32] revealed that GT-MAS:gk possesses a greater quantity and unique composition of kernel wax, which may serve as a barrier to *A. flavus* infection [33]. Although cutinase produced by *A. flavus* appears to facilitate active infection of corn kernels [32]. *A. flavus* secretes extracellular cutinase when growing on cutin-containing medium, suggesting *A. flavus* acts as an opportunistic pathogen utilizing cutinase as a virulent factor for establishing infection under field conditions. To evaluate the potential role of kernel wax as a physical barrier to *A. flavus* infection and colonization, Russin et al. (1997) dissolved wax from various maize genotypes in chloroform or acetone and mixed it with autoclaved A and M medium [33]. Remarkably, only wax extracts from GT-MAS:gk exhibited antifungal activity. Thin-layer chromatography further revealed a unique compound present exclusively in GT-MAS:gk but also lacking a peak common to all others.

Another interesting phenomenon related to kernel germination or sprouting was observed when kernels of both resistant and susceptible genotypes were preincubated for three days at 100% relative humidity (RH) prior to inoculation with *A. flavus*; germination levels increased dramatically compared to kernels that were not preincubated [34]. In preincubated kernels aflatoxin levels remained consistently low in GT-MAS:gk but decreased markedly (61%) in Pioneer 3154. When eight susceptible hybrids were evaluated for aflatoxin accumulation under the same preincubation conditions, seven exhibited significantly lower toxin levels compared to kernels that were not preincubated. On average, aflatoxin reduction across all tests was 83%, ranging from 68% to 96% [34]. This preincubation-induced germination, or "physiological sprouting", was associated with a reduction in aflatoxin accumulation, which might be attributed to the induction of specific antifungal proteins, such as zeamatin and ribosome-inactivating protein (RIP) [35]. The distributions of these two specific antifungal proteins in maize kernel tissues indicate that RIP-like protein was present at higher levels within endosperm than in embryo tissues, whereas zeamatin-like protein was more concentrated in embryo than in endosperm [36].

The "living embryo" theory further suggests that resistant corn kernels lose their resistance to *A. flavus* and subsequent aflatoxin accumulation when the embryo is damaged or inactivated, pointing to an active, metabolic defense system involving the production of specific proteins and other protective metabolic compounds. Research has identified several resistance-associated proteins (RAPs) that contribute to the resistance observed in corn. In summary, there appear to be two primary levels of disease resistance: one at the pericarp, where the pericarp waxes play a critical physical role in preventing infection [20], and another at the sub-pericarp level, where RAPs function as biochemical defenses against *A. flavus* colonization [30,37,38]. Several RAPs, especially those constitutively expressed in corn kernels, have been identified as the second layer of defense. These include maize RIP and zeamatin that concentrate in the aleurone layer to protect the endosperm and embryo, respectively [36], in addition to storage proteins such as globulin 1 (GLB1) [39]; stress-responsive proteins such as glyoxalase 1 (GLX1) [40]; antifungal proteins such as the 14 kDa trypsin inhibitor protein (TI); pathogenesis-related protein 10 (PR10) [41]; and a novel β-1,3-glucanase [42].

The germination-induced resistance as reported by Guo et al. [34] suggests that the process of germination, a metabolic activity of the living embryo, activates defense mechanisms [34]. This finding aligns with reports that *A. flavus*-resistant maize tends to accumulate higher antioxidant enzymes, such as peroxidase, and exhibit greater tolerance to drought and heat stress compared to susceptible varieties. This phenomenon may be explained by the findings of Hite et al. (1999), who demonstrated an inverse correlation between catalase activity and hydrogen peroxide (H_2O_2) levels in maize during seed germination [43]. In all examined maize lines, H_2O_2 levels were highest during the early 1–2 days post-imbibition (or preincubation) and decreased thereafter, but the total antioxidant enzyme catalase activity was lowest during the early 1–2 days post-imbibition and reached maximal activity at 4–6 days post-imbibition. Given the fact that oxidative stress caused by increased reactive oxygen species (ROS) such as H_2O_2 accumulates to maximum quantities at the first two days post-imbibition followed by increased antioxidative catalase activity beginning at three days in maize kernels [43], a combination of host-derived resistance and antioxidant proteins and reduced ROS production at the time of inoculation may have contributed to the reduction in aflatoxin production [34], which also leads to the next section, "Key Largo" theory [18], to investigate the potential role of drought stress, particularly oxidative stress caused by excessive ROS in host-drought-*A. flavus* interactions, the role of ROS in aflatoxin production regulation, how ROS may function in signaling between host plants and *A. flavus* during infections under drought conditions and their effects on aflatoxin contamination.

Together, these findings clarify two complementary layers of resistance—physical pericarp barriers and embryo-driven biochemical defenses—and provide the biological foundation for Section 3, which examines how drought and oxidative stress reshape host–pathogen interactions.

3. The "Key Largo" Theory, Host—Drought—*A. flavus* Interactions and Oxidative Stress

A large body of host–pathogen studies shows that drought and heat elevate oxidative and nitrosative stress in maize, and genotypes that maintain stronger antioxidant capacity tend to be less prone to aflatoxin contamination [44]. A coordinated series of studies from Yang et al. [30,44] further elucidated the tissue-specific redox responses to drought stress. Proteomic analyses of maize kernels revealed broad stress-signaling changes under drought [30]; histochemical and quantitative assays showed that drought-sensitive lines accumulate higher ROS and reactive nitrogen species (RNS) in leaves and developing kernels than drought-tolerant lines, and kernel metabolomics mapped drought-induced shifts in antioxidant and stress-metabolite pathways, with sensitive lines mounting more intense responses consistent with susceptibility patterns [44].

On the fungal side, oxidative stress functions as a key prerequisite for aflatoxin biosynthesis. In *A. parasiticus*, the transition from trophophase to idiophase in toxigenic strains is characterized by increased oxygen demand and enhanced antioxidant defenses precisely as aflatoxin production begins [45]. Complementarily, mutants that stall at successive precursor steps show a graded increase in ROS relative to a nontoxigenic strain, and modest exogenous H_2O_2 further elevates AFB_1 production—linking redox load to pathway induction [46]. Together, these findings position ROS both as a trigger for pathway activation and as a condition to which aflatoxin (and its precursors) contributes adaptive redox homeostasis.

More direct evidence for redox regulation of aflatoxin biosynthesis arose from pathway genetics. In *A. parasiticus*, a comparison of wild type (SU-1) and an *aflR*-disruptant (AFS10) showed that total ROS declines between 24 and 48 h in SU-1 coincident with peak aflatoxin accumulation, whereas AFS10 does not show the same reduction. Notably, exogenous aflatoxin treatment lowers ROS in AFS10 at 24 h without inducing superoxide dismutase (SOD) transcripts, indicating the presence of both *aflR*-dependent and toxin-dependent ROS mitigation mechanisms [47]. Finotti et al. (2021) also showed that aflatoxin B1 can actively scavenge H_2O_2 in direct reactions and provide antioxidant protection to *E. coli* when exogenously supplied, providing further evidence for the role of aflatoxins in oxidative stress alleviation [48]. In *A. flavus*, oxidative signals co-regulate development and secondary metabolism, antioxidants that modulate ROS and thiol redox balance suppress sclerotial differentiation, and aflatoxin B1 (AFB1) production tracks with oxidative status [49]. A *veA* deletion mutant lacks both sclerotia and AFB1, underscoring the redox-sensitive developmental control of the pathway [21].

Population-level comparisons reinforce the functional link between aflatoxin capacity and oxidative-stress tolerance. Across highly aflatoxigenic, moderate, commercial atoxigenic, and naturally atoxigenic *A. flavus* isolates, conidia from high-AF producers survive higher H_2O_2 than low/atoxigenic isolates, consistent with aflatoxin production (or tightly linked mechanisms) buffering oxidative stress. Complementary transcriptomics revealed oxidative challenges to coordinate changes in development regulators, antioxidant systems, and secondary-metabolism genes [50].

In summary, drought and heat elevate host ROS and RNS, while the fungus senses and integrates oxidative signals to drive development and aflatoxin biosynthesis. Recently, Fountain et al. (2025) summarized this phenomenon, coined the "Key Largo" theory, and described contrasting field scenarios: under non-stress conditions—reminiscent of "sitting on the beach in Key Largo"—with adequate irrigation and optimal temperatures, aflatoxin accumulation remains low due to lack of physiological stress on both host crops and the infecting pathogen *A. flavus* [18]. However, under stressful environmental conditions, particularly drought and high temperatures, aflatoxin contamination tends to increase due to elevated physiological stress in both the host and the fungus. This hypothesis is based on observed responses in sensitive hosts, where elevated ROS under drought and heat stress are perceived by infecting *A. flavus*, leading to exacerbated aflatoxin production. Alternatively, reduced ROS accumulation in drought-tolerant hosts, either under stressful conditions or normal growth, can lead to normal or even reduced aflatoxin contamination. The differences in overall oxidative stress tolerance seen among strains of *A. flavus* with contrasting aflatoxin production capabilities also point to the possible role of aflatoxin production in alleviating oxidative stress in *A. flavus*, with aflatoxin synthesis being further exacerbated by host- or environment-derived oxidative stress.

To test the "Key Largo" theory, a series of experiments examining the responses of various isolates of *A. flavus* with differing levels of oxidative stress tolerance and aflatoxin production capability to H_2O_2-derived oxidative stress in vitro was conducted using several different approaches, including transcriptomics [50,51], proteomics [52], and metabolomics [53]. These studies have shed light on isolate-specific responses to oxidative stress correlated with their aflatoxin production levels and identified additional secondary metabolite pathways stimulated by oxidative stresses. Highly aflatoxigenic isolates such as AF13 showed less vigorous responses to stress, while moderate aflatoxin producers such as NRRL3357 and atoxigenic isolates such as K54A exhibit stronger oxidative-stress responses than highly aflatoxigenic strains at equivalent time points, and the biological-control strains showed more vigorous responses across all associated omics studies at the examined time points. Therefore, the role of aflatoxin production as a stress-alleviating mechanism also factors into the overall "Key Largo" theory, as highly aflatoxigenic isolates exhibit a greater level of tolerance to oxidative stress than less aflatoxigenic or non-aflatoxigenic isolates due to more aflatoxin biosynthesis-associated oxidase activity leading to more secondary ROS bursts and subsequent increases in antioxidant expression [54].

These host–pathogen interactions occur within environmental contexts defined by seasonal drought severity, soil-moisture deficits, canopy temperature, and nighttime humidity. Historical records from the southeastern United States show that high-aflatoxin years consistently align with mid-season moisture stress followed by late-season heat [55,56], reinforcing the environmental foundation of the Key Largo hypothesis.

While the primary focus is aflatoxin, it is important to consider whether altering drought-response or antioxidant pathways may inadvertently influence the accumulation of other mycotoxins such as fumonisins or DON [57–59]. Comparisons of resistant vs. susceptible germplasm will be required to ensure that preharvest aflatoxin mitigation does not shift risk toward other toxins.

4. Integrating CRISPR-Based Genome Editing and Tissue Culture for Drought Tolerance and Aflatoxin Resistance in Crops

To complement the historical and mechanistic perspectives described above, recent advances in CRISPR-based genome editing allow direct manipulation of pathways central to both the living embryo and Key Largo frameworks. These tools provide a molecular bridge from classical resistance mechanisms to modern crop improvement strategies.

Genome-wide activation, knockout, and inhibition are powerful CRISPR-based genome editing approaches to study gene function and identify key regulators of biological processes. Genome-wide activation is a gain-of-function study that uses a modified CRISPR system to upregulate the expression of genes. Genome-wide knockout is a loss-of-function study that ablates gene expression to study the resulting phenotypic changes. Genome-wide inhibition is another loss-of-function study that represses gene expression at the transcriptional level, without altering the underlying DNA sequence. Clevenger et al. (2016) reported identification of a potential susceptibility factor, *ABR1*, as a repressor of ABA signaling that may play a role in permitting preharvest aflatoxin contamination (PAC) [60]. Recent advancements in CRISPR-based genome editing, combined with plant tissue culture techniques, offer transformative solutions. These technologies enable precise genetic modifications, accelerating the development of resilient crop varieties. Given *A. flavus*' saprophytic nature, an optimal strategy would be to elevate broad immunity within the plant host by enhancing the gene expression of RAPs (resistance-associated proteins) and other effective immunity genes, by suppressing negative regulators of disease resistance such as *2-oxoglutarate Fe(II)-dependent oxygenase* (*2OGO*) [61], and by improving the plant's fitness under drought and other abiotic stresses. This section explores the integration of CRISPR-mediated genome editing and tissue culture for enhancing drought tolerance and aflatoxin resistance, highlighting key breakthroughs, challenges, and prospects.

The CRISPR/Cas9 system has revolutionized genetic engineering by allowing targeted modifications of plant genomes with unprecedented precision. The system relies on a guide RNA (gRNA) to direct the Cas9 endonuclease to specific genomic loci, inducing double-stranded breaks (DSBs) [62]. These breaks are subsequently repaired via non-homologous end joining (NHEJ), often resulting in gene knockouts, or homology-directed repair (HDR), enabling precise edits. Beyond conventional knockouts, advanced CRISPR variants such as base editing and CRISPR activation (CRISPRa) facilitate single-nucleotide substitutions and transcriptional modulation without DSBs [63]. The groundbreaking and yet relatively underexplored potential of CRISPRa systems offers powerful opportunities for gain-of-function (GOF) studies in plant biology. We advocate for the broader adoption of CRISPRa as a transformative approach to discover and harness genetic variation, ultimately accelerating the development of crops with enhanced disease resistance [64]. These innovations broaden the scope of genome editing, enabling fine-tuned regulation of stress-responsive genes. The CRISPR/Cas9 system has emerged as a powerful and versatile tool for crop genetic improvement, enabling precise genome editing to enhance disease resistance, abiotic stress tolerance, and yield-related traits. Recent advances have demonstrated the potential of CRISPR in peanuts, including targeting *AhMULE9A* to enhance tolerance to aluminum toxicity, a key factor limiting growth on acidic soils [65,66]. In addition, the editing of *AhNFR1* and *AhNFR5* genes via hairy root transformation provided new insights into nodulation mechanisms [67]. Several of the CRISPR targets discussed—such as antioxidant genes, cuticle biosynthesis pathways, and flavonoid regulators—directly intersect the mechanisms highlighted in the living embryo and Key Largo models.

Tissue culture and transformation methods are central to developing aflatoxin-resistant crops. Plant tissue culture has long been a cornerstone of agricultural biotechnology, enabling the cultivation of plants under sterile conditions to address goals such as crop improvement, disease resistance, and conservation of germplasm. In addition, it is a crucial step for successful genetic transformation, serving as the regenerative system for delivering CRISPR components and recovering edited plant lines [68]. Core techniques include somatic embryogenesis and organogenesis, which rely on responsive explants such as immature embryos, cotyledons, hypocotyls, or shoot apices [69]. These methods enable dedifferentiation and subsequent regeneration of whole plants from transformed cells, making tissue culture indispensable for crop biotechnology and functional genomics. There are two major approaches widely used for gene delivery: Agrobacterium tumefaciens-mediated transformation and biolistic (particle bombardment) methods. Agrobacterium-mediated transformation is favored for its high efficiency, low transgene copy number, and minimal genomic disruption, making it ideal for stable gene integration in many species [70]. In contrast, biolistic delivery is particularly valuable for crops that are recalcitrant to Agrobacterium, such as certain peanut genotypes or monocots such as maize [68]. Regardless of the delivery method, optimizing tissue culture conditions, including media composition, growth regulators (such as auxins and cytokinins), explant age, and genotype selection is essential for enhancing transformation efficiency and regeneration rates.

When conducting research on aflatoxin mitigation in plants, tissue culture serves as a fundamental component, as it supports various research approaches. For instance, investigating developmental processes under controlled conditions often relies on organogenesis, where maintaining excised roots or shoots in vitro enables researchers to study plant-pathogen interactions during *A. flavus* colonization and evaluate the effects of transgenes or genome edits on organ-specific resistance [71]. Another valuable technique is protoplast culture, which plays a crucial role in functional genomics and gene editing [72]. Isolated protoplasts allow for direct DNA or RNA delivery, supporting transient assays to test candidate genes involved in aflatoxin resistance. Additionally, protoplast fusion enables the combination of genetic material from different species, potentially leading to novel hybrids with enhanced defense traits. Callus culture also provides a versatile platform for studying stress responses, performing genetic transformation, and producing secondary metabolites. In the context of aflatoxin research, callus-based systems facilitate high-throughput screening of maize or peanut lines for resistance-associated traits, such as drought stress tolerance and enhanced antifungal metabolite production.

Therefore, callus induction combined with in vitro screening approaches expands the potential for resistance discovery [73]. One widely used method involves supplementing tissue culture media with polyethylene glycol (PEG) to simulate drought stress, a major predisposing factor for *A. flavus* infection and aflatoxin accumulation. PEG imposes osmotic stress by lowering water potential, enabling researchers to identify calli that maintain growth and regeneration under water-limited conditions [74,75]. Surviving tissues often exhibit physiological and molecular hallmarks of drought tolerance, such as proline accumulation and induction of stress-responsive genes, traits that are tightly linked to reduced aflatoxin contamination in the field.

Hence, advances in tissue culture and transformation not only enable the precise introduction of resistance alleles through CRISPR-based or transgenic strategies but also provide controlled systems for screening stress resilience traits that indirectly mitigate aflatoxin risk. As tissue culture technologies continue to evolve, their integration with in vitro screening methods promises to accelerate the identification, testing, and deployment of resistant germplasm, moving the field closer to a durable "Silver Shotgun" strategy against aflatoxin contamination.

CRISPR-mediated engineering of drought tolerance. Drought response in plants is governed by intricate genetic networks regulating osmotic balance, antioxidant responses, calcium efflux, and morphological adaptations such as root architecture and stomatal closure and opening [76,77]. CRISPR gene editing has enabled precise manipulation of these complex pathways, offering a targeted strategy to enhance drought tolerance without compromising growth or yield [78].

Therefore, CRISPR/Cas9 technology has been instrumental in uncovering gene functions and enhancing drought tolerance in major crops. A major focus has been on editing transcription factors such as *DREB*, *NAC*, and *bZIP* families, which act as master regulators of stress-inducible gene expression [78,79]. By activating or repressing downstream genes involved in osmolyte accumulation, membrane stability, and protective protein production, these transcription factors can fine-tune the plant's response to water deficit. We have recently found success in editing the *AsDREBL* (*Agrotis stolenifera DREB-like*) gene in creeping bentgrass to improve drought tolerance [80]. On the other hand, CRISPRa has demonstrated that manipulating these factors can significantly improve drought resilience in model and crop species like sugarcane [81]. Advances in tissue-specific genome editing have further refined CRISPR applications in plants. In *Arabidopsis*, a highly efficient editing system combining Cas9 and guide RNAs driven by the *AtEF1* promoter enabled precise mutation of *OST2/AHA1*, genes involved in abiotic stress response [82]. This approach yielded new *OST2/AHA1* alleles with improved stomatal regulation and no detectable pleiotropic side effects. These findings demonstrate the potential of spatially controlled gene editing to fine-tune plant responses to environmental stress. Collectively, these studies underscore how CRISPR/Cas9 can be harnessed to enhance agricultural productivity and engineer crops with robust, multi-stress resistance [72].

CRISPR approaches for aflatoxin resistance. Aflatoxin contamination is exacerbated by abiotic stresses like drought and high temperatures, which compromise plant defense mechanisms and favor fungal colonization [83]. CRISPR-based gene editing provides a promising avenue for developing aflatoxin-resistant varieties by targeting both host susceptibility factors and fungal infection processes. CRISPR can be used to enhance host resistance by modifying genes that strengthen physical and biochemical defenses. Editing genes associated with pericarp structure and kernel development can improve physical barriers, reducing the likelihood of fungal penetration. For instance, mutations in genes that regulate lipid transfer proteins or cuticle formation may lead to tighter, more resistant seed coats [84]. Also, targeting regulatory enzymes in flavonoid and phenylpropanoid biosynthesis can increase the accumulation of antifungal secondary metabolites [85]. These compounds not only inhibit *A. flavus* growth but may also interfere with aflatoxin biosynthesis [86]. Importantly, reactive oxygen species accumulation under drought stress weakens plant immunity and promotes fungal infection [87,88]. Editing antioxidant-related genes such as those encoding glutathione S-transferases or superoxide dismutases can enhance the plant's oxidative stress tolerance and indirectly limit aflatoxin accumulation [18]. Further efforts integrating CRISPR with host transcriptomic responses and QTL mapping for aflatoxin resistance could accelerate the identification of new, durable gene targets. A comprehensive, multi-gene editing strategy may ultimately be required to achieve reliable field-level resistance.

Challenges and future directions. Despite the significant advancements in CRISPR-based crop improvement, several challenges continue to hinder widespread application. One major obstacle is transformation efficiency, particularly in recalcitrant crops like peanuts, where genotype-dependent tissue culture responses limit the regeneration of edited lines [89,90]. Developing genotype-independent transformation protocols remains a top priority to expand CRISPR accessibility across diverse plant species. Off-target effects also present a concern, potentially leading to unintended mutations that compromise plant fitness or trigger regulatory scrutiny. Advances in guide RNA (gRNA) design algorithms and high-fidelity Cas9 variants have significantly improved targeting specificity, reducing off-target activity and enhancing biosafety [91]. Furthermore, regulatory uncertainty and public acceptance remain key impediments to the deployment of genome-edited crops. While some countries have begun to differentiate gene-edited organisms from traditional GMOs in their regulatory frameworks, global harmonization and transparent communication with stakeholders will be crucial for the responsible commercialization of CRISPR-derived crops [92–94].

Emerging technologies offer promising solutions to these challenges. Ribonucleoprotein (RNP) delivery systems, which introduce preassembled Cas9-gRNA complexes directly into plant cells, eliminate foreign DNA integration and reduce regulatory burdens [95]. Likewise, viral vector-mediated CRISPR delivery is gaining traction as a scalable, DNA-free alternative for transient gene editing in planta [96,97]. As these technologies mature, they are expected to broaden the scope and efficiency of CRISPR applications in crop improvement.

5. The Path Forward Toward a "Silver Shotgun" Strategy

Since the paradigm shift in the 1970s—from post-harvest prevention to preharvest genetic evaluation and breeding of resistant crops—over 50 years of research have revealed much about genetic resistance and the factors that affect the complex process of host and *A. flavus*, interaction with recent studies revealing the potential ROS-mediated crosstalk between hosts and *A. flavus*. The current data supports an underlying aflatoxin production, which involves *A. flavus* self-protection and survival within a high-ROS environment, including other secondary metabolites like kojic acid. CRISPR is a powerful tool for creating disease-resistant crops, and the integration of CRISPR genome editing and plant tissue culture has opened new frontiers in the development of crops resilient to climate-induced stresses and mycotoxin contamination. Targeted editing of drought-responsive genes and the engineering of host–pathogen resistance mechanisms illustrate the precision and versatility of CRISPR for addressing real-world agricultural challenges. As researchers continue to refine transformation techniques and uncover novel gene targets, these tools will become even more powerful in enabling climate-adapted agriculture. Realizing their full potential will require not only technical advancements but also field validation, regulatory clarity, and proactive engagement with farmers and consumers.

Together, these findings and approaches represent a newly described direction for aflatoxin research. For decades, the research community has sought the proverbial "Silver Bullet"—a single intervention that could reliably and consistently eliminate preharvest aflatoxin contamination. No individual solution is likely to succeed in isolation. Instead, durable progress will require coordinated, multi-component strategies that combine knowledge of host resistance and breeding, fungal biology, and environmental influences with modern tools such as CRISPR genome editing, biotechnology, nanotechnology, and improved forecasting and detection systems. In this context, the success of aflatoxin mitigation must be measured not by percentage reduction alone but by the consistent achievement of aflatoxin concentrations below national and international maximum residue limits (MRLs). Within this broader multi-strategy, atoxigenic *A. flavus* biocontrol remains an important tool; however, their safety must be evaluated not only based on aflatoxin deficiency but also regarding ecological behavior, secondary metabolite profiles, and long-term field persistence. These considerations are increasingly important as biological interventions become more widely adopted and highlight the need for integrated approaches to ensure progress toward a secure, resilient, and aflatoxin-safe food supply.

Author Contributions: B.G., R.D. and J.C.F.: contributed to the conceptualization and organization and editing of the manuscript. All authors contributed the writing. All authors have read and agreed to the published version of the manuscript.

Funding: This review received no external funding.

Institutional Review Board Statement: Not applicable.

Informed Consent Statement: Not applicable.

Data Availability Statement: No new data were created or analyzed in this study. Data sharing is not applicable to this article.

Acknowledgments: We have received decades of support for our research on aflatoxin and related topics from the US Department of Agriculture Agricultural Research Service (USDA-ARS), the USDA Annual Aflatoxin Elimination Workshop, Georgia Corn Grower Association, the Peanut Research Foundation, the National Corn Growers Association Aflatoxin Mitigation Center of Excellence (AMCOE), the National Peanut Board, and the Georgia Peanut Commission.

Conflicts of Interest: The authors declare no conflicts of interest.

References

1. Kendra, D.F.; Dyer, R.B. Opportunities for biotechnology and policy regarding mycotoxin issues in international trade. *Int. J. Food Microbiol.* **2007**, *119*, 147–151. [CrossRef] [PubMed]
2. Blount, W.P. A new turkey disease problem in England characterized by heavy mortality. *Q. Poult. Bull.* **1960**, *27*, 1–3.
3. Nesbitt, B.F.; O'Kelly, J.; Sargeant, K.; Sheridan, A. *Aspergillus flavus* and turkey X disease: Toxic metabolites of *Aspergillus flavus*. *Nature* **1962**, *195*, 1062–1063. [CrossRef] [PubMed]

4. Williams, J.H.; Phillips, T.D.; Jolly, P.E.; Stiles, J.K.; Jolly, C.M.; Aggarwal, D. Human aflatoxicosis in developing countries: A review of toxicology, exposure, potential health consequences, and interventions. *Am. J. Clin. Nutr.* **2004**, *80*, 1106–1122. [CrossRef]
5. Anderson, H.W.; Nehring, E.W.; Wichser, W.R. Aflatoxin contamination of corn in the field. *J. Agric. Food Chem.* **1975**, *23*, 775–782. [CrossRef]
6. Smith, J.S.; Williams, W.P.; Windham, G.L. Aflatoxin in maize: A review of the early literature from "moldy-corn toxicosis" to the genetics of aflatoxin accumulation resistance. *Mycotoxin Res.* **2019**, *35*, 111–128. [CrossRef]
7. Scully, B.T.; Krakowsky, M.D.; Ni, X.; Wilson, J.P.; Lee, R.D.; Guo, B.Z. Preharvest aflatoxin contamination of corn and other grain crops grown on the U.S. Southeastern Coastal Plain. *Toxin Rev.* **2009**, *28*, 169–179. [CrossRef]
8. Payne, G.A.; Widstrom, N.W. Aflatoxin in maize. *Crit. Rev. Plant Sci.* **1992**, *10*, 423–440. [CrossRef]
9. Cotty, P.J.; Mellon, J.E. Ecology of aflatoxin producing fungi and biocontrol of aflatoxin contamination. *Mycotoxin Res.* **2006**, *22*, 110–117. [CrossRef]
10. Soni, P.; Gangurde, S.S.; Ortega-Beltran, A.; Kumar, R.; Parmar, S.; Sudini, H.K.; Lei, Y.; Ni, X.; Huai, D.; Fountain, J.C.; et al. Functional biology and molecular mechanisms of host-pathogen interactions for aflatoxin contamination in groundnut (*Arachis hypogaea* L.) and maize (*Zea mays* L.). *Front. Microbiol.* **2020**, *11*, 227. [CrossRef]
11. Windham, G.L.; Williams, W.P. Evaluation of Corn Inbreds and Advanced Breeding Lines for Resistance to Aflatoxin Contamination in the Field. *Plant Dis.* **2002**, *86*, 232–234. [CrossRef]
12. Pandey, M.K.; Kumar, R.; Pandey, A.K.; Soni, P.; Gangurde, S.S.; Sudini, H.K.; Fountain, J.C.; Liao, B.S.; Desmae, H.; Okori, P.; et al. Mitigating aflatoxin contamination in groundnut through a combination of genetic resistance and post-harvest management practices. *Toxins* **2019**, *11*, 315. [CrossRef]
13. Wahl, N.; Murray, S.C.; Isakeit, T.; Krakowsky, M.; Windham, G.L.; Williams, W.P.; Guo, B.Z.; Ni, X.Z.; Knoll, J.; Xu, W.W.; et al. Identification of resistance to aflatoxin accumulation and yield potential in maize hybrids in the southeast regional aflatoxin trials (SERAT). *Crop Sci.* **2017**, *57*, 202–215. [CrossRef]
14. Pekar, J.J.; Murray, S.C.; Isakeit, T.S.; Scully, B.T.; Guo, B.Z.; Knoll, J.E.; Ni, X.Z.; Abbas, H.K.; Williams, P.; Xu, W.W. Evaluation of elite maize inbred lines for reduced *Aspergillus flavus* infection, aflatoxin accumulation, and agronomic traits. *Crop Sci.* **2019**, *59*, 2562–2571. [CrossRef]
15. Torres, A.M.; Barros, G.G.; Palacios, S.A.; Chulze, S.N.; Battilani, P. Review on pre- and post-harvest management of peanuts to minimize aflatoxin contamination. *Food Res. Int.* **2014**, *62*, 11–19. [CrossRef]
16. Shabeer, S.; Asad, S.; Jamal, A.; Ali, A. Aflatoxin contamination, its impact and management strategies: An updated review. *Toxins* **2022**, *14*, 307. [CrossRef]
17. Pokhrel, S.; Kharel, P.; Pandey, S.; Botton, S.; Nugraha, G.T.; Holbrook, C.; Ozias-Akins, P. Understanding the impacts of drought on peanuts (*Arachis hypogaea* L.): Exploring physio-genetic mechanisms to develop drought-resilient peanut cultivars. *Front. Genet.* **2025**, *15*, 1492434. [CrossRef]
18. Fountain, J.C.; Gangurde, S.S.; Pandey, M.K.; Varshney, R.K.; Guo, B. The Key Largo hypothesis: Recent advances in understanding aflatoxin contamination in peanut with omics and biotechnology. In *Peanut Genomics and Biotechnology Status and Prospects for Sustainability*; Zhuang, W., Varshney, R.K., Wang, X., Zhang, X., Eds.; Taylor & Francis Group, LLC: Boca Raton, FL, USA, 2025.
19. Brown, R.L.; Cotty, P.J.; Cleveland, T.E.; Widstrom, N.W. Living maize embryo influences accumulation of aflatoxin in maize kernels. *J. Food Prot.* **1993**, *56*, 967–971. [CrossRef] [PubMed]
20. Guo, B.Z.; Russin, J.S.; Cleveland, T.E.; Brown, R.L.; Widstrom, N.W. Wax and cutin layers in maize kernels associated with resistance to aflatoxin production by *Aspergillus flavus*. *J. Food Prot.* **1995**, *58*, 296–300. [CrossRef]
21. Amare, M.G.; Keller, N.P. Molecular mechanisms of secondary metabolism and development. *Fungal Genet. Biol.* **2014**, *66*, 11–18. [CrossRef]
22. Wild, C.P.; Gong, Y.Y. Mycotoxins and human disease: A largely ignored global health issue. *Carcinogenesis* **2010**, *31*, 71–82. [CrossRef]
23. Marchese, S.; Polo, A.; Ariano, A.; Velotto, S.; Costantini, S.; Severino, L. Aflatoxin B1 and M1: Biological properties and their involvement in cancer development. *Toxins* **2018**, *10*, 214. [CrossRef]
24. Schrenk, D.; Bignami, M.; Bodin, L.; Chipman, J.K.; del Mazo, J.; Grasl-Kraupp, B.; Hogstrand, C.; Hoogenboom, L.; Leblanc, J.C.; Nebbia, C.S.; et al. Risk assessment of aflatoxins in food. *EFSA J.* **2020**, *18*, e06040. [CrossRef]
25. Commission, C.A. General Standard for Contaminants and Toxins in Food and Feed (CXS 193-1995; Amended 2019). Available online: https://www.fao.org/fao-who-codexalimentarius/sh-proxy/en/?lnk=1&url=https%253A%252F%252Fworkspace.fao.org%252Fsites%252Fcodex%252Fstandards%252FCXS%2B193-1995%252FCXS_193e.pdf (accessed on 21 November 2025).
26. Zuber, M.S.; Calvert, O.H.; Kwolek, W.F.; Lillehoj, E.B.; Kang, M.S. Aflatoxin B_1 production in an eight-line diallel of *Zea mays* infected with *Aspergillus flavus*. *Phytopathology* **1978**, *68*, 1346–1349. [CrossRef]
27. Guo, B.Z.; Li, R.G.; Widstrom, N.W.; Lynch, R.E.; Cleveland, T.E. Genetic variation within maize population GT-MAS:gk and the relationship with resistance to *Aspergillus flavus* and aflatoxin production. *Theor. Appl. Genet.* **2001**, *103*, 533–539. [CrossRef]

28. Guo, B.; Widstrom, N.W.; Wilson, D.M.; Lee, R.D.; Coy, A.E. Registration of maize germplasm GT601 (AM-1) and GT602 (AM-2). *J. Plant Regist.* **2007**, *1*, 155–156. [CrossRef]
29. Guo, B.; Widstrom, N.W.; Wilson, D.M.; Lee, R.D.; Coy, A.E. Registration of maize inbred line GT603. *J. Plant Regist.* **2011**, *5*, 233–234. [CrossRef]
30. Yang, L.M.; Jiang, T.B.; Fountain, J.C.; Scully, B.T.; Lee, R.D.; Kemerait, R.C.; Chen, S.X.; Guo, B.Z. Protein profiles reveal diverse responsive signaling pathways in kernels of two maize inbred lines with contrasting drought sensitivity. *Int. J. Mol. Sci.* **2014**, *15*, 18892–18918. [CrossRef]
31. Guo, B. Mechanisms of Resistance to Aflatoxin Accumulation by *Aspergillus flavus* in Maize Genotype GT-MAS:gk. Ph.D. Thesis, Louisiana State University, Baton Rouge, LA, USA, 1995.
32. Guo, B.Z.; Russin, J.S.; Cleveland, T.E.; Brown, R.L.; Damann, K.E. Evidence for cutinase production by *Aspergillus flavus* and its possible role in infection of corn kernels. *Phytopathology* **1996**, *86*, 824–829. [CrossRef]
33. Russin, J.S.; Guo, B.Z.; Tubajika, K.M.; Brown, R.L.; Cleveland, T.E.; Widstrom, N.W. Comparison of kernel wax from corn genotypes resistant or susceptible to *Aspergillus flavus*. *Phytopathology* **1997**, *87*, 529–533. [CrossRef]
34. Guo, B.Z.; Russin, J.S.; Brown, R.L.; Cleveland, T.E.; Widstrom, N.W. Resistance to aflatoxin contamination in corn as influenced by relative humidity and kernel germination. *J. Food Prot.* **1996**, *59*, 276–281. [CrossRef]
35. Guo, B.Z.; Chen, Z.Y.; Brown, R.L.; Lax, A.R.; Cleveland, T.E.; Russin, J.S.; Mehta, A.D.; Selitrennikoff, C.P.; Widstrom, N.W. Germination induces accumulation of specific proteins and antifungal activities in corn kernels. *Phytopathology* **1997**, *87*, 1174–1178. [CrossRef]
36. Guo, B.Z.; Cleveland, T.E.; Brown, R.L.; Widstrom, N.W.; Lynch, R.E.; Russin, J.S. Distribution of antifungal proteins in maize kernel tissues using immunochemistry. *J. Food Prot.* **1999**, *62*, 295–299. [CrossRef] [PubMed]
37. Chen, Z.; Brown, R.L.; Lax, A.R.; Guo, B.; Cleveland, T.E.; Russin, J.S. Resistance to *Aspergillus flavus* in corn kernels is associated with a 14-kDa protein. *Phytopathology* **1998**, *88*, 276–281. [CrossRef] [PubMed]
38. Guo, B.Z.; Brown, R.L.; Lax, A.R.; Cleveland, T.E.; Russin, J.S.; Widstrom, N.W. Protein profiles and antifungal activities of kernel extracts from corn genotypes resistant and susceptible to *Aspergillus flavus*. *J. Food Prot.* **1998**, *61*, 98–102. [CrossRef]
39. Chen, Z.Y.; Brown, R.L.; Damann, K.E.; Cleveland, T.E. Identification of unique or elevated levels of kernel proteins in aflatoxin-resistant maize genotypes through proteome analysis. *Phytopathology* **2002**, *92*, 1084–1094. [CrossRef]
40. Chen, Z.Y.; Brown, R.L.; Damann, K.E.; Cleveland, T.E. Identification of a maize kernel stress-related protein and its effect on aflatoxin accumulation. *Phytopathology* **2004**, *94*, 938–945. [CrossRef] [PubMed]
41. Chen, Z.Y.; Brown, R.L.; Damann, K.E.; Cleveland, T.E. PR10 expression in maize and its effect on host resistance against *Aspergillus flavus* infection and aflatoxin production. *Mol. Plant Pathol.* **2010**, *11*, 69–81. [CrossRef]
42. Liang, X.; Holbrook, C.C.; Lynch, R.E.; Guo, B. β-1,3-glucanase activity in peanut seed (*Arachis hypogaea*) is induced by inoculation with *Aspergillus flavus* and copurifies with a conglutin-like protein. *Phytopathology* **2005**, *95*, 506–511. [CrossRef]
43. Hite, D.R.C.; Auh, C.; Scandalios, J.G. Catalase activity and hydrogen peroxide levels are inversely correlated in maize scutella during seed germination. *Redox Rep.* **1999**, *4*, 29–34. [CrossRef]
44. Yang, L.M.; Fountain, J.C.; Ji, P.S.; Ni, X.Z.; Chen, S.X.; Lee, R.D.; Kemerait, R.C.; Guo, B.Z. Deciphering drought-induced metabolic responses and regulation in developing maize kernels. *Plant Biotechnol. J.* **2018**, *16*, 1616–1628. [CrossRef]
45. Jayashree, T.; Subramanyam, C. Oxidative stress as a prerequisite for aflatoxin production by *Aspergillus parasiticus*. *Free Radic. Bio. Med.* **2000**, *29*, 981–985. [CrossRef]
46. Narasaiah, K.V.; Sashidhar, R.B.; Subramanyam, C. Biochemical analysis of oxidative stress in the production of aflatoxin and its precursor intermediates. *Mycopathologia* **2006**, *162*, 179–189. [CrossRef]
47. Kenne, G.J.; Gummadidala, P.M.; Omebeyinje, M.H.; Mondal, A.M.; Bett, D.K.; McFadden, S.; Bromfield, S.; Banaszek, N.; Velez-Martinez, M.; Mitra, C.; et al. Activation of aflatoxin biosynthesis alleviates total ROS in *Aspergillus parasiticus*. *Toxins* **2018**, *10*, 57. [CrossRef]
48. Finotti, E.; Parroni, A.; Zaccaria, M.; Domin, M.; Momeni, B.; Fanelli, C.; Reverberi, M. Aflatoxins are natural scavengers of reactive oxygen species. *Sci. Rep.* **2021**, *11*, 16024. [CrossRef]
49. Grintzalis, K.; Vernardis, S.I.; Klapa, M.I.; Georgiou, C.D. Role of oxidative stress in Sclerotial differentiation and aflatoxin B1 biosynthesis in *Aspergillus flavus*. *Appl. Environ. Microbiol.* **2014**, *80*, 5561–5571. [CrossRef]
50. Fountain, J.C.; Bajaj, P.; Pandey, M.; Nayak, S.N.; Yang, L.M.; Kumar, V.; Jayale, A.S.; Chitikineni, A.; Zhuang, W.J.; Scully, B.T.; et al. Oxidative stress and carbon metabolism influence *Aspergillus flavus* transcriptome composition and secondary metabolite production. *Sci. Rep.* **2016**, *6*, 38747. [CrossRef]
51. Fountain, J.C.; Pandey, A.K.; Nayak, S.N.; Bajaj, P.; Wang, H.; Kumar, V.; Chitikineni, A.; Abbas, H.K.; Scully, B.T.; Kemerait, R.C.; et al. Transcriptional responses of toxigenic and atoxigenic isolates of *Aspergillus flavus* to oxidative stress in aflatoxin-conducive and non-conducive media. *World Mycotoxin J.* **2020**, *13*, 443–457. [CrossRef]

52. Fountain, J.C.; Koh, J.; Yang, L.M.; Pandey, M.K.; Nayak, S.N.; Bajaj, P.; Zhuang, W.J.; Chen, Z.Y.; Kemerait, R.C.; Lee, D.; et al. Proteome analysis of *Aspergillus flavus* isolate-specific responses to oxidative stress in relationship to aflatoxin production capability. *Sci. Rep.* **2018**, *8*, 3430. [CrossRef] [PubMed]
53. Fountain, J.C.; Yang, L.M.; Pandey, M.K.; Bajaj, P.; Alexander, D.; Chen, S.X.; Kemerait, R.C.; Varshney, R.K.; Guo, B.Z. Carbohydrate, glutathione, and polyamine metabolism are central to *Aspergillus flavus* oxidative stress responses over time. *BMC Microbiol.* **2019**, *19*, 209. [CrossRef] [PubMed]
54. Roze, L.V.; Laivenieks, M.; Hong, S.Y.; Wee, J.; Wong, S.S.; Vanos, B.; Awad, D.; Ehrlich, K.C.; Linz, J.E. Aflatoxin biosynthesis is a novel source of reactive oxygen species—A potential redox signal to initiate resistance to oxidative stress. *Toxins* **2015**, *7*, 1411–1430. [CrossRef]
55. Battilani, P.; Leggieri, M.C. Predictive modelling of aflatoxin contamination to support maize chain management. *World Mycotoxin J.* **2015**, *8*, 161–170. [CrossRef]
56. Dolezal, A.L.; Shu, X.; OBrian, G.R.; Nielsen, D.M.; Woloshuk, C.P.; Boston, R.S.; Payne, G.A. *Aspergillus flavus* infection induces transcriptional and physical changes in developing maize kernels. *Front. Microbiol.* **2014**, *5*, 384. [CrossRef]
57. Munkvold, G.P. Epidemiology of Fusarium Diseases and their Mycotoxins in Maize Ears. *Eur. J. Plant Pathol.* **2003**, *109*, 705–713. [CrossRef]
58. Medina, Á.; Rodríguez, A.; Magan, N. Climate change and mycotoxigenic fungi: Impacts on mycotoxin production. *Curr. Opin. Food Sci.* **2015**, *5*, 99–104. [CrossRef]
59. Brown, M.P.; Brown-Jenco, C.S.; Payne, G.A. Genetic and Molecular Analysis of Aflatoxin Biosynthesis. *Fungal Genet. Biol.* **1999**, *26*, 81–98. [CrossRef]
60. Clevenger, J.; Marasigan, K.; Liakos, V.; Sobolev, V.; Vellidis, G.; Holbrook, C.; Ozias-Akins, P. RNA sequencing of contaminated seeds reveals the state of the seed permissive for pre-harvest aflatoxin contamination and points to a potential susceptibility factor. *Toxins* **2016**, *8*, 317. [CrossRef]
61. Low, Y.C.; Lawton, M.A.; Di, R. Validation of barley 2OGO gene as a functional orthologue of *Arabidopsis* DMR6 gene in *Fusarium* head blight susceptibility. *Sci. Rep.* **2020**, *10*, 9935. [CrossRef] [PubMed]
62. Kumar, R.; Das, S.P.; Choudhury, B.U.; Kumar, A.; Prakash, N.R.; Verma, R.; Chakraborti, M.; Devi, A.G.; Bhattacharjee, B.; Das, R.; et al. Advances in genomic tools for plant breeding: Harnessing DNA molecular markers, genomic selection, and genome editing. *Biol. Res.* **2024**, *57*, 80. [CrossRef] [PubMed]
63. Ding, X.; Yu, L.; Chen, L.; Li, Y.J.; Zhang, J.L.; Sheng, H.Y.; Ren, Z.W.; Li, Y.L.; Yu, X.H.; Jin, S.X.; et al. Recent progress and future prospect of CRISPR/Cas-derived transcription activation (CRISPRa) system in plants. *Cells* **2022**, *11*, 3045. [CrossRef] [PubMed]
64. McLaughlin, J.E.; Foka, I.C.K.; Lawton, M.A.; Di, R. CRISPR activation: Identifying and using novel genes for plant disease resistance breeding. *Front. Genome Ed.* **2025**, *7*, 1596600. [CrossRef]
65. Neelakandan, A.K.; Wright, D.A.; Traore, S.M.; Ma, X.L.; Subedi, B.; Veeramasu, S.; Spalding, M.H.; He, G.H. Application of CRISPR/Cas9 system for efficient gene editing in peanut. *Plants* **2022**, *11*, 1361. [CrossRef]
66. Li, A.L.; Zhou, M.; Liao, G.T.; Li, X.Y.; Wang, A.Q.; Xiao, D.; He, L.F.; Zhan, J. CRISPR/Cas9 gene editing in peanut by *Agrobacterium tumefaciens*-mediated pollen tube transformation. *Plant Cell Tissue Organ Cult.* **2023**, *155*, 883–892. [CrossRef]
67. Shu, H.M.; Luo, Z.L.; Peng, Z.; Wang, J.P. The application of CRISPR/Cas9 in hairy roots to explore the functions of AhNFR1 and AhNFR5 genes during peanut nodulation. *BMC Plant Biol.* **2020**, *20*, 417. [CrossRef]
68. Alam, T. Advances in tissue culture-free genetic engineering and genome editing of peanut. *Mol. Biotechnol.* **2025**, *2025*, 1–15. [CrossRef]
69. Desai, P.; Desai, S.; Rafaliya, R.; Patil, G. Plant tissue culture: Somatic embryogenesis and organogenesis. In *Advances in Plant Tissue Culture*; Elsevier: Amsterdam, The Netherlands, 2022; pp. 109–130.
70. Azizi-Dargahlou, S.; Pouresmaeil, M. *Agrobacterium tumefaciens*-mediated plant transformation: A review. *Mol. Biotechnol.* **2024**, *66*, 1563–1580. [CrossRef]
71. Hicks, G.S. Shoot induction and organogenesis in vitro: A developmental perspective. *Vitr. Cell. Dev. Biol. Plant* **1994**, *30*, 10–15. [CrossRef]
72. Abdelrahman, M.; Al-Sadi, A.M.; Pour-Aboughadareh, A.; Burritt, D.J.; Tran, L.S.P. Genome editing using CRISPR/Cas9-targeted mutagenesis: An opportunity for yield improvements of crop plants grown under environmental stresses. *Plant Physiol. Biochem.* **2018**, *131*, 31–36. [CrossRef] [PubMed]
73. Wani, S.; Sofi, P.; Gosal, S.; Singh, N. In vitro screening of rice (*Oryza sativa* L.) callus for drought tolerance. *Commun. Biometry Crop Sci.* **2010**, *5*, 108–115.
74. Kacem, N.S.; Delporte, F.; Muhovski, Y.; Djekoun, A.; Watillon, B. In vitro screening of durum wheat against water-stress mediated through polyethylene glycol. *J. Genet. Eng. Biotechnol.* **2017**, *15*, 239–247. [CrossRef] [PubMed]
75. Zebarjadi, A.; Borjian, L.; Ghasempour, H.; Noori, A.; Kahrizi, D.; Chaghakaboodi, Z. Growth and physiological characterization in five genotypes of *Brassica napus* callus culture under drought–induced osmotic stress. *Agrotech. Ind. Crops* **2024**, *4*, 171–179. [CrossRef]

76. Haghpanah, M.; Hashemipetroudi, S.; Arzani, A.; Araniti, F. Drought tolerance in plants: Physiological and molecular responses. *Plants* **2024**, *13*, 2962. [CrossRef] [PubMed]
77. Zahedi, S.M.; Karimi, M.; Venditti, A.; Zahra, N.; Siddique, K.H.M.; Farooq, M. Plant adaptation to drought stress: The role of anatomical and morphological characteristics in maintaining the water status. *J. Soil Sci. Plant Nutr.* **2025**, *25*, 409–427. [CrossRef]
78. Sami, A.; Xue, Z.; Tazein, S.; Arshad, A.; Zhu, Z.H.; Chen, Y.P.; Hong, Y.; Zhu, X.T.; Zhou, K.J. CRISPR-Cas9-based genetic engineering for crop improvement under drought stress. *Bioengineered* **2021**, *12*, 5814–5829. [CrossRef]
79. Shelake, R.M.; Kadam, U.S.; Kumar, R.; Pramanik, D.; Singh, A.K.; Kim, J.Y. Engineering drought and salinity tolerance traits in crops through CRISPR-mediated genome editing: Targets, tools, challenges, and perspectives. *Plant Commun.* **2022**, *3*, 100417. [CrossRef]
80. Di, R.; Ravikumar, S.; Daddio, R.; Bonos, S. CRISPR-editing AsDREBL improved creeping bentgrass abiotic stress tolerance. *Int. J. Plant Biol.* **2025**, *16*, 89. [CrossRef]
81. Pandey, H.; Misra, V.; Mall, A.K.; Sharma, A.; Hillary, V.E.; Ceasar, S.A. Enhancing sugar crop resilience to abiotic stress using CRISPR/Cas tools. *Sugar Tech* **2025**, *27*, 985–1002. [CrossRef]
82. Martignago, D.; Rico-Medina, A.; Blasco-Escáez, D.; Fontanet-Manzaneque, J.B.; Cano-Delgado, A.I. Drought resistance by engineering plant tissue-specific responses. *Front. Plant Sci.* **2020**, *10*, 1676. [CrossRef]
83. Kebede, H.; Abbas, H.K.; Fisher, D.K.; Bellaloui, N. Relationship between aflatoxin contamination and physiological responses of corn plants under drought and heat stress. *Toxins* **2012**, *4*, 1385–1403. [CrossRef]
84. Wang, W.; Heitschmidt, G.W.; Windham, W.R.; Feldner, P.; Ni, X.; Chu, X. Feasibility of detecting aflatoxin B1 on inoculated maize kernels surface using Vis/NIR hyperspectral imaging. *J. Food Sci.* **2015**, *80*, M116–M122. [CrossRef] [PubMed]
85. Shetty, R.; Fretté, X.; Jensen, B.; Shetty, N.P.; Jensen, J.D.; Jorgensen, H.J.L.; Newman, M.A.; Christensen, L.P. Silicon-induced changes in antifungal phenolic acids, flavonoids, and key phenylpropanoid pathway genes during the interaction between miniature roses and the biotrophic pathogen *Podosphaera pannosa*. *Plant Physiol.* **2011**, *157*, 2194–2205. [CrossRef] [PubMed]
86. Castano-Duque, L.; Gilbert, M.K.; Mack, B.M.; Lebar, M.D.; Carter-Wientjes, C.H.; Sickler, C.M.; Cary, J.W.; Rajasekaran, K. Flavonoids modulate the accumulation of toxins from *Aspergillus flavus* in maize kernels. *Front. Plant Sci.* **2021**, *12*, 761446. [CrossRef]
87. Qi, J.S.; Song, C.P.; Wang, B.S.; Zhou, J.M.; Kangasjärvi, J.; Zhu, J.K.; Gong, Z.Z. Reactive oxygen species signaling and stomatal movement in plant responses to drought stress and pathogen attack. *J. Integr. Plant Biol.* **2018**, *60*, 805–826. [CrossRef] [PubMed]
88. Dikilitas, M.; Karakas, S.; Hashem, A.; Abd Allah, E.F.; Ahmad, P. Oxidative stress and plant responses to pathogens under drought conditions. In *Water Stress and Crop Plants*; John Wiley & Sons, Ltd.: Hoboken, NJ, USA, 2016; pp. 102–123.
89. Sharma, K.K.; Anjaiah, V. An efficient method for the production of transgenic plants of peanut (*Arachis hypogaea* L.) through *Agrobacterium tumefaciens*-mediated genetic transformation. *Plant Sci.* **2000**, *159*, 7–19. [CrossRef]
90. Chen, M.N.; Yang, Q.L.; Wang, T.; Chen, N.; Pan, L.J.; Chi, X.Y.; Yang, Z.; Wang, M.A.; Yu, S.L. Agrobacterium-mediated genetic transformation of peanut and the efficient recovery of transgenic plants. *Can. J. Plant Sci.* **2015**, *95*, 735–744. [CrossRef]
91. Guo, C.T.; Ma, X.T.; Gao, F.; Guo, Y.X. Off-target effects in CRISPR/Cas9 gene editing. *Front. Bioeng. Biotech.* **2023**, *11*, 1143157. [CrossRef]
92. Asquer, A.; Krachkovskaya, I. Uncertainty, institutions and regulatory responses to emerging technologies: CRISPR Gene editing in the US and the EU (2012–2019). *Regul. Gov.* **2021**, *15*, 1111–1127. [CrossRef]
93. Shew, A.M.; Nalley, L.L.; Snell, H.A.; Nayga, R.M.; Dixon, B.L. CRISPR versus GMOs: Public acceptance and valuation. *Glob. Food Secur.* **2018**, *19*, 71–80. [CrossRef]
94. Ahmad, S.; Shahzad, R.; Jamil, S.; Tabassum, J.; Chaudhary, M.A.M.; Atif, R.M.; Iqbal, M.M.; Monsur, M.B.; Lv, Y.; Sheng, Z.; et al. Chapter 31-Regulatory aspects, risk assessment, and toxicity associated with RNAi and CRISPR methods. In *CRISPR and RNAi Systems*; Abd-Elsalam, K.A., Lim, K.-T., Eds.; Elsevier: Amsterdam, The Netherlands, 2021; pp. 687–721.
95. Lin, Y.; Wagner, E.; Lächelt, U. Non-viral delivery of the CRISPR/Cas system: DNA versus RNA versus RNP. *Biomater. Sci.* **2022**, *10*, 1166–1192. [CrossRef]
96. Kujur, S.; Senthil-Kumar, M.; Kumar, R. Plant viral vectors: Expanding the possibilities of precise gene editing in plant genomes. *Plant Cell Rep.* **2021**, *40*, 931–934. [CrossRef]
97. Mahmood, M.A.; Naqvi, R.Z.; Rahman, S.U.; Amin, I.; Mansoor, S. Plant virus-derived vectors for plant genome engineering. *Viruses* **2023**, *15*, 531. [CrossRef] [PubMed]

toxins

MDPI

Review

The Difficulties in Demonstrating That Aflatoxin Reduction Improves Stunting in Developing World Regions

Paul C. Turner [1,*] and Erica Phillips [2]

[1] School of Public Health, University of Maryland, College Park, MD 20742, USA
[2] Ross and Carol Nese College of Nursing, The Pennsylvania State University, State College, PA 16802, USA; elp28@cornell.edu
* Correspondence: pturner3@umd.edu

Abstract

Aflatoxins are highly toxic secondary metabolites that contaminate dietary staples in many developing world regions, with hundreds of millions of people estimated to be chronically exposed. In this review, we summarize the evidence about AF exposure assessment and its relationship to stunting. Despite multiple attempts, this question has eluded a strong scientific conclusion due to the nature of the toxin and exposure, the disparate methods used for assessment, and the ethical difficulties of studying a toxin in low-resource settings. We highlight current challenges in defining these relationships, how this has reduced the ability to draw conclusions in this area, and approaches to overcome these to advance the field. Current reviews tend to report mixed associations, but typically lack critique of the study designs, and a limited understanding of patterns of aflatoxin exposure coupled with a probable variable threshold for effect. We highlight the potential diverse patterns of AF exposure over time and how that may influence study design to address this critical public health issue.

Keywords: aflatoxin; infant; stunting; growth; exposure; aflatoxin-lysine; aflatoxin-albumin

Key Contribution: (i). Inverse relationships between aflatoxin and linear growth faltering are observed where large distributions of aflatoxin exposure occur, despite many reviews suggesting mixed outcomes. (ii). Large-scale interventions from the in utero to late infancy period are critical to mitigate the adverse effects of aflatoxin on growth. (iii). Such studies need to be powered by the understanding that the majority of infants are unlikely to be exposed to aflatoxin at levels likely to cause stunting, and that significant variations in exposure levels will occur by season and age group.

1. Introduction

Malnutrition refers to both the excesses and the deficiencies in nutrient intake, leading to an imbalance in growth and/or function. Undernutrition in children is characterized by anthropometry, such as stunting, wasting, underweight, and micronutrient deficiencies [1]. Stunted infants and children have a low height (or length) for age (HAZ or LAZ). Here, the term HAZ will be used throughout. Being stunted is defined as a HAZ of more than two standard deviations below the World Health Organization (WHO) median, typically expressed as a HAZ of <-2; while extreme stunting has a HAZ of <-3. The WHO describes stunting as the consequence of chronic or recurrent undernutrition, usually associated with poverty, poor maternal health and nutrition, frequent illness, and/or inappropriate feeding and care in early life. Stunting is more than just being shorter than average, and a low HAZ is associated with children and then adults failing to reach their physical and cognitive potential; specifically, the condition is associated with a higher risk of morbidity and mortality [2–6]. Globally, 14–17% of child deaths under 5 years are associated with stunting, and child undernutrition remains a significant public health concern [1,4–11] affecting about 148 million children under 5 years of age [1].

For several decades, the focus on mitigation of early life stunting has been on improved infant and young child feeding interventions (with or without micronutrient supplementation), and/or water, sanitation, and hygiene interventions, and while of value, especially to mitigate acute malnutrition, they appear to only provide modest improvements in stunting [12–17]. This lack of impact between well-established risk factors and efficacy of intervention to reduce stunting with strong and meaningful mitigation approaches suggests that other factors contribute to poor linear growth. One contribution that is frequently overlooked is the putative role of mycotoxins and, in particular, aflatoxins [18–20]. The aim of this review is to explore the potential role of aflatoxin in early life growth by; (a) introducing key concepts from several epidemiological studies, (b) illustrating the complexity of exposure assessment for aflatoxin, (c) highlighting a possible threshold of exposure for stunting, and (d) indicating complex patterns of exposure to aflatoxins in the first few years of life. Combined, these observations suggest a difficulty in demonstrating that aflatoxin interventions will lead to improved infant growth.

2. Mycotoxins

Under the right conditions of temperature and humidity, fungal contamination of foods by some species of *Aspergillus*, *Fusarium*, and *Penicillium* can lead to the production of a wide range of poisons known as mycotoxins [21–23]. Among thousands of these secondary metabolites, a handful contaminate key dietary staples at levels of contamination, frequency of contamination, and regularity of consumption to be of a public health concern [19,22,24–26]. Mycotoxins of major concern include aflatoxins produced from *Aspergillus flavus* and *A. parasiticus*; fumonisins, deoxynivalenol, and zearalenone produced from various *Fusarium* species, and ochratoxin A produced by both *Aspergillus* and *Penicillium* species [21–23]. Aflatoxins and fumonisins are typically more frequent contaminants of corn (maize) in hot and humid climates such as sub-Saharan Africa, Central America, and tropical Asia. Aflatoxins can additionally occur at high concentrations in groundnuts (peanuts) in tropical regions [19,21–23]. For aflatoxins, both field growth and long-term storage contribute to the burden of contamination, while fumonisins are predominantly a field-produced toxin of maize [19,21]. The other mycotoxins mentioned are more prevalent in temperate climates, though mixtures of all these toxins are observed in biofluids in both temperate and tropical countries [27,28]. Mycotoxins tend to be resistant to processing, and their stability during cooking also contributes to dietary exposure [21,22]. More developed regions of the world tend to have both the regulation and the infrastructure to enforce relevant laws, while the required infrastructure in developing-world regions is lacking, especially in subsistence or small-hold farm settings. Thus, individuals who are particularly vulnerable face a combination of limited dietary variation, heavy reliance on one or two high-risk dietary staples, and no useful regulation that influences or protects against exposure.

3. Aflatoxins

Aflatoxins are a family of closely related poisons that occur naturally in certain grains and nuts, and include aflatoxin B1 (AFB1), AFB2, AFG1, and AFG2 (Figure 1a). AFB1 occurs

https://doi.org/10.3390/toxins18010032

most frequently and is the most toxic [19,21,22,29,30], and as such, AFB1 will be the focus of this review. Aflatoxin contamination of foods and subsequent human exposure vary by climate, season, geography, agricultural practice, and dietary behavior [18,19,31–35]. In many settings where crops are at risk of Aspergillus contamination and aflatoxin production, extended storage times in high humidity with insufficiently dried crops further increase contamination and risk of exposure [19,35].

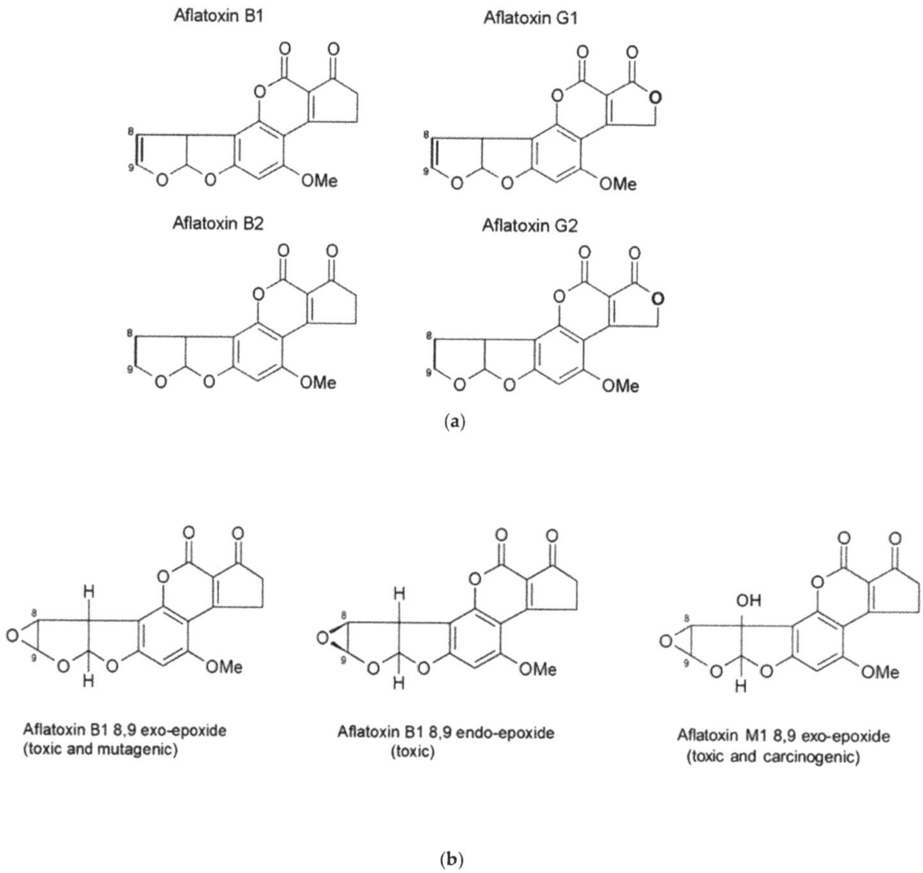

Figure 1. (**a**) Structures of the four naturally occurring aflatoxins. The -8,9- position is where the reactive epoxide can be readily formed across the double bond. (**b**) Structures of the aflatoxin B1 exo- and endo-epoxides, and aflatoxin M1 exo-epoxide.

Once ingested, AFB1 is metabolized by cytochrome P450 enzymes (CYPs) in many organs, as reviewed by [24,30,36,37], leading to an array of metabolites, including the toxic AFM1, and less toxic AFQ1 and AFP1; and two highly reactive epoxides, AFB1 exo-8,9-epoxide and AFB1 endo-8,9-epoxide (Figure 1b) [38,39]. The reactive epoxides cause toxicity via the formation of covalent adducts with multiple macromolecules, including nucleic acids and proteins [40,41]. The metabolite AFM1 can also undergo further transformation to form a reactive AFM1-epoxide, which is also toxic and carcinogenic [42]. Non-specific oxidative stress caused by aflatoxin biotransformation also contributes to toxicity [24].

Mechanism(s) of aflatoxin-induced stunting have been hypothesized and likely involve, in part, aflatoxin activation by CYPs to these damaging epoxides [18,19]. The main target organ for aflatoxin toxicity is the liver, and modulation of liver function may disrupt

https://doi.org/10.3390/toxins18010032

general nutritional homeostasis [18,43]. In addition, a reduction in insulin-like growth factor (particularly IGF-1) production and release by the liver, and/or other sites, may contribute to poor linear growth. Intestinal enterocytes contain CYPs that can also produce aflatoxin epoxides, and damage here leads to a reduction in both the functional surface of the intestine for nutrient absorption and the integrity of the intestine [44]. Given that early-life intestinal enteropathy, typically associated with gastrointestinal infections, is a well-established driver of infant stunting [45–47], it is reasonable to consider interactions of aflatoxin and intestinal infections that perhaps prolong the intestinal enteropathy, leading to a worsening of malnutrition. Aflatoxin also suppresses the immune system [48,49], including a demonstrated reduction in the protective secretory IgA in the saliva of Gambian children [50]; thus, aflatoxin may further contribute to this suggested interaction via a suppression of immune defenses. AFB1 also has epigenetic potential [51], with suggested modulation of genes such as IGF-1 that are associated with infant growth [52,53].

AFB1 is a proven human carcinogen [19,29], yet global efforts to reduce exposure remain limited. Exposures that critically impact infants often carry more power to drive action. However, despite multiple attempts, demonstrating strong scientific evidence for the suggested role of aflatoxin on poor linear growth has not been achieved. This is in part due to the variable nature of the toxin contamination and exposure profile, the disparate methods used for assessment, the limited sizes of many studies, and the ethical difficulties of studying this toxin in low-resource settings. Here, we highlight current challenges in defining these relationships, how this has reduced the ability to draw conclusions in this area, and approaches to overcome these to advance the field.

4. Aflatoxin Exposure Assessment

While several foods are potentially contaminated, the major foods causing aflatoxin exposure in high-risk settings typically involve one or two limited dietary sources: maize (corn) and/or groundnuts (peanuts); foods that are typically dietary staples and used as complementary feeding in many tropical world regions [19]. Robust and accurate exposure tools are essential to conduct epidemiological research and to assess the efficacy of mitigation efforts to reduce aflatoxin exposure [27,28,54,55]. Aflatoxin can be readily detected in food samples; however, food is a precious commodity, and thus, food sampling for toxins becomes problematic in many low-resource settings. In addition, aflatoxins are extremely heterogeneously distributed within foods, typically making exposure assessment imprecise unless sampling regimes are extensive. By contrast, the measurement of body fluids can capture the concentration of either the parent toxin (or a metabolite) more accurately, and thus, provide an improved estimate of exposure [27,28,54–56]. All four of the naturally occurring aflatoxins have been observed in urine, indicative of exposure. However, our understanding of the toxicokinetics of aflatoxin reveals more quantitative indicators in the form of AFM1 and AF-N7-guanine in urine [57–60].

A longer-term biomarker of exposure to aflatoxin is found by measuring the concentration of aflatoxin covalently bound to albumin, typically reported as the aflatoxin-lysine equivalent per mg of albumin, also known as the aflatoxin-albumin (AF-alb) adduct [61–66]. All three of these biomarkers demonstrate a strong quantitative relationship between intake of aflatoxin and the biological measurement, providing much improved exposure estimates for epidemiological studies (more detail on biomarker development and validation can be found in reviews [26–28,54]. As LC-MS/MS technology has advanced [67–72], some researchers have discussed reporting aflatoxin-lysine concentrations only [73], and personal communication, avoiding adjustment for albumin by arguing that different assays for albumin provide a slightly different denominator for the AF-alb calculation, and thus, they argue that the use of the albumin adjustment does not refine the exposure estimate. While

https://doi.org/10.3390/toxins18010032

this observation is valid, it does create difficulty when examining epidemiological studies (and or interventions involving aflatoxin exposure) when trying to compare aflatoxin exposures between studies. A crude estimate can be created with a conversion based on infant age and the serum concentration of albumin. Infants under the age of 1 year have a serum albumin concentration of 0.019–0.048 mg/μL [74]; thus, 1 pg AF-lysine/ul of serum is equivalent to 21–53 pg/mg of AF-alb. After the first year, the normal range of albumin is 0.034–0.042 mg/μL, while after 3 years is 0.035–0.056 mg/μL. This converts a 1 pg/μL measure to a range of 24–29 pg/mg, and 18–29 pg/mg, respectively, with a caveat that this does not include individuals with protein malnutrition, potentially further complicating these estimates.

Where individuals are chronically exposed to aflatoxin, the physiological half-life of the AF-alb adduct can be interpreted such that any given measurement of the adduct provides an integrated estimate of exposure over 2–3 months, smoothing within and across day variations in exposure [41,61,64]. This characteristic means that AF-alb is extremely useful to examine the relationship between exposure to aflatoxin and stunting in regions with a high frequency and variation in aflatoxin contamination of the diet. Typically, more developed world regions, such as Western Europe and North America, will not have detectable AF-alb, while many developing world regions, such as those within sub-Saharan Africa, parts of Central America, and Asia, frequently observe AF-alb in sera [19,24,26,27,65]. In some regions, greater than 90% of individuals, randomly recruited from rural populations in sub-Saharan Africa, have detectable AF-alb, and sometimes across a 3-log range of exposure [75–77], while in Canada and the USA, the majority of the samples are below the LOD [27]. Regions such as Brazil and Egypt are thought to be intermediate in exposure [18,19,26,27]. Of note, these historic patterns are likely to shift over time, based on predictive modeling of climate change [78–80].

5. Associations Between Aflatoxin Exposure and Early Life Stunting

Several animal models have clearly demonstrated the negative effects of aflatoxins on growth, including stunting [81]. Over the last 25 years, several groups have investigated the role of aflatoxin in stunting in human populations. Current reviews tend to report mixed associations, but typically lack critique of the study designs, and a limited understanding of patterns of aflatoxin exposure coupled with a probable variable threshold, discussed later. In this review, Tables 1 and 2 report several of the published surveys of aflatoxin exposure and stunting, noting, however, that these are representative examples for illustrative purposes and not a systematic review of the evidence. Several studies use stunting as a response outcome with reference to aflatoxin, while others report HAZ (or LAZ) with reference to aflatoxin. Studies are divided into cross-sectional, Table 1 (weaker design), longitudinal, Table 2 (intermediate design), and two interventions, no table (stronger design).

Table 1. Key Cross-sectional studies investigating aflatoxin and either HAZ or being stunted.

Country	Age and n		AF-alb/pg/mg Range and Average		HAZ Stunted p-Value		Standard Used ^	Analysis ^^	Ref.
BeninTogo	9–60 mth	479	nd–1000	GM 33	<0.001	n/d	UoL	ELISA	[75,76]
Gambia	6–9 yrs	472	nd–256	GM 22	>0.05	n/d	UoL	ELISA	[50]
Egypt	1–54 mth	46	Serum AFB1	n/r	n/a		Comm *	TLC	[82]
Kenya	7–19 yrs	199	nd–750	GM 111	**		UoL	ELISA	[83]

https://doi.org/10.3390/toxins18010032

Table 1. *Cont.*

Country	Age and n		AF-alb/pg/mg Range and Average		HAZ Stunted p-Value		Standard Used ^	Analysis ^^	Ref.
Zambia	6–24	311	1–315	GM 6	n/d	$p = 0.02$	CDC ***	LC-MS/MS	[84]
Pakistan	1–11 yrs	238	1–56	Med 11	n/d	$p > 0.05$	UoG	HPLC-F	[85]

mth—month, yrs—years, nd—non-detect, n/d—non-determined, GM—Geometric mean. Med—Median, n/r—not relevant ^ Standard used—AF-lysine is not commercially available and was synthesized by individual research groups: UoL—University of Leeds, UK, CDC—Center for Disease Control, USA; UoG—University of Georgia, USA. ^^ ELISA Enzyme-linked Immunosorbent Assay—in-house; TLC—Thin Layer Chromatography; LC-MS/MS—Liquid Chromatography with Mass Spectrometry; HPLC-F—High Performance Liquid Chromatography with Fluorescence, * Comm—commercial purchase—but AFB1 is a measure that exposure has occurred, but cannot be used to quantify exposure. ** height was compared to AF exposure—which is not relevant. *** Uncertain of the source of the standard.

Table 2. Longitudinal studies of aflatoxin and stunting 40.4 pg/mg (range 4.8–260.8 pg/mg).

Country	Age and n		AF-alb Range pg/mg and Average	HAZ Stunted p-Value		Standard Used ^	Analysis ^^	Ref.
Benin	24–36	200	T1 * T2 nd–1500 5 T3	<0.001	n/d	UoL	ELISA	[77]
Gambia	<12	138	Preg 5–261 40 16 Wk 5–30 9	<0.05	n/d	UoL	ELISA	[86]
Tanzania	6–14	166	T1 n/d 5 T2 n/d 13 T3 n/d 24	>0.05	n/d	UoL	ELISA	[87]
Nepal	12–36	85	T1 n/d 4 T2 n/d 3 T3 n/d 4	>0.05	n/d	JHU	LC-MS/MS	[88]
Gambia	6–18	374	T1 n/d 3 T2 n/d 25 T3 n/d 52	<0.05	n/d	UoL	ELISA	[89]
Bangladesh	7–36	228	T1 <0.1–6 Mn 1 T2 <0.1–6 2 T3 <0.1–66 3 T4 <0.1–127 4	Overall $p > 0.05$		JHU	LC-MS/MS	[90]
Ethiopia	6–35	102	75th percentile < LOD	>0.05	n/d	UoC	LC-MS/MM	[91]
Nepal	3–22	1484	Preg <0.4–147 2 T1 <0.4–25 1 T2 <0.4–54 1 T3 <0.4–85 1 T4 <0.4–128 1	$p = 0.003$	$p = 0.005$	UoG	HPLC-F	[92]
MALAWI	<30	241	AF-lysine pg/uL	<0.05	n/d	JHU	LC-MS/MS	[73]

T = time point for multiple collections, Preg—during pregnancy, * Average of three > 98% of Ts had detectable AF-alb. nd—non-detect, n/d—no data. Average is the Geometric mean unless stated. Mn—arithmetic mean. ^ Standard used—AF-lysine is not commercially available and was synthesized by individual research groups: UoL—University of Leeds, UK; UoG—University of Georgia, USA; JHU—Johns Hopkins University, USA. ^^ ELISA Enzyme-linked Immunosorbent Assay—in-house; LC-MS/MS—Liquid Chromatography with Mass Spectrometry; HPLC-F—High Performance Liquid Chromatography with Fluorescence.

6. Cross-Sectional Studies

The seminal biomarker-driven epidemiological study to assess the relationship between aflatoxin exposure and stunting was a cross-sectional design, conducted in Benin and Togo, that examined anthropometry and serum AF-alb in nearly 500 young children, aged 9–60 months [75,76]. It is important to note that the AF-alb concentration was assessed by ELISA at the University of Leeds (UoL). A strong inverse dose–response relationship was observed between the aflatoxin biomarker and HAZ ($p < 0.001$). Figure 2 identifies a possible threshold below which a log fold variation in AF-alb provides no observable effect on stunting, while a dose–response effect is observed at higher doses. The range of

https://doi.org/10.3390/toxins18010032

detectable AF-alb in this survey was <3 pg/mg to >1000 pg/mg, and an AF-alb threshold level at perhaps 50 pg/mg. This putative point of deviation has not formerly been determined, and if such a threshold exists, it is likely to vary individually and by study location based on additional gene-environment-nutritional factors for any given population. Linear growth retardation in the early years of life is especially important because the majority of stunted children do not regain a healthy growth trajectory and are likely to suffer irreversible developmental effects. In Benin, the strongest effect of aflatoxin on HAZ was in those three years or less [75,76].

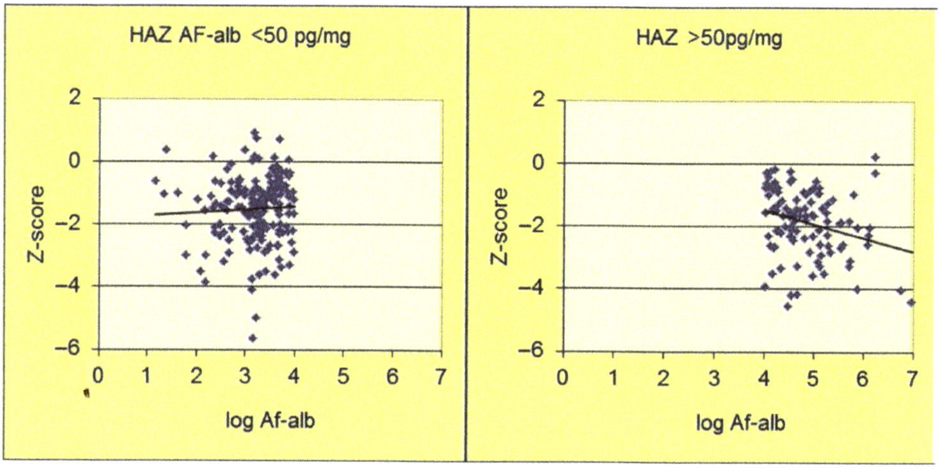

Figure 2. AF-alb versus HAZ scatterplot (adapted from Gong et al., [77]). Scatterplot divided into two sections to highlight a potential point of departure at an AF-alb of about 50 pg/mg. HAZ—Height for Age Z score. AF-alb—aflatoxin-albumin.

Other cross-sectional studies [50,82–85] are often reported in the literature reviews, and a modest examination of Table 1 reveals significant design differences. For example, when child growth was examined in The Gambia in relation to aflatoxin exposure [50], the authors reported no statistically significant relationship with stunting. However, the age is significantly greater (6–9 yrs), and notably, the Benin and Togo study [75,76] suggested the effect on growth is more prevalent in those 3 yrs and younger. In the Gambian study, the aflatoxin exposure, again measured as above by ELISA, is high and of concern (some individuals at >100 pg/mg), but does not reach the very high levels in Benin and Togo. To put this into context, no detection of this biomarker was observed in sera from 200 Canadian individuals [18,26], where the limit of detection (LOD) was 3 pg/mg using the same ELISA assay; and less than 1% of individual from a US-NHANES survey of >2000 samples [93] were above the LOD of 0.4 pg/mg using an LC-MS/MS assay. Additionally, the Gambian study involved children who were part of a nutritional supplementation initiative, thus, further complicating any comparisons between aflatoxin and growth. The study in Egypt [82] has been cited in reviews, though it appears to measure AFB1 directly in blood samples. This is not a validated quantitative biomarker of aflatoxin exposure and can only really identify recently exposed versus recently non-exposed individuals; thus, this provides little value in assessing a relationship between typical aflatoxin exposure and stunting.

Aflatoxin exposure measures were added to a pre-existing Kenyan survey involving children and adolescents [83] in an attempt to provide a mechanism for aflatoxin-induced stunting; again, AF-alb concentrations were determined by the previously mentioned ELISA. However, the authors response variable is height rather than HAZ, which has lim-

 https://doi.org/10.3390/toxins18010032

ited value in a cross-sectional study of children over a 12-year age range (6–17 years of age). Younger children consume more per kg bodyweight compared to older adolescents, and thus, an artificial gradient of AF-alb and height across this range may appear statistically significant, but not toxicologically relevant, nor useful. The group also proposed changes in insulin-like growth binding protein-3 (IGFBP-3) as a potential mechanism. IGFBP-3 is a protein that controls the availability of insulin-like growth factor (IGF), and its availability is critical to child growth and development. However, over this same 12-year age range, it would be predicted to change in line with height, so again provides no usable evaluation to suggest a mechanism.

Other cross-sectional studies used an alternate assay for AF-alb; thus, it is important to note that only three labs have conducted cross-comparison studies of their analytical assay for AF-alb. In the first study, sera were analyzed at the UoL by ELISA, the US Center for Disease Control by HPLC-F, and Johns Hopkins University (JHU) by LC-MS/MS; in a second, distinct survey, sera were analyzed by two of the same assays but only involved UoL and JHU. While there was a strong correlation of both data sets, the ELISA, on average, reports levels roughly 5× higher than the LC-MS/MS [67,69]; thus, adjustment for this difference is suggested when comparing studies. A study in Zambia [84] provides a statistically significant relationship between AF-alb biomarker concentration (by LC-MS/MS) and being stunted. Moreover, AF-alb concentrations appear much lower in this survey compared to the Benin and Togo study [75,76]; this apparent discrepancy does not remain after adjustment for differences in analytical approach. In addition, only three of the laboratories have reported any collaborative comparison of standards used. This is particularly critical as the AF-lysine standard used by all laboratories is not commercially available and tends to be synthesized separately in each laboratory. This presents a major hurdle for any review of the evidence of aflatoxin and stunting to overcome and is often ignored in such review papers.

Finally, a cross-sectional study of children aged 1–11 years failed to find an association between AF-alb and stunting [85]. AF-alb was frequent and appeared to be at similar levels to that of the Gambian study [50]. Again, this modest-sized cross-sectional study of children over an extensive 11-year age range is poorly designed to identify causes of stunting, as there are such profound changes over such a disparate physiological range of other growth drivers; and as previously indicated, stunting was most strongly associated with aflatoxin exposure in those three and under [75,76].

In summary, it is difficult to reach any solid conclusions looking at the cross-sectional data presented, not because associations do not agree, but rather, because few studies are even closely related in terms of design, age, and/or use of an exposure tool. Where a strong effect was reported, this was in the 3-year and under category, where a 3-log range of AF-alb occurred.

7. Longitudinal Studies

The team at the UoL followed up on their cross-sectional study in Benin and Togo with a novel cohort to conduct a longitudinal survey in 200 Beninese children aged 1–3 years, assessing growth velocity over 8 months [77]. AF-alb was measured in all children on three occasions, start, middle, and end; again, noting each AF-alb measurement is an integrated estimate of exposure over the previous 2–3 months. AF-alb was observed in all children on at least two occasions, and contamination occurred over a 3-log range. Those infants in the highest quartile of AF-alb concentration were observed to be on average 1.7 cm shorter than those in the lowest quartile of AF-alb, after 8 months ($p < 0.001$). This study represents one of the strongest associations between aflatoxin exposure and growth faltering (as stunting) to date.

 https://doi.org/10.3390/toxins18010032

A longitudinal study followed the growth of Gambian infants from age 6 to 18 months (n = 374), with serum AF-alb measured by ELISA at 6, 12, and 18 months [89]. Anthropometry was obtained at these time points and at 6 months post-blood collection. Inverse relationships were observed between AF-alb and HAZ ($p = 0.015$). AF-alb at 12 months was associated with changes in HAZ between 12 and 18 months of age $p = 0.003$. AF-alb at 6 months was also associated with IGFBP-3 at 12 months ($p = 0.04$), but not for any of the other comparisons they report. A more recent study of Gambian infants identified a relationship between aflatoxin exposure and epigenetic patterns, including changes in methylation of genes involving in part several growth factors [52]. Thus, AF induced modulation of growth by changes in growth factors remains a plausible mechanism of AF induced growth faltering.

A study in Tanzania investigated AF-alb exposure, using ELISA, in relation to growth by following infants for 1 year [87]. Infants (n = 166) were recruited at 6–14 months of age with measures at this baseline and subsequently after 6 and 12 months. Overall AF exposure increased on average as the infants aged in the study; a statistically significant relationship between AF-alb exposure and HAZ was not observed, although a trend was noted. AF-alb detection was frequent but of the order of about a log lower than in the Benin study, perhaps explaining the lack of an observed association.

In a distinct study design, maternal AF-alb was used as a proxy for in utero exposure to aflatoxin [86]. This survey in The Gambia assessed in utero aflatoxin exposure (via two maternal blood draws during pregnancy) in relation to infant growth from birth to age one year, n = 138. Infant anthropometry was recorded from birth and then every 4 weeks up to age 1 year, and these data were compared to maternal average AF-alb measurements. The maternal AF-alb concentration (geometric mean 40 pg/mg, range 5–261 pg/mg) was strongly inversely associated with both weight ($p = 0.012$) and height ($p = 0.044$) gain. The authors predicted that a reduction in maternal AF-alb from 110 pg/mg to 10 pg/mg would lead to a 0.8 kg increase in weight and a 2 cm increase in height by age 1 year. Turner et al. [83] also noted that complementary foods were introduced to 11% of the infants prior to 16 weeks of age, and a 16-week blood draw highlighted that these infants were the only ones to have detectable AF-alb. This additional early life aflatoxin exposure further strongly predicted growth faltering in these infants up to 1 year of age. AF-alb frequency in these Gambian mothers was similar, but adduct concentration was slightly lower than that in Benin infants discussed above. These data suggest that in utero AF may lead to stunting in infancy and that this is further impacted by early introduction of AF contaminated complementary foods; foods that were introduced significantly in advance of WHO recommendations on infant feeding [1]. The relatively small size of this Gambian study, however, limits its generalizability. A separate survey suggested that aflatoxin appears to modulate growth-related gene methylation in infants, where mothers were exposed during pregnancy [53]; thus, supporting early suggestions of a mechanism.

Two studies, one in Bangladesh and one in Ethiopia, found no association between aflatoxin exposure and infant growth, though in both studies the AF-alb adduct was relatively modest [90,91]. The lack of a significant gradient of exposure likely explains the lack of association, as discussed for several cross-sectional analyses. Somewhat surprisingly, a longitudinal survey in Nepal reported statistically significant associations between aflatoxin exposure and infants being stunted, despite very modest aflatoxin exposure in this population [92]. Noting, however, the study is large (n = 1484), providing greater statistical power compared to most, and has multiple exposure measures (four) over the first 18 months post birth. Here, the ranges of exposure are non-detect to only 147 pg/mg, but the geometric means at each collection are all < 2 pg/mg. The AF-lysine here was measured by HPLC with fluorescence (HPLC-F), and no data comparison from that lab in

https://doi.org/10.3390/toxins18010032

Athens, not CDC, with other methods is reported in the literature. Again, this serves to highlight a major hurdle when comparing studies. Noting where two labs perform their own distinct digestion/extraction and then quantify AF-lys using their own synthesized standards, readers cannot assume the data to be identical just because they both state detection by HPLC-F, which may also have distinct characteristics. However, there is about a 2–3 log variation in biomarker concentration reported in the Nepal study [92]. If HPLC-F and ELISA were providing similar estimates of exposure, then one possible explanation, though speculative, is that Nepalese infants are more sensitive to aflatoxin than sub-Saharan African infants.

The modeling of data in all these longitudinal studies also creates some difficulty. Given the duration and repetition of sampling, it becomes reasonable to think about models that adjust for age and perhaps season. However, age and season are not necessarily independent. Additionally, in some high-risk regions for stunting and aflatoxin exposure, in the first couple of years of life, there are seasonal variations in aflatoxin and food availability. There are also age-dependent changes in intestinal enteropathy and linear growth; thus, in models looking for associations between aflatoxin exposure and stunting, adjustment for age and season may be confounding on both the exposure and the outcome. As these studies evolve to become larger, models that additionally involve subgroup characterization will be valuable. In the Nepalese study, authors also adjusted their statistical model for detect versus non-detect, and the purpose is not clear, given that non-detects were assigned a value.

One study in Malawi involving large numbers of infants followed over a period of 2 years reports a high frequency and range of aflatoxin exposure, and they observe a significant correlation between aflatoxin exposure and stunting. Authors report using pg AF-lysine per ul serum using LC-MS/MS, and crude estimates indicate that 25% of the study population likely exceeds an equivalent of >125 pg/mg (after adjustment) in comparison to the ELISA data [67,69].

A study in Mexico (not included in Table 2) that recruited infants at about 8 months of age and followed for 4 months (including a blood draw for AF-alb) and again at 10 months post-baseline (without a blood draw) [94]. In one model, authors observed a modest improvement in infant growth in relation to aflatoxin at 4 months but not at 10 months, and suggest a hormesis response. Other models in their supplementary section do not see any strong effects. While the detection frequency for AF-alb was high, the concentrations were very modest (0.84 pg/mg, SD 0.7 pg/mg), and the range likely falls within sampling and extraction error when it comes to the ability to accurately estimate exposure using this biomarker. This typical error in exposure estimate is only relevant in studies with very modest AF-alb variation; in general, this remains un-discussed in most aflatoxin papers [18,27]. Here, it creates some uncertainty in interpreting this finding as hormesis. However, aflatoxin-driven hormesis has been suggested in animals [95], and perhaps this modest effect is typically missed in studies with larger aflatoxin distributions. The Mexican study also includes dietary supplementation, and it is unclear if this has influenced the aflatoxin hormesis effect.

Overall, longitudinal studies are somewhat more informative, and studies with larger gradients of aflatoxin exposure are more likely to reveal an effect.

8. Intervention Designs

A cluster randomized controlled study in Kenya used 28 intervention and 28 control clusters to examine the effect of aflatoxin intervention on improving infant growth [96]. In the intervention arm, local (predicted contaminated) maize was replaced with aflatoxin-safe maize throughout the study. Women in the fifth to final month of pregnancy were invited

 https://doi.org/10.3390/toxins18010032

to enroll in the study, and infants were assessed at mid-point (age 11 months) and end point (19 months). The main health outcome was HAZ in relation to the study arm at the end point. At the end point, authors claim a significant difference in aflatoxin exposure but not HAZ. Conversion of their Ln transformed AF-alb data reveals geometric means AF-alb of 5.9 pg/mg (95%CI: 5.3, 6.7, n = 436) in the intervention, and 7.5 pg/mg (95%CI: 6.5, 8.5, n = 362) in the control, thus while statistically significant (using $p < 0.05$), toxicologically we would not expect to see differences across this small range. The study seems well designed from an epidemiological standpoint but failed to create a sufficient gradient of exposure across arms. It may also have had a level of aflatoxin exposure that was irrelevant in stunting—see next section. A similar but larger study design in Tanzania aimed to provide aflatoxin-safe flours to 1500 infants from 6 to 18 months and examine the effect of this intervention compared to a control population consuming their normal household flours. The flours consisted of either maize, groundnut, or a mix of maize and groundnut, used in the production of complementary foods in this region [97,98]. Both arms additionally received nutritional and hygiene guidance throughout, with the aim to balance these across arms [99,100]. Several preliminary studies were conducted and revealed (i) a variable and sometimes high level of aflatoxin in typical dietary staples, (ii) a strong acceptance by the infants of the supplied flours, and (iii) a significant reduction in a urinary biomarker (urinary AFM1) after 1 week involving a transition to the aflatoxin-safe flours [101,102]. The study recruited infants into an intervention or control arm (n = 25 hubs for each) based on accessibility to a health center hub. Control and intervention arm hubs were matched for population size and elevation above sea level. The study recruited into both arms monthly over 12 months when infants were <6 months old, and the main study started at 6 months. Mean HAZ was not statistically different between arms at 6 months, and in both arms decreased (HAZ became worse) over the next year, as infants reached 18 months of age. A statistically significant difference in HAZ was not observed at the mid-point, nor at the study end point (though 12-month WAZ and 12- and 18-month MUAC did show statistically significant differences). Food measures for aflatoxin in a subgroup revealed only a modest, albeit statistically significant reduction in maize and groundnut flour contamination [103]. However, in the main study, the use of AF-alb biomarkers (using a novel LC-MS/MS) did not reveal a sufficient gradient in aflatoxin exposure had been achieved between arms [104]. Thus, this second randomized controlled study was ethically designed to target the infant diet and isolate the effect of aflatoxin consumption; however, the natural variation in AF contamination over several years in this region meant the study failed to create an exposure gradient that could test the central hypothesis.

9. Complexity of Demonstrating Effective Interventions That Reduce Aflatoxin and Modify Linear Growth

The studies described above that examined the relationship between aflatoxin and either HAZ (or stunting) or attempted to modify the effect on growth via intervention clearly brought up issues on study design and implementation. One highlighted issue is the use of an appropriate biomarker of exposure. In most of the examples discussed, this has been the well-established AF-alb, where in chronically exposed populations a single measurement effectively provides an integrated measure of exposure over several months. At this point, this is the ideal quantitative measure, and while AFM1 in urine could be used, it is more susceptible to shorter-term variation, and urinary AFB1 itself is not useful [18,27,54]. In accepting the AF-alb biomarker, part of the complexity in trying to examine and compare the data within these studies is simply the lack of standardization of two of the analytes typically used, namely a mono-adducted AF-alb as a control material for enzymic digestion, and the AF-lysine residue used for quantitation. Both are typically

 https://doi.org/10.3390/toxins18010032

synthesized in-house, and with a couple of exceptions, no comparative assessments have been made. In one evaluation a specific LC-MS/MS method was compared with an ELISA, and though there was a strong correlation with the two methods, the ELISA typically gave about a 5 x higher adduct measure, possibly as it was influenced by additional AF-residues such as AFG1-lysine and/or incomplete AF-alb digestion that may contain AF-lysine but attached to one or more additional amino acids. Neither residue would be identified by LC-MS/MS due to the specificity of that assay [18,54]. Therefore, where these two assays are used, data adjustment can be attempted. However, there may be alternate assay-specific components that explain this difference, and thus, caution is needed in using this comparison adjustment for other/novel LC-MS/MS approaches. Thus, a concerted effort among multiple players is required to better amalgamate the exposure tools, and this remains a major hurdle. In this respect, the extent of data reporting could be improved. Some studies report GM and 95%CI, others mean and SD, some give ranges, and others, median and IQR. Some of the early studies reported more fully the distribution of data, and this may be valuable as outlined below. Often, we do not know what the distribution of data is, and a simple addition of an appendix showing box and whisker plots or simple distribution bar charts would be useful.

Figure 3 suggests two possible distributions of aflatoxin exposure (as measured by AF-alb) in relation to an aflatoxin-suggested role in the modification of linear growth. Readers are urged not to overinterpret the minor details of the figures. The hypothetical figures are based on the idea that there is going to be a distribution of HAZ scores in any population, but here, a gradient of AF exposure is highlighted as a major driver of changes in HAZ. The y-axis represents HAZ, and the extended diamond shapes represent possible distributions of HAZ. The x-axis is the AF-alb by group across multiple log increases. The values are based crudely on the ELISA data reported, but readers could envisage adjustment, where available, for other analytical tools as described above. The width of the diamonds is meant to crudely represent the number of individuals in that AF-alb group, which is also indicated by "n" at the top of each group. The widest part of the diamond is at the median HAZ for that group. The background shading of the groups is simply to reinforce the idea of moving to a higher AF-alb group as you go from left to right. Both scenarios suggest there may be a threshold below which aflatoxin has no clear effect. The threshold suggested here is for illustrative purposes, though it is roughly in line with data suggested by surveys in Benin and Togo [75–77], where the ELISA was used.

In scenario 1, each exposure group would have roughly equal numbers of infants with the given exposure across a wide range, noting that such a scenario has never been reported in any study to our knowledge. However, if this were the distribution that existed in a high-risk part of the globe, then we could readily observe a large percentage of the population with aflatoxin exposures that have no effect on HAZ, but also a large percentage where aflatoxin had quite a strong effect. In those where aflatoxin had an effect, there is an apparent dose–response component, but also a large amount of variation in HAZ in any given exposure group that is independent and/or additional to the aflatoxin effect. Thus, one could predict that a modest-sized study population may allow a statistically significant association between aflatoxin and HAZ to be observed. It also would indicate that an intervention to reduce AF exposure would be well-positioned to see a reduction in average AF-alb, and if causal, a reduction that then modifies HAZ. This figure also can be used to illustrate that in a region with more modest range of aflatoxin, perhaps only involving exposure in the lower three groups, that a high frequency of exposure could be observed, a gradient of aflatoxin exposure could be observed, and an intervention that successfully reduced exposure could be demonstrated, but crucially, no effect on growth occurs; i.e., a threshold is not reached in the control to create a toxicologically relevant

 https://doi.org/10.3390/toxins18010032

gradient, despite a gradient existing. Many studies report a high frequency of exposure, but perhaps a non-effect of aflatoxin on growth is simply indicative of failing to reach this suggested threshold.

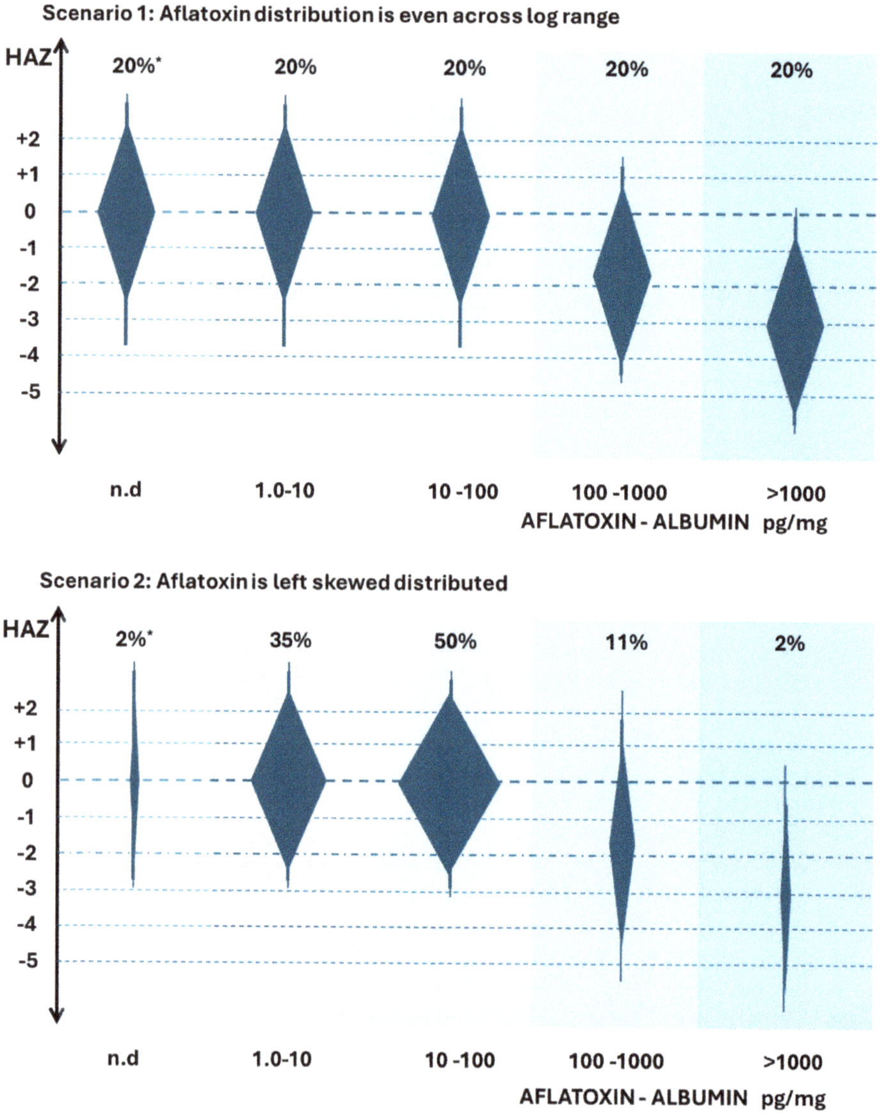

Figure 3. Hypothetical distributions of HAZ in relation to Aflatoxin exposure by group. AF exposure in groups is indicated by aflatoxin-albumin (pg/mg), noting groups log increments. The extended diamond shapes are indicators of HAZ distribution, width is indicative of the suggested distribution of individuals in any group of that aflatoxin exposure, * indicative of the % distribution. All scenarios are based on aflatoxin being a major driver of stunting. Readers are advised not to overinterpret the precision of the data—but rather focus on the changes in distributions. Data are based on the author's interpretation of studies demonstrating a broad range of aflatoxin exposure in studies on stunting, while the AF-alb values suggested are crudely based on ELISA estimates [75–77]. n.d. means non detected.

https://doi.org/10.3390/toxins18010032

In Scenario 2, a more realistic distribution of AF-alb groups is proposed, a distribution based on a high-risk aflatoxin region, but highly left-skewed. Many studies show this left skew of aflatoxin exposure data, as reviewed [18]. In this scenario, the vast majority of the exposure fails to meet a suggested threshold that would impact HAZ, and the exposure concentrations associated with stunting are restricted to a relatively small percentage of the population. Modestly sized studies would likely not observe a statistically significant effect of aflatoxin on stunting, and the early sections of this review are typically only reporting associations where there was both a large gradient of exposure and a large study size. It could also be expected that intervention studies involving a control arm and an intervention arm would need to be extremely large in order to determine an effect, and that a study with a more modest range of exposure could demonstrate a successful reduction with no impact on HAZ, as described for scenario 1.

The aflatoxin exposure situation is, however, more complex. Figure 4 attempts to additionally portray changes in aflatoxin exposure over time with both ages (food behavior aspect) and seasonality of exposure due to additional accumulation of aflatoxin in food that is in prolonged storage post-harvest [19]. The frequently observed pattern is that aflatoxin accumulates both in the field and in storage, but settings with poor and prolonged storage strongly drive the risk. At birth, infants may be exposed to relatively modest amounts of aflatoxin as the lipophilic toxin can transfer to breast milk if present in the mother's diet. Typically, as complementary foods are introduced, exposure significantly increases, and during the first two years of life, AF exposure slowly transitions to levels and frequencies seen in older children and adults, and unless the diet and agricultural practices around the diet change, essentially remains similar throughout life, as previously reviewed [18]. Seasonality plays a significant role, typically with the period around harvest having significantly lower (albeit unacceptable levels), and around 4–8 months post-harvest, levels significantly rise. Several studies report on such typical patterns (reviewed by [18]).

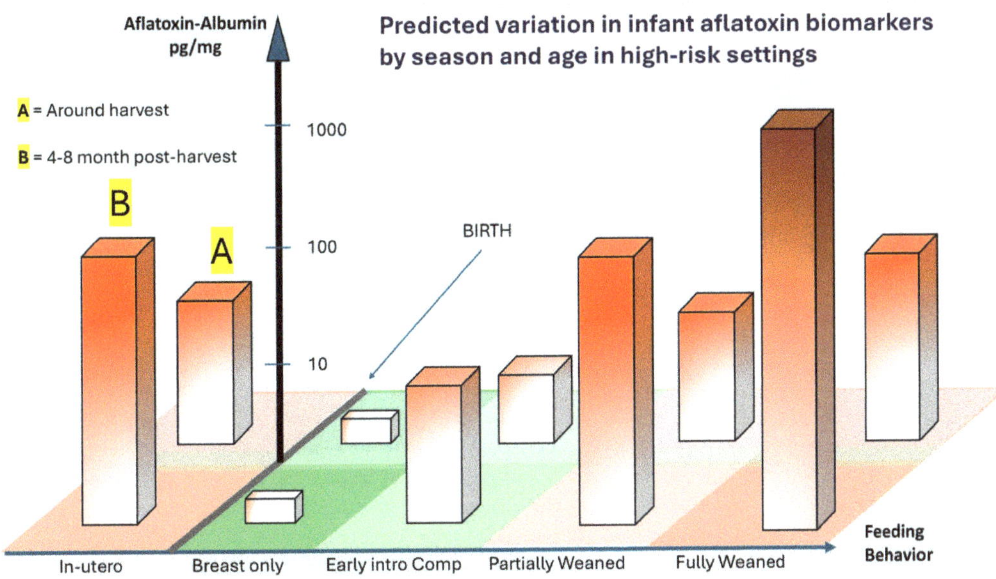

Figure 4. Hypothetical age and seasonal variation in AF-alb in a high-risk setting. Early intro Comp = Early introduction to complementary foods. Proposed scenario of AF exposure estimated by

https://doi.org/10.3390/toxins18010032

AF-alb measures in early life in a high-risk setting, such as for subsistence or small-hold farmers in sub-Saharan Africa, from in utero through to the infant being fully weaned. The exclusive breastfeeding period is proposed to be highly protective of exposure. The bars are deliberately shaded to indicate that, in any given time frame, there is a range of likely exposures. The probable magnitude of those distributions increases with age, as diets increasingly move away from breast milk and onto high-risk foods, including groundnuts and maize. Seasonal variation is suggested using a crude dichotomy—*back section* (A) harvest is lower risk, and *front section* (B) at 4–8 months post-harvest with a higher risk. Noting that the bars are distributions, some younger infants will have higher levels of AF-alb than older; and some infants in section A will have higher AF-alb than those in section B. A checkered base to the figure is in place simply to assist the reader in identifying groups. Figure is suggested by one interpretation of data from multiple studies, and AF-alb estimates using ELISA [50,75–77,86]. Readers are encouraged to focus on the pattern rather than overinterpret the precision of any individual suggested data point in terms of AF-alb values.

Figure 4 serves to visually describe this transition at birth from being relatively aflatoxin-free to being at risk of exposure, but that exposure is dependent upon both diet and the timing of consumption. The units of AF-alb are roughly based on those using ELISA to quantify [50,75–77,86]. The figure deliberately uses shading of color to imply a higher exposure at certain stages. The bars should be interpreted as infants having the potential to fall somewhere within the bar, not that all will be at the maximum. Rather, there will be a distribution of data as implied by Figure 3, scenario 2. Thus, in utero exposure can be high, but has quite a potential range, and such high exposures have been associated with infant growth faltering. Then, following birth, there may be quite a significant fluctuation in exposure.

Given the seasonality of exposure, it will be important to understand if there are any critical windows in which exposure to high levels causes greater toxicity. For example, it is plausible to think of two groups of infants that from 6 months to 18 months have the same average level of aflatoxin exposure, but if critical windows exist, is it perhaps more harmful if most of that exposure occurs at 6–10 months of age versus 14–18 months of age; simply based on timing of birth and local harvest timing of the groundnut and maize crops, this remains unexplored. Intervention approaches need to be sufficiently large to account for aflatoxin distribution at any given time, how that varies by season, and how that may be impacted by the timing of the introduction of at-risk foods. The patterns of aflatoxin contamination and, therefore, exposure should not be taken as constant. Annual variation in these patterns can occur and was suggested as a major issue in a recent randomized case–control study [104]. In that pilot study, data indicated significant frequency and levels of exposure, though a suggested change in climate conditions during the 18 months of the main study negatively impacted conditions for aflatoxin production in the control arm; thus, it impacted the ability of the study to show a gradient of exposure between the two arms.

10. Recommendations

Aflatoxin has been associated with poor linear growth in several settings and typically occurs where there is a wide gradient of exposure. There are other components that will influence linear growth, including diet and gastrointestinal disease, as well as genetics. When considering diet and hygiene, these may either confound the studies or may be notable components to examine interactions. Such interactions may be important to understand, as modest changes to all three may have a larger-than-expected effect on improving growth. Recommendations from this review include the following:

I. A network is established among aflatoxin researchers to share standards and compare methods, as suggested by Prof David Miller, Dr Mark Sumarah, and other colleagues during one of the Gordon Research Conferences (personal communication)

 https://doi.org/10.3390/toxins18010032

II. When AF-alb data related (or unrelated) to stunting is generated, authors better describe the distribution of the data. Such data should be shared in a public repository, as it is becoming more of the standard of funders and publication best practice.

III. When designing studies, researchers consider the wide variation in aflatoxin exposures and that aflatoxin biomarker detection is not necessarily toxicologically relevant to stunting as an outcome, unless a suggested threshold is reached. That threshold is not clearly established at this point and may vary by study location and be based on exposure to other drivers of stunting. Establishment of this threshold through statistical studies of previously collected data would be beneficial.

IV. As indicated in Figure 4, researchers consider a larger life course in aflatoxin exposure and its intervention in relation to reducing the burden of stunting. This includes both in utero and over the first few years.

V. Aflatoxin is not the only chemical exposure associated with stunting. Fumonsins are an additional family of mycotoxin that are found in maize in regions that have aflatoxin issues, and may play an additional role, though studies remain limited on co-exposures [87,91].

11. Conclusions

Since the seminal studies by Gong and colleagues [75–77] that demonstrated strong dose–response relationships between aflatoxin exposure and poor linear growth in infants, many additional studies have been undertaken with mixed results. This review highlights that some at least are due to low exposure, inappropriate biomarkers, and possibly the wrong target population. In studies where an inverse effect between exposure and growth is observed, it could be argued, particularly in the cross-sectional studies, that AF-alb may only be a surrogate measure of malnutrition in an aflatoxin-exposed population; however, the strong evidence in animal studies would counter that argument [81]. Additional cross-sectional or longitudinal studies remain of interest, but causality will only really be established through large-scale intervention studies, where seasonality and other dietary components are well accounted for, as discussed by [104].

The requirement remains "if aflatoxin mitigation efforts in high-risk settings require infant stunting to be demonstrated in order to gain sufficient global traction to be effective in protecting the 100 of millions of people exposed to aflatoxin, larger scale studies covering an extensive in utero through early childhood period are essential". However, "gold-standard" level of evidence from a randomized trial is often preferred for decision making, we believe that ethical, nonexperimental, interventions are more appropriate for future studies assessing aflatoxin exposures during critical developmental periods. Given the well-documented negative health effects of aflatoxin, mitigating its consumption should be a public health priority.

Author Contributions: P.C.T. and E.P. conceptualized, wrote and reviewed this review. All authors have read and agreed to the published version of the manuscript.

Funding: This research received no external funding.

Institutional Review Board Statement: Not applicable.

Informed Consent Statement: Not applicable.

Data Availability Statement: No new data were created or analyzed in this study.

Conflicts of Interest: The authors declare no conflicts of interest.

 https://doi.org/10.3390/toxins18010032

References

1. United Nations Children's Fund (UNICEF); World Health Organization (WHO); International Bank for Reconstruction and Development/The World Bank. *Levels and Trends in Child Malnutrition: UNICEF/WHO/World Bank Group Joint Child Malnutrition Estimates: Key Findings of the 2023 Edition*; UNICEF: New York, NY, USA; WHO: Geneva, Switzerland, 2023.
2. Adair, L.S.; Fall, C.H.; Osmond, C.; Stein, A.D.; Martorell, R.; Ramirez-Zea, M.; Sachdev, H.S.; Dahly, D.L.; Bas, I.; Norris, S.A.; et al. Associations of linear growth and relative weight gain during early life with adult health and human capital in countries of low and middle income: Findings from five birth cohort studies. *Lancet* **2013**, *382*, 525–534. [CrossRef] [PubMed]
3. Prendergast, A.J.; Humphrey, J.H. The stunting syndrome in developing countries. *Paediatr. Int. Child Health* **2014**, *34*, 250–265. [CrossRef]
4. Black, R.E.; Victora, C.G.; Walker, S.P.; Bhutta, Z.A.; Christian, P.; de Onis, M.; Ezzati, M.; Grantham-McGregor, S.; Katz, J.; Martorell, R.; et al. Maternal and Child Nutrition Study Group. Maternal and child undernutrition and overweight in low-income and middle-income countries. *Lancet* **2013**, *382*, 427–451. [CrossRef]
5. Vaivada, T.; Akseer, N.; Akseer, S.; Somaskandan, A.; Stefopulos, M.; Bhutta, Z.A. Stunting in childhood: An overview of global burden, trends, determinants, and drivers of decline. *Am. J. Clin. Nutr.* **2020**, *112*, 777S–791S. [CrossRef]
6. WHO Multicentre Growth Reference Study Group (WHO); de Onis, M. WHO Child Growth Standards based on length/height, weight and age. *Acta Paediatr.* **2006**, *95*, 76–85. [CrossRef]
7. Luby, S.P.; Rahman, M.; Arnold, B.F.; Unicomb, L.; Ashraf, S.; Winch, P.J.; Stewart, C.P.; Begum, F.; Hussain, F.; Benjamin-Chung, J.; et al. Effects of water quality, sanitation, handwashing, and nutritional interventions on diarrhoea and child growth in rural Bangladesh: A cluster randomised controlled trial. *Lancet Glob. Health* **2018**, *6*, e302–e315. [CrossRef]
8. Humphrey, J.H.; Mbuya, M.N.N.; Ntozini, R.; Moulton, L.H.; Stoltzfus, R.J.; Tavengwa, N.V.; Mutasa, K.; Majo, F.; Mutasa, B.; Mangwadu, G.; et al. Sanitation Hygiene Infant Nutrition Efficacy (SHINE) Trial Team. Independent and combined effects of improved water, sanitation, and hygiene, and improved complementary feeding, on child stunting and anaemia in rural Zimbabwe: A cluster-randomised trial. *Lancet Glob. Health* **2019**, *7*, e132–e147. [CrossRef] [PubMed]
9. Null, C.; Stewart, C.P.; Pickering, A.J.; Dentz, H.N.; Arnold, B.F.; Arnold, C.D.; Benjamin-Chung, J.; Clasen, T.; Dewey, K.G.; Fernald, L.C.H.; et al. Effects of water quality, sanitation, handwashing, and nutritional interventions on diarrhoea and child growth in rural Kenya: A cluster-randomised controlled trial. *Lancet Glob. Health* **2018**, *6*, e316–e329. [CrossRef] [PubMed]
10. Victora, C.G.; Christian, P.; Vidaletti, L.P.; Gatica-Domínguez, G.; Menon, P.; Black, R.E. Revisiting maternal and child undernutrition in low-income and middle-income countries: Variable progress towards an unfinished agenda. *Lancet* **2021**, *397*, 1388–1399. [CrossRef]
11. Stevens, G.A.; Beal, T.; Mbuya, M.N.N.; Luo, H.; Neufeld, L.M. Global Micronutrient Deficiencies Research Group. Micronutrient deficiencies among preschool-aged children and women of reproductive age worldwide: A pooled analysis of individual-level data from population-representative surveys. *Lancet Glob. Health* **2022**, *10*, e1590–e1599. [CrossRef]
12. Bhutta, Z.A.; Das, J.K.; Rizvi, A.; Gaffey, M.F.; Walker, N.; Horton, S.; Webb, P.; Lartey, A.; Black, R.E. Lancet Nutrition Interventions Review Group, the Maternal and Child Nutrition Study Group. Evidence-based interventions for improvement of maternal and child nutrition: What can be done and at what cost? *Lancet* **2013**, *382*, 452–477. [CrossRef]
13. Keats, E.C.; Das, J.K.; Salam, R.A.; Lassi, Z.S.; Imdad, A.; Black, R.E.; Bhutta, Z.A. Effective interventions to address maternal and child malnutrition: An update of the evidence. *Lancet Child Adolesc. Health* **2021**, *5*, 367–384. [CrossRef]
14. Lassi, Z.S.; Das, J.K.; Zahid, G.; Imdad, A.; Bhutta, Z.A. Impact of education and provision of complementary feeding on growth and morbidity in children less than 2 years of age in developing countries: A systematic review. *BMC Public Health* **2013**, *13*, S13. [CrossRef] [PubMed]
15. Lassi, Z.S.; Rind, F.; Irfan, O.; Hadi, R.; Das, J.K.; Bhutta, Z.A. Impact of Infant and Young Child Feeding (IYCF) Nutrition Interventions on Breastfeeding Practices, Growth and Mortality in Low- and Middle-Income Countries: Systematic Review. *Nutrients* **2020**, *12*, 722. [CrossRef]
16. Panjwani, A.; Heidkamp, R. Complementary Feeding Interventions Have a Small but Significant Impact on Linear and Ponderal Growth of Children in Low- and Middle-Income Countries: A Systematic Review and Meta-Analysis. *J. Nutr.* **2017**, *147*, 2169S–2178S. [CrossRef] [PubMed]
17. Dewey, K.G.; Adu-Afarwuah, S. Systematic review of the efficacy and effectiveness of complementary feeding interventions in developing countries. *Matern. Child Nutr.* **2008**, *4*, 24–85. [CrossRef]
18. Turner, P.C. The Molecular Epidemiology of Chronic Aflatoxin Driven Impaired Child growth. *Scientifica* **2013**, *2013*, 152879. [CrossRef]
19. International Agency for Research on Cancer (IARC). Human exposure to aflatoxins and fumonisins. In *Mycotoxin Control in Low- and Middle-Income Countries*; Wild, C.P., Groopman, J.D., Eds.; International Agency for Research on Cancer: Lyon, France, 2015.
20. Smith, L.E.; Prendergast, A.J.; Turner, P.C.; Mbuya, M.N.; Mutasa, K.; Kembo, G.; Stoltzfus, R.J. The Potential Role of Mycotoxins as a Contributor to Stunting in the SHINE Trial. *Clin. Infect. Dis.* **2015**, *61*, S733–S737. [CrossRef] [PubMed]

https://doi.org/10.3390/toxins18010032

21. Council for Agricultural Science and Technology (CAST). Mycotoxins: Risks in Plant, Animal and Human Systems. In *Potential Economic Costs of Mycotoxins in the United States*; Task Force Report; Council for Agricultural Science and Technology: Ames, IA, USA, 2003; pp. 136–142.
22. Miller, J.D. Fungi and Mycotoxins in Grain: Implications for Stored Product Research. *J. Stored Prod. Res.* **1995**, *31*, 1–16. [CrossRef]
23. Pitt, J.I.; Miller, J.D. A Concise History of Mycotoxin Research. *J. Agric. Food Chem.* **2017**, *65*, 7021–7033. [CrossRef]
24. Kensler, T.W.; Roebuck, B.D.; Wogan, G.N.; Groopman, J.D. Aflatoxin: A 50-Year Odyssey of Mechanistic and Translational Toxicology. *Toxicol. Sci.* **2011**, *120*, S28–S48. [CrossRef]
25. Eskola, M.; Kos, G.; Elliott, C.T.; Hajšlová, J.; Mayar, S.; Krska, R. Worldwide Contamination of Food-Crops with Mycotoxins: Validity of the Widely Cited 'FAO Estimate' of 25%. *Crit. Rev. Food Sci. Nutr.* **2020**, *60*, 2773–2789. [CrossRef]
26. Turner, P.C.; Flannery, B.; Isitt, C.; Ali, M.; Pestka, J. The Role of Biomarkers in Evaluating Human Health Concerns from Fungal contaminants in food. *Nutr. Res. Rev.* **2012**, *25*, 162–179. [CrossRef]
27. Turner, P.C.; Snyder, J.A. Development and Limitations of Exposure Biomarkers to Dietary Contaminants Mycotoxins. *Toxins* **2021**, *13*, 314. [CrossRef] [PubMed]
28. Habschied, K.; Šarić, G.K.; Krstanović, V.; Mastanjević, K. Mycotoxins: Biomonitoring and Human Exposure. *Toxins* **2021**, *13*, 113. [CrossRef] [PubMed]
29. International Agency for Research on Cancer (IARC). Some Naturally Occurring Substances: Food Items and Constituents, Heterocyclic Aromatic Amines and Mycotoxins. In *Monographs on the Evaluation of Carcinogenic Risks to Humans*; International Agency for Research on Cancer: Lyon, France, 1993; Volume 56.
30. Wild, C.P.; Turner, P.C. The Toxicology of Aflatoxins as a Basis for Public Health Decisions. *Mutagenesis* **2002**, *17*, 471–481. [CrossRef]
31. Cotty, P.J.; Jaime-Garcia, R. Influences of climate on aflatoxin producing fungi and aflatoxin contamination. *Int. J. Food Microbiol.* **2007**, *119*, 109–115. [CrossRef]
32. Hell, K.; Mutegi, C. Aflatoxin Control and prevention strategies in key crops of Sub-Saharan Africa. *Afr. J. Microbiol. Res.* **2011**, *5*, 459–466.
33. Mutiga, S.K.; Were, V.; Hoffmann, V.; Harvey, J.W.; Milgroom, M.G.; Nelson, R.J. Extent and drivers of mycotoxin contamination: Inferences from a survey of kenyan maize mills. *Phytopathology* **2014**, *104*, 1221–1231. [CrossRef] [PubMed]
34. Smith, L.; Stasiewicz, M.; Hestrin, R.; Morales, L.; Mutiga, S.; Nelson, R.J. Examining environmental drivers of spatial variability in aflatoxin accumulation in Kenyan maize: Potential utility in risk prediction models. *Afr. J. Food Agric. Nutr. Dev.* **2016**, *16*, 11086–11105. [CrossRef]
35. Bruns, H.A. Controlling Aflatoxin and Fumonisin in Maize by Crop Management. *J. Toxicol. Toxin Rev.* **2003**, *22*, 153–173. [CrossRef]
36. Wogan, G.N.; Kensler, T.W.; Groopman, J.D. Present and future directions of translational research on aflatoxin and hepatocellular carcinoma. A review. *Food Addit. Contam. Part A* **2012**, *29*, 249–257. [CrossRef]
37. Eaton, D.L.; Gallagher, E.P. Mechanisms of aflatoxin carcinogenesis. *Annu. Rev. Pharmacol. Toxicol.* **1994**, *34*, 135–172. [CrossRef] [PubMed]
38. Guengerich, F.P.; Ueng, Y.-F.; Kim, B.-R.; Langouet, S.; Coles, B.; Iyer, R.S.; Thier, R.; Harris, T.M.; Shimada, T.; Yamazaki, H.; et al. Activation of Toxic Chemicals by Cytochrome P450 Enzymes: Regio- and Stereoselective Oxidation of Aflatoxin B1. In *Biological Reactive Intermediates V*; Snyder, R., Sipes, I.G., Jollow, D.J., Monks, T.J., Kocsis, J.J., Kalf, G.F., Greim, H., Witmer, C.M., Eds.; Advances in Experimental Medicine and Biology; Springer: Boston, MA, USA, 1996; Volume 387, pp. 7–15.
39. Essigmann, J.M.; Croy, R.G.; Nadzan, A.M.; Busby, W.F.; Reinhold, V.N.; Büchi, G.; Wogan, G.N. Structural Identification of the Major DNA Adduct Formed by Aflatoxin B1 in Vitro. *Proc. Natl. Acad. Sci. USA* **1977**, *74*, 1870–1874. [CrossRef] [PubMed]
40. Raney, V.M.; Harris, T.M.; Stone, M.P. DNA Conformation Mediates Aflatoxin B1-DNA Binding and the Formation of Guanine N7 Adducts by Aflatoxin B1 8,9-Exo-Epoxide. *Chem. Res. Toxicol.* **1993**, *6*, 64–68. [CrossRef]
41. Sabbioni, G. Chemical and Physical Properties of the Major Serum Albumin Adduct of Aflatoxin B1 and Their Implications for the Quantification in Biological Samples. *Chem. Biol. Interact.* **1990**, *75*, 1–15. [CrossRef]
42. Neal, G.E.; Eaton, D.L.; Judah, D.J.; Verma, A. Metabolism and toxicity of aflatoxins M1 and B1 in human-derived in vitro systems. *Toxicol. Appl. Pharmacol.* **1998**, *151*, 152–158. [CrossRef] [PubMed]
43. Smith, L.E.; Prendergast, A.J.; Turner, P.C.; Humphrey, J.H.; Stoltzfus, R.J. Aflatoxin Exposure During Pregnancy, Maternal Anemia, and Adverse Birth Outcomes. *Am. J. Trop. Med. Hyg.* **2017**, *96*, 770–776. [CrossRef]
44. Choi, H.; Garavito-Duarte, Y.; Gormley, A.R.; Kim, S.W. Aflatoxin B1: Challenges and Strategies for the Intestinal Microbiota and Intestinal Health of Monogastric Animals. *Toxins* **2025**, *17*, 43. [CrossRef]
45. Lunn, P.G.; Northrop-Clewes, C.A.; Downes, R.M. Intestinal permeability, mucosal injury, and growth faltering in Gambian infants. *Lancet* **1991**, *338*, 907–910. [CrossRef]
46. Lunn, P.G. The impact of infection and nutrition on gut function and growth in childhood. *Proc. Nutr. Soc.* **2000**, *59*, 147–154. [CrossRef]

 https://doi.org/10.3390/toxins18010032

47. Campbell, D.I.; Lunn, P.G.; Elia, M. Age-related association of small intestinal mucosal enteropathy with nutritional status in rural Gambian children. *Br. J. Nutr.* **2002**, *88*, 499–505. [CrossRef]
48. Pierron, A.; Alassane-Kpembi, I.; Oswald, I.P. Impact of mycotoxin on immune response and consequences for pig health. *Anim. Nutr.* **2016**, *2*, 63–68. [CrossRef]
49. Chałaśkiewicz, K.; Kępka-Borkowska, K.; Starzyński, R.R.; Ogłuszka, M.; Borkowski, M.; Poławska, E.; Lepczyński, A.; Lichwiarska, E.; Sultana, S.; Kalra, G.; et al. Impact of Aflatoxins on the Digestive, Immune, and Nervous Systems: The Role of Microbiota and Probiotics in Toxicity Protection. *Int. J. Mol. Sci.* **2025**, *26*, 8258. [CrossRef]
50. Turner, P.C.; Moore, S.E.; Hall, A.J.; Prentice, A.M.; Wild, C.P. Modification of immune function through exposure to dietary aflatoxin in Gambian children. *Environ. Health Perspect.* **2003**, *111*, 217–220. [CrossRef] [PubMed]
51. Dai, Y.; Huang, K.; Zhang, B.; Zhu, L.; Xu, W. Aflatoxin B1-induced epigenetic alterations: An overview. *Food Chem. Toxicol.* **2017**, *109*, 683–689. [CrossRef]
52. Ghantous, A.; Novoloaca, A.; Bouaoun, L.; Cuenin, C.; Cros, M.P.; Xu, Y.; Hernandez-Vargas, H.; Darboe, M.K.; Prentice, A.M.; Moore, S.E.; et al. Aflatoxin Exposure during Early Life Is Associated with Differential DNA Methylation in Two-Year-Old Gambian Children. *Int. J. Mol. Sci.* **2021**, *22*, 8967. [CrossRef] [PubMed]
53. Hernandez-Vargas, H.; Castelino, J.; Silver, M.J.; Dominguez-Salas, P.; Cros, M.P.; Durand, G.; Le Calvez-Kelm, F.; Prentice, A.M.; Wild, C.P.; Moore, S.E.; et al. Exposure to aflatoxin B1 in utero is associated with DNA methylation in white blood cells of infants in The Gambia. *Int. J. Epidemiol.* **2015**, *44*, 1238–1248. [CrossRef]
54. Cramer, B.; Visintin, L.; Maris, E.; Kuhn, M.; Degen, G.H.; Turner, P.C.; Humpf, H.-U.; De Saeger, S. Human Biomonitoring of Mycotoxins: Key Challenges and Future Directions. *Mycotoxin Res.* **2025**, *accepted*. [CrossRef] [PubMed]
55. Arce-López, B.; Lizarraga, E.; Vettorazzi, A.; González-Peñas, E. Human Biomonitoring of Mycotoxins in Blood, Plasma and Serum in Recent Years: A Review. *Toxins* **2020**, *12*, 147. [CrossRef]
56. Wild, C.P.; Turner, P.C. Exposure Biomarkers in Chemoprevention Studies of Liver Cancer. *IARC Sci. Publ.* **2001**, *154*, 215–222.
57. Groopman, J.D.; Hall, A.J.; Whittle, H.; Hudson, G.J.; Wogan, G.N.; Montesano, R.; Wild, C.P. Molecular Dosimetry of Aflatoxin-N_7-Guanine in Human Urine Obtained in The Gambia, West Africa. *Cancer Epidemiol. Biomark. Prev.* **1992**, *1*, 221–227.
58. Groopman, J.D.; Zhu, J.Q.; Donahue, P.R.; Pikul, A.; Zhang, L.S.; Chen, J.S.; Wogan, G.N. Molecular Dosimetry of Urinary Aflatoxin-DNA Adducts in People Living in Guangxi Autonomous Region, People's Republic of China. *Cancer Res.* **1992**, *52*, 45–52.
59. Groopman, J.D.; Wild, C.P.; Hasler, J.; Junshi, C.; Wogan, G.N.; Kensler, T.W. Molecular Epidemiology of Aflatoxin Exposures: Validation of Aflatoxin-N_7-Guanine Levels in Urine as a Biomarker in Experimental Rat Models and Humans. *Environ. Health Perspect.* **1993**, *99*, 107–113. [CrossRef] [PubMed]
60. Zhu, J.Q.; Zhang, L.S.; Hu, X.; Xiao, Y.; Chen, J.S.; Xu, Y.C.; Fremy, J.; Chu, F.S. Correlation of Dietary Aflatoxin B1 Levels with Excretion of Aflatoxin M1 in Human Urine. *Cancer Res.* **1987**, *47*, 1848–1852.
61. Gan, L.-S.; Skipper, P.L.; Peng, X.; Groopman, J.D.; Chen, J.; Wogan, G.N.; Tannenbaum, S.R. Serum Albumin Adducts in the Molecular Epidemiology of Aflatoxin Carcinogenesis: Correlation with Aflatoxin B1 Intake and Urinary Excretion of Aflatoxin M1. *Carcinogenesis* **1988**, *9*, 1323–1325. [CrossRef] [PubMed]
62. Sabbioni, G.; Ambs, S.; Wogan, G.N.; Groopman, J.D. The Aflatoxin-Lysine Adduct Quantified by High-Performance Liquid Chromatography from Human Serum Albumin Samples. *Carcinogenesis* **1990**, *11*, 2063–2066. [CrossRef]
63. Wild, C.P.; Hudson, G.J.; Sabbioni, G.; Chapot, B.; Hall, A.J.; Wogan, G.N.; Whittle, H.; Montesano, R.; Groopman, J.D. Dietary Intake of Aflatoxins and the Level of Albumin-Bound Aflatoxin in Peripheral Blood in The Gambia, West Africa. *Cancer Epidemiol. Biomark. Prev.* **1992**, *1*, 229–234.
64. Wild, C.P.; Jiang, Y.Z.; Sabbioni, G.; Chapot, B.; Montesano, R. Evaluation of Methods for Quantitation of Aflatoxin-Albumin Adducts and Their Application to Human Exposure Assessment. *Cancer Res.* **1990**, *50*, 245–251.
65. Wild, C.P.; Jiang, Y.-Z.; Allen, S.J.; Jansen, L.A.M.; Hall, A.J.; Montesano, R. Aflatoxin—Albumin Adducts in Human Sera from Different Regions of the World. *Carcinogenesis* **1990**, *11*, 2271–2274. [CrossRef]
66. Cupid, B.C.; Lightfoot, T.J.; Russell, D.; Gant, S.J.; Turner, P.C.; Dingley, K.H.; Curtis, K.D.; Leveson, S.H.; Turteltaub, K.W.; Garner, R.C. The formation of AFB_1-macromolecular adducts in rats and humans at dietary levels of exposure. *Food Chem. Toxicol.* **2004**, *42*, 559–569. [CrossRef]
67. Scholl, P.F.; Turner, P.C.; Sutcliffe, A.E.; Sylla, A.; Diallo, M.S.; Friesen, M.D.; Groopman, J.D.; Wild, C.P. Quantitative Comparison of Aflatoxin B1 Serum Albumin Adducts in Humans by Isotope Dilution Mass Spectrometry and ELISA. *Cancer Epidemiol. Biomark. Prev.* **2006**, *15*, 823–826. [CrossRef]
68. McCoy, L.F.; Scholl, P.F.; Schleicher, R.L.; Groopman, J.D.; Powers, C.D.; Pfeiffer, C.M. Analysis of Aflatoxin B1-Lysine Adduct in Serum Using Isotope-Dilution Liquid Chromatography/Tandem Mass Spectrometry. *Rapid Commun. Mass Spectrom.* **2005**, *19*, 2203–2210. [CrossRef] [PubMed]

69. McCoy, L.F.; Scholl, P.F.; Sutcliffe, A.E.; Kieszak, S.M.; Powers, C.D.; Rogers, H.S.; Gong, Y.Y.; Groopman, J.D.; Wild, C.P.; Schleicher, R.L. Human Aflatoxin Albumin Adducts Quantitatively Compared by ELISA, HPLC with Fluorescence Detection, and HPLC with Isotope Dilution Mass Spectrometry. *Cancer Epidemiol. Biomark. Prev.* **2008**, *17*, 1653–1657. [CrossRef]
70. Renaud, J.B.; Sabourin, L.; Topp, E.; Sumarah, M.W. Spectral Counting Approach to Measure Selectivity of High-Resolution LC–MS Methods for Environmental Analysis. *Anal. Chem.* **2017**, *89*, 2747–2754. [CrossRef]
71. McMillan, A.; Renaud, J.B.; Burgess, K.M.N.; Orimadegun, A.E.; Akinyinka, O.O.; Allen, S.J.; Miller, J.D.; Reid, G.; Sumarah, M.W. Aflatoxin Exposure in Nigerian Children with Severe Acute Malnutrition. *Food Chem. Toxicol.* **2018**, *111*, 356–362. [CrossRef] [PubMed]
72. Collins, S.L.; Walsh, J.P.; Renaud, J.B.; McMillan, A.; Rulisa, S.; Miller, J.D.; Reid, G.; Sumarah, M.W. Improved Methods for Biomarker Analysis of the Big Five Mycotoxins Enables Reliable Exposure Characterization in a Population of Childbearing Age Women in Rwanda. *Food Chem. Toxicol.* **2021**, *147*, 111854. [CrossRef]
73. Matchado, A.; Smith, J.W.; Schulze, K.J.; Groopman, J.D.; Kortekangas, E.; Chaima, D.; Arnold, C.D.; Maleta, K.; Ashorn, U.; Ashorn, P.; et al. Child Aflatoxin Exposure is Associated with Poor Child Growth Outcomes: A Prospective Cohort Study in Rural Malawi. *Curr. Dev. Nutr.* **2023**, *7*, 101962. [CrossRef] [PubMed]
74. Ari, H.F.; Turanli, E.E.; Yavuz, S.; Guvenc, K.; Avci, A.; Keskin, A.; Aslan, N.; Yildizdas, D. Association between serum albumin levels at admission and clinical outcomes in pediatric intensive care units: A multi-center study. *BMC Pediatr.* **2024**, *24*, 844. [CrossRef]
75. Gong, Y.Y.; Cardwell, K.; Hounsa, A.; Egal, S.; Turner, P.C.; Hall, A.J.; Wild, C.P. Dietary aflatoxin exposure and impaired growth in young children from Benin and Togo: Cross sectional study. *BMJ* **2002**, *325*, 20–21. [CrossRef]
76. Gong, Y.Y.; Hounsa, A.; Egal, S.; Turner, P.C.; Sutcliffe, A.E.; Hall, A.J.; Cardwell, K.; Wild, C.P. Postweaning exposure to aflatoxin results in impaired child growth: A longitudinal study in Benin, West Africa. *Environ. Health Perspect.* **2004**, *112*, 1334–1338. [CrossRef]
77. Gong, Y.Y.; Egal, S.; Hounsa, A.; Turner, P.C.; Hall, A.J.; Cardwell, K.F.; Wild, C.P. Determinants of aflatoxin exposure in young children from Benin and Togo, West Africa: The critical role of weaning. *Int. J. Epidemiol.* **2003**, *32*, 556–562. [CrossRef]
78. Battilani, P.; Toscano, P.; Van Der Fels-Klerx, H.J.; Moretti, A.; Camardo Leggieri, M.; Brera, C.; Rortais, A.; Goumperis, T.; Robinson, T. Aflatoxin B1 contamination in maize in Europe increases due to climate change. *Sci. Rep.* **2016**, *6*, 24328. [CrossRef] [PubMed]
79. Medina, Á.; Rodríguez, A.; Magan, N. Climate change and mycotoxigenic fungi: Impacts on mycotoxin production. *Curr. Opin. Food Sci.* **2015**, *5*, 99–104. [CrossRef]
80. Medina, Á.; Rodríguez, A.; Sultan, Y.; Magan, N. Climate change factors and Aspergillus flavus: Effects on gene expression, growth and aflatoxin production. *World Mycotoxin J.* **2015**, *8*, 171–180. [CrossRef]
81. Khlangwiset, P.; Shephard, G.S.; Wu, F. Aflatoxins and growth impairment: A review. *Crit. Rev. Toxicol.* **2011**, *41*, 740–755. [CrossRef] [PubMed]
82. Shouman, B.O.; El Morsi, D.; Shabaan, S.; Abdel-Hamid, A.H.; Mehrim, A. Aflatoxin B1 level in relation to child's feeding and growth. *Indian J. Pediatr.* **2012**, *79*, 56–61. [CrossRef] [PubMed]
83. Castelino, J.M.; Routledge, M.N.; Wilson, S.; Dunne, D.W.; Mwatha, J.K.; Gachuhi, K.; Wild, C.P.; Gong, Y.Y. Aflatoxin exposure is inversely associated with IGF1 and IGFBP3 levels in vitro and in Kenyan schoolchildren. *Mol. Nutr. Food Res.* **2015**, *59*, 574–581. [CrossRef]
84. Alamu, E.O.; Gondwe, T.; Akello, J.; Maziya-Dixon, B.; Mukanga, M. Relationship between serum aflatoxin concentrations and the nutritional status of children aged 6–24 months from Zambia. *Int. J. Food Sci. Nutr.* **2020**, *71*, 593–603. [CrossRef]
85. Ashraf, W.; Rehman, A.; Ahmad, M.U.; Rabbani, M.; Mushtaq, M.H.; Aamir, K.; Xue, K.S.; Wang, J.S. Assessment of aflatoxin B_1-lysine adduct in children and its effect on child growth in Lahore, Pakistan. *Food Addit. Contam. Part A* **2022**, *39*, 1463–1473. [CrossRef]
86. Turner, P.C.; Collinson, A.C.; Cheung, Y.B.; Gong, Y.; Hall, A.J.; Prentice, A.M.; Wild, C.P. Aflatoxin Exposure in Utero Causes Growth Faltering in Gambian Infants. *Int. J. Epidemiol.* **2007**, *36*, 1119–1125. [CrossRef]
87. Shirima, C.P.; Kimanya, M.E.; Routledge, M.N.; Srey, C.; Kinabo, J.L.; Humpf, H.U.; Wild, C.P.; Tu, Y.K.; Gong, Y.Y. A prospective study of growth and biomarkers of exposure to aflatoxin and fumonisin during early childhood in Tanzania. *Environ. Health Perspect.* **2015**, *123*, 173–178. [CrossRef] [PubMed]
88. Mitchell, N.J.; Hsu, H.H.; Chandyo, R.K.; Shrestha, B.; Bodhidatta, L.; Tu, Y.K.; Gong, Y.Y.; Egner, P.A.; Ulak, M.; Groopman, J.D.; et al. Aflatoxin exposure during the first 36 months of life was not associated with impaired growth in Nepalese children: An extension of the MAL-ED study. *PLoS ONE* **2017**, *12*, e0172124. [CrossRef]
89. Watson, S.; Moore, S.E.; Darboe, M.K.; Chen, G.; Tu, Y.K.; Huang, Y.T.; Eriksen, K.G.; Bernstein, R.M.; Prentice, A.M.; Wild, C.P.; et al. Impaired growth in rural Gambian infants exposed to aflatoxin: A prospective cohort study. *BMC Public Health* **2018**, *18*, 1247. [CrossRef] [PubMed]

https://doi.org/10.3390/toxins18010032

90. Mahfuz, M.; Hasan, S.M.T.; Alam, M.A.; Das, S.; Fahim, S.M.; Islam, M.M.; Gazi, M.A.; Hossain, M.; Egner, P.A.; Groopman, J.D.; et al. Aflatoxin exposure was not associated with childhood stunting: Results from a birth cohort study in a resource-poor setting of Dhaka, Bangladesh. *Public Health Nutr.* **2021**, *24*, 3361–3370. [CrossRef]
91. Tessema, M.; De Groote, H.; Brouwer, I.D.; De Boevre, M.; Corominas, A.V.; Stoecker, B.J.; Feskens, E.J.; Belachew, T.; Karakitsou, A.; Gunaratna, N.S. Exposure to aflatoxins and fumonisins and linear growth of children in rural Ethiopia: A longitudinal study. *Public Health Nutr.* **2021**, *24*, 3662–3673. [CrossRef] [PubMed]
92. Andrews-Trevino, J.Y.; Webb, P.; Shively, G.; Kablan, A.; Baral, K.; Davis, D.; Paudel, K.; Shrestha, R.; Pokharel, A.; Acharya, S.; et al. Aflatoxin exposure and child nutrition: Measuring anthropometric and long-bone growth over time in Nepal. *Am. J. Clin. Nutr.* **2021**, *113*, 874–883. [CrossRef]
93. Schleicher, R.L.; McCoy, L.F.; Powers, C.D.; Sternberg, M.R.; Pfeiffer, C.M. Serum concentrations of an aflatoxin-albumin adduct in the National Health and Nutrition Examination Survey (NHANES) 1999–2000. *Clin. Chim. Acta* **2013**, *423*, 46–50. [CrossRef]
94. Leroy, J.L.; Sununtnasuk, C.; García-Guerra, A.; Wang, J.S. Low level aflatoxin exposure associated with greater linear growth in southern Mexico: A longitudinal study. *Matern. Child Nutr.* **2018**, *14*, e12619. [CrossRef]
95. Diaz, G.J.; Calabrese, E.; Blain, R. Aflatoxicosis in chickens (*Gallus gallus*): An example of hormesis? *Poult. Sci.* **2008**, *87*, 727–732. [CrossRef]
96. Hoffmann, V.; Jones, K.; Leroy, J.L. The impact of reducing dietary aflatoxin exposure on child linear growth: A cluster randomised controlled trial in Kenya. *BMJ Glob. Health* **2018**, *3*, e000983. [CrossRef]
97. Phillips, E.L.; Kassim, N.; Smith, L.E.; Ngure, F.M.; Makule, E.; Turner, P.C.; Nelson, R.J.; Kimanya, M.E.; Stoltzfus, R. Protocol for the trial to establish a causal linkage between mycotoxin exposure and child stunting: A cluster randomized trial. *BMC Public Health* **2020**, *20*, 598. [CrossRef]
98. Ngure, F.M.; Makule, E.; Mgongo, W.; Phillips, E.; Kassim, N.; Stoltzfus, R.; Nelson, R. Processing complementary foods to reduce mycotoxins in a medium scale Tanzanian mill: A hazard analysis critical control point (HACCP) approach. *Food Control* **2024**, *162*, 110463. [CrossRef]
99. Kayanda, R.A.; Kassim, N.; Ngure, F.M.; Stoltzfus, R.J.; Phillips, E. Nutrient Intake and Dietary Adequacy Among Rural Tanzanian Infants Enrolled in the Mycotoxin Mitigation Trial. *Nutrients* **2024**, *17*, 131. [CrossRef] [PubMed]
100. Phillips, E.; Kayanda, R.A.; Kassim, N.; Ngure, F.M.; Turner, P.C.; Stoltzfus, R.J. Comparison of Methods to Assess Adherence to Infant and Young Child Feeding Practices and Provision of Low-Aflatoxin Porridge Flours in a Community-Based Intervention Trial. *Nutrients* **2024**, *16*, 4315. [CrossRef] [PubMed]
101. Ngure, F.M.; Kassim, N.; Phillips, E.L.; Turner, P.C. Infant and Young Child Feeding Practices and Mycotoxin Contamination of Complementary Food Ingredients in Kongwa District, Tanzania. *Curr. Dev. Nutr.* **2023**, *7*, 100030. [CrossRef]
102. Kassim, N.; Ngure, F.; Smith, L.; Turner, P.C.; Stoltzfus, R.; Makule, E.; Makori, N.; Phillips, E. Provision of low-aflatoxin local complementary porridge flour reduced urinary aflatoxin biomarker in children aged 6–18 months in rural Tanzania. *Matern. Child Nutr.* **2023**, *19*, e13499. [CrossRef] [PubMed]
103. Kayanda, R.; Kassim, N.; Phillips, E.; Turner, P.C.; Stoltzfus, R.J.; Ngure, F.M. Comparison of aflatoxin contamination and dietary exposure from complementary foods among rural Tanzanian infants enrolled in the mycotoxin mitigation trial. *Food Sci. Nutr.* **2026**, *accepted*.
104. Phillips, E.; Ngure, F.M.; Kassim, N.; Turner, P.C.; Makule, E.; Smith, L.E.; Makori, N.; Cramer, B.; Humpf, H.U.; Nelson, R.J.; et al. The effect of an intervention to reduce aflatoxin consumption from 6 to 18 mo of age on length-for-age z-scores in rural Tanzania: A cluster-randomized trial. *Am. J. Clin. Nutr.* **2025**, *121*, 333–342. [CrossRef]

 https://doi.org/10.3390/toxins18010032

toxins

MDPI

Review

Aflatoxin Exposure and Human Health with a Focus on Northern Latin America

Karen A. Corleto [1,2], Christian S. Alvarez [3], Manuel Ramirez-Zea [4], John D. Groopman [5] and Katherine A. McGlynn [2,*]

1 Division of Cancer Prevention, National Cancer Institute, Rockville, MD 20850, USA; karen.corleto@nih.gov
2 Division of Cancer Epidemiology and Genetics, National Cancer Institute, Rockville, MD 20850, USA
3 Division of Intramural Research, National Institute on Minority Health and Health Disparities, Rockville, MD 20852, USA; christian.alvarez@nih.gov
4 Center for the Prevention of Chronic Diseases, Institute of Nutrition of Central America and Panama, Guatemala City 1188, Guatemala; mramirez@incap.int
5 Departments of Environmental Health and Engineering and Epidemiology, Bloomberg School of Public Health, Johns Hopkins University, Baltimore, MD 21205, USA; jgroopm1@jhu.edu
* Correspondence: mcglynnk@nih.gov; Tel.: +1-240-276-7297

Abstract

Aflatoxins, mycotoxins produced by *Aspergillus flavus* and *Aspergillus parasiticus*, were discovered sixty-five years ago and remain a significant public health threat, particularly amid increasing instances of extreme weather events. Of the four principal forms of aflatoxins found in foods (B_1, B_2, G_1, and G_2), aflatoxin B_1 is the most potent carcinogen. Aflatoxins commonly contaminate a variety of foodstuffs, with maize being among the most susceptible. Chronic exposure to aflatoxins has been linked to liver cancer, childhood stunting, gallbladder cancer, and other adverse health effects. Due to public health concerns related to the consumption of aflatoxin-contaminated foods, most countries have established regulatory limits. Here, we present estimated aflatoxin exposure per day derived from human biomarker data across many studies around the world spanning more than forty years. We specifically focus on the impact of dietary aflatoxin in northern Latin America, where assessment of the total problem remains limited. These findings suggest a multipronged toolkit could mitigate aflatoxin exposure in the region, which would help to decrease the health burden.

Keywords: aflatoxin; maize; liver cancer; Latin America

Key Contribution: Aflatoxin contamination of food items is well-known to be a major health threat in parts East Asia and sub-Saharan Africa. Less well-appreciated is the role that aflatoxin may play in Latin American countries that consume high levels of maize.

1. Introduction

Aflatoxins, identified as disease-causing mycotoxins sixty-five years ago [1,2], continue to be significant public health issues due to their toxic, mutagenic, and carcinogenic properties [3]. Primarily produced by the fungi *Aspergillus flavus* and *Aspergillus parasiticus* [4,5], approximately twenty aflatoxins have been described [2], but the four principal forms that dominate human exposure are aflatoxin B_1 (AFB_1), B_2 (AFB_2), G_1 (AFG_1), and G_2 (AFG_2) [4]. Of these forms, AFB_1 is the major aflatoxin driving health concerns [6].

Although other routes of exposure occur, human exposure to AFB_1 occurs predominantly through the consumption of contaminated foods. Various foodstuffs have tested positive for aflatoxin contamination, including spices, pulses, beans, tea, cocoa, milk, grains, and groundnuts [3,6,7]. The major sources of aflatoxin in the human diet, however, are maize, groundnuts and other grains [4,6,8]. AFB_1 contamination can be challenging to combat as it can develop both pre- and post-harvest, with weather conditions including rainfall, temperature, and humidity converging to produce environmental conditions optimal for mold growth [6,8].

Due to widespread environmental contamination by aflatoxins and the negative health implications for both humans and other animal species, a number of countries have established regulatory limits on aflatoxins in foodstuffs, but there is no global consensus on regulatory standards.

2. Regulatory Limits on Aflatoxins

Regulatory limits for aflatoxins vary widely by country and food item. For example, the European Union (EU) regulations are some of the most stringent, with limits for both total aflatoxins (4–15 parts per billion, ppb), and for AFB_1 (2–12 ppb) [9]. The EU regulations vary by commodity but are most strict for ready-to-eat foods. In contrast, the United States has only one limit (20 ppb) for all food items [10], while Mexico has a limit of 20 ppb for maize grain but a lower level (12 ppb) for nixtamalized maize products [11,12]. Guatemala also has a limit of 20 ppb (total aflatoxins) for maize and maize products [12,13].

Despite the existence of regulatory limits, aflatoxin contamination remains a concern in many countries. A risk assessment that evaluated the effectiveness of aflatoxin regulatory standards in protecting against liver cancer concluded that most standards limited lifetime risk to below 1 case per 10,000 individuals [14]. However, the report also found that in some parts of Latin America, regulatory standards did not meet this level of protection [14]. In addition, regulatory standards are only effective if they are enforced and many countries lack the capacity to do so.

Table 1 shows the estimated intake of total aflatoxins depending on the regulatory standard and the grams of a dietary item consumed. To calculate daily aflatoxin exposure, 3% of the intake of contaminated food was used to estimate AFB_1 μg/day. The calculation assumes a steady state of adduct accumulation over 30 days, as previous work indicates that 2.9% of the daily dietary exposure is converted to the aflatoxin albumin adduct.

Table 1. Estimated daily aflatoxin exposure by regulatory limits and intake of contaminated foods.

Contaminated Food Consumption Level per Day (g)	Total Aflatoxins Regulatory Limits (ppb)	Estimated Aflatoxin Intake (ug)
25	4	0.10
	10	0.25
	15	0.38
	20	0.50
50	4	0.20
	10	0.50
	15	0.75
	20	1.00
100	4	0.40
	10	1.00
	15	1.50
	20	2.00
250	4	1.00
	10	2.50
	15	3.75
	20	5.00

https://doi.org/10.3390/toxins18010058

Table 1. *Cont.*

Contaminated Food Consumption Level per Day (g)	Total Aflatoxins Regulatory Limits (ppb)	Estimated Aflatoxin Intake (ug)
350	4	1.40
	10	3.50
	15	5.25
	20	7.00

3. Evaluating Aflatoxin Exposure

While global exposure to aflatoxins from contaminated foods is well documented, estimating the putative dose to humans has been a goal of aflatoxin biomarker research. Knowledge of the metabolism and formation of specific covalent aflatoxin adducts in DNA and proteins has been deployed in many epidemiologic studies. In recent years the recognition that the aflatoxin-lysine adduct formed in albumin is an integrative biomarker of exposure has been of great significance in the field [15]. To put the AFB_1 levels in northern Latin America in context, Table 2 summarizes studies of Groopman and colleagues of AFB_1-lys adduct levels and converts those levels to estimated daily aflatoxin exposure in μg, using the formula mentioned above [16,17].

As seen in Table 2, the lowest mean daily aflatoxin exposure (0.01 ± 0.02 μg/day) seen in these studies was in 2012 in Qidong, China. This low level was achieved after the implementation in Qidong of the switch in dietary staple from maize to rice. In comparison, the highest exposure (91.1 ± 201.42 μg/day) in Table 2 occurred during an outbreak of acute aflatoxicosis in Kenya in 2004 [33–35]. Figure 1 displays the results of many of these studies plotted side by side.

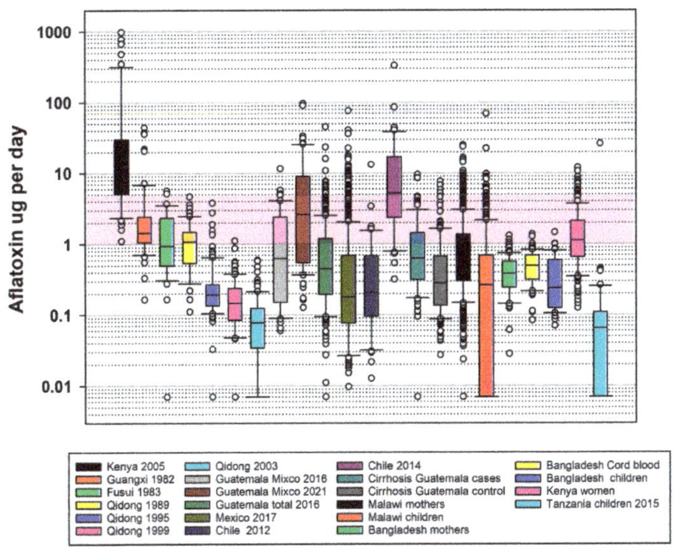

Figure 1. Graphical representation of daily aflatoxin exposure in μg for studies in Kenya (2005) [25,26]; Guangxi, Fusui, and Qidong [17,21]; Guatemala [23,24]; Mexico [29,30]; Chile [36,37]; cirrhosis in Guatemala [22]; Malawi [18]; Bangladesh [18–20]; Kenyan women [27,28]; and Tanzanian children [31,32]. The area highlighted represents the 1 μg to 5 μg per day range where many human health effects have been documented. The open circles represent individual data points that are either below the 5th percentile or above the 95th percentile.

https://doi.org/10.3390/toxins18010058

Table 2. Daily aflatoxin exposure (μg) for various studies.

Country	Year	Details	n	Aflatoxin (SD)	95% CI	Min.	Max.	%ND *	Ref.
Bangladesh	2008–2011	Preg. women 1st trimester	63	0.35 (0.22)	(0.29, 0.41)	ND	1.14	6.4	[18–20]
		Preg. women 3rd trimester	63	0.48 (0.25)	(0.42, 0.55)	ND	1.31	1.6	
		Cord blood	63	0.51 (0.27)	(0.44, 0.57)	0.08	1.38	0	
		Child 24 mos.	63	0.37 (0.30)	(0.30, 0.45)	ND	1.47	1.6	
China	1982	Guangxi	76	4.01 (8.30)	(2.11, 5.91)	0.17	44.38	0	[17,21]
	1983	Fusui	31	1.55 (1.40)	(1.04, 2.06)	ND	5.66	3.2	
	1989	Qidong	74	1.20 (0.88)	(1.00, 1.40)	0.11	4.66	0	
	1995	Qidong	100	0.33 (0.52)	(0.22, 0.43)	ND	3.79	2	
	1999	Qidong	100	0.20 (0.19)	(0.16, 0.23)	ND	1.12	8	
	2003	Qidong	100	0.10 (0.12)	(0.08, 0.13)	ND	0.6	24	
	2009	Qidong	100	0.06 (0.14)	(0.03, 0.09)	ND	0.81	77	
	2012	Qidong	100	0.01 (0.02)	(0.01, 0.02)	ND	0.16	92	
Guatemala	2015	Cirrhosis cases	99	1.18 (1.54)	(0.87, 1.49)	ND	9.52	1	[22]
		Controls	200	0.67 (1.11)	(0.52, 0.83)	0.03	7.62	0	
	2016	Escuintla	93	7.73 (12.82)	(5.09, 10.37)	ND	87.38	4.3	[23,24]
		Mixco	60	1.50 (2.06)	(0.97, 2.03)	0.06	11.57	0	
		Sololá	60	1.97 (3.13)	(1.16, 2.78)	0.18	23.51	0	
		Suchitepéquez	82	2.02 (2.43)	(1.49, 2.56)	0.09	16.12	0	
		Quiche	101	1.33 (4.93)	(0.36, 2.31)	ND	45.2	1	
Kenya	2005	Aflatoxicosis outbreak	55	91.1 (201.42)	(36.65, 145.55)	1.11	981.1	0	[25,26]
	2015–2016	Women baseline	120	1.93 (1.95)	(1.58, 2.29)	0.13	10.61	0	[27,28]
		Women 12-mo. follow-up	115	1.55 (1.62)	(1.25, 1.85)	0.14	11.93	0	
Malawi	2011–2015	Preg. women baseline	255	1.04 (1.43)	(0.87, 1.22)	ND	15.57	4.7	[18]
		Preg. women GA 36 wks.	255	1.20 (1.77)	(0.98, 1.41)	ND	10.73	4.7	
		Women 6 mos. postpartum	230	1.86 (3.31)	(1.43, 2.29)	0.04	25.04	0	
		Infant 6 mos. old	230	0.41 (1.00)	(0.28, 0.54)	ND	8.53	43.5	
		Infant 18 mos. old	231	1.49 (4.98)	(0.85, 2.14)	ND	69.28	8.7	
Mexico	2018–2019	South and eastern Mexico	855	1.03 (3.77)	(0.78, 1.28)	0.01	76.23	0	[29,30]
Tanzania	2018	Haydom (rural)	545	1.76 (3.00)	(1.51, 2.02)	ND	42.98	0.2	[31,32]

Aflatoxin is represented in μg/day; calculations were estimated from plasma serum AFB1-albumin adducts. Abbreviations: pregnant (Preg.), month (mo.), months (mos.), gestational age (GA), standard deviation (SD), confidence interval (CI), nondetectable (ND), minimum (Min.), maximum (Max.), and references (refs.). * ND = nondetectable.

4. Maize Consumption as a Vehicle for Aflatoxin Exposure

In northern Latin America, maize has been a dietary staple for millenia. Numerous foods, such as tortillas, tamales, gorditas, and pupusas, are made from nixtamalized maize flour, which is maize grain that has been cooked in a solution of calcium hydroxide prior to being ground [38–40]. Environmental conditions (temperature, humidity, and rainfall) in the region can facilitate pre- and post-harvest AFB contamination [3]. Extreme weather events, including droughts and unseasonal rains, further increase the risk of AFB contamination, and rising temperatures and humidity are projected to enhance pre-harvest aflatoxin contamination of susceptible crops [8,41].

Of the food items made from maize, tortillas are consumed in the greatest quantity. For example, in Veracruz City, Mexico, reports indicate that tortilla intake averages 118.4 g

https://doi.org/10.3390/toxins18010058

(person/day) [42]. In a recent report from Mexico that evaluated maize consumption using the country's National Health and Nutrition Survey (ENSANUT), the median intake of maize was 307 g/d, mainly attributed to tortilla intake (77%) [29]. The high consumption of tortillas is of particular concern as tortillas have been demonstrated by several studies to be contaminated with AFB. In the Mexican state of San Luis Potosí, an evaluation of tortillas revealed that 18% of the samples exceeded Mexico's limit (12 ppb) for AFB_1 [43], while in Mexico City, 4.5% of nixtamalized maize samples were reported to have detectable levels of aflatoxins [39].

In Guatemala, a cross-sectional evaluation of 461 adults found median AFB_1 levels of 7.5 pg/mg albumin among women and 11.4 pg/mg albumin among men [44]. For reference, a level of 17.5 pg/mg albumin is an adduct burden arising from a daily exposure to 1 μg AFB_1 per day for 30 days [17]. In the cross-sectional study, the median AFB_1 levels were higher among individuals in rural areas (14.0 pg/mg albumin) than in urban areas (4.9 pg/mg) [44]. The study also found a significant relationship between tortilla consumption and levels of AFB_1-albumin adducts [45]. A separate study of Guatemalan women who worked as tortilla makers reported an average weekly consumption of maize to be 3470.5 g, primarily in the form of tortillas. Tortilla sampling found that 11% had detectable levels AFB_1 [46]. In a study from Honduras, 65% of maize and maize products were contaminated with aflatoxin, with the mean total aflatoxins ranging from 1.06 μg/kg to 6.23 μg/kg [47].

A 2014 examination of global maize consumption estimated that the highest levels of consumption in the western hemisphere were in Mexico (267 g/person/day), Guatemala (187 g/person/day), and Honduras (169 g/person/day) [48]. Thus, with the aflatoxin regulatory limit in Mexico of 20 ppb (20 μg per kg), the consumption of 267 g/person/day in Mexico would result in an aflatoxin exposure of roughly 3.2 μg/day. A similar calculation for Guatemala results in an aflatoxin exposure of roughly 3.7 μg/day. In addition, localized reports from many areas have found that maize products are being consumed at a level of more than 260 g/day [29,45–47]. These data indicate that contamination levels in several regions exceed the regulatory limits, making these regulations insufficient/ineffective to protect human health.

5. Health Burden of Aflatoxin Exposure in Latin America

Aflatoxin has been associated with a number of health-related conditions, with liver cancer, after acute aflatoxicosis, being one of the most fatal. Liver cancer is the sixth most commonly diagnosed cancer worldwide and the third largest contributor to cancer mortality [49]. The relationship between aflatoxin exposure and liver cancer is well documented, leading the International Agency for Research on Cancer to classify aflatoxin as a group 1 human carcinogen [5,17,50–53]. In Latin America, while there are few established cancer registries, it is estimated that Guatemala has the highest age-standardized liver cancer incidence rate (15.5 per 100,000 persons) in the western hemisphere [24]. In contrast, the age-standardinzed liver cancer incidence rate in the U.S. is 6.8/100,000 persons

Aflatoxin is not only a risk factor itself but can be an even more potent risk factor when it co-occurs with other factors, including alcohol, obesity, and type II diabetes, as well as chronic infections with hepatitis C virus and hepatitis B virus (HBV) [24,54–57]. The synergism between aflatoxin and HBV was well demonstarted in a study conducted in Shanghai, China, that found the risk of liver cancer was 3.4-fold higher among persons exposed to AFB_1, 7-fold higher among persons who were HBV(+), and 59-fold higher among persons with both factors [58]. This synergistic relationship was also subsequently observed in other cohorts [51]. In Latin America, HBV prevalence estimates tend to be lower than in other areas of the world, although comprehensive prevalence data for the

https://doi.org/10.3390/toxins18010058

region are very limited [59]. For example, a study conducted in Guatemala that examined both aflatoxin and HBV found that the prevalence of aflatoxin was high but the prevalence of HBV was low [22–24].

Although HBV may not play a significant role in liver cancer in Latin America, factors such as obesity and type II diabetes [24,57] may also increase the risk of liver cancer among persons exposed to aflatoxin. In Latin America, it is estimated that 30.5% of adults live with obesity, and 64% are overweight [60]. With the increase in obesity rates, type II diabetes has also increased, with estimates that in the next 20 years there will be a 50% increase in type II diabetes in the region [60]. Obesity and type II diabetes also are risk factors for metabolic dysfunction-associated steatotic liver disease (MASLD), which itself is a risk factor for liver cancer [61]. In Guatemala, a study reported a significant association between AFB_1-albumin adduct levels and diabetes [44]. Although the mechanism by which AFB_1 increases risk of diabetes is uncertain, the relationship may be due to AFB_1 causing inflammation and oxidative stress, impairing insulin secretion and disrupting carbohydrate metabolism. More research is needed to improve the understanding of the relationship between aflatoxins, metabolic disorders, and other factors in affecting liver cancer risk in Latin America.

In addition to liver cancer and metabolic disorders, aflatoxin has been associated with childhood stunting, both independently and in conjunction with other risk factors [4]. Hypotheses on the mechanism by which aflatoxin influences stunting include impairment of the immune system, effects on the IGF-1 axis, and an effect on environmental enteric dysfunction (EED) [4,62]. Among Latin American countries, Guatemala has a notably high level of stunting, with a prevalence $\geq$ 40% [62], and aflatoxin exposure has been negatively correlated with child height-for-age-z-scores [63]. A cross-sectional study conducted in low-income African countries found that children with both stunting and underweight had the highest levels of aflatoxin albumin adducts as measured by enzyme-linked immunosorbent assay (ELISA) (132.27 pg/mg albumin), followed by children with stunting alone (109.41 pg/mg albumin), followed by children without stunting (75.01 pg/mg albumin) [64]. In addition, a study in Malawi that used mass spectrometry reported that aflatoxin exposure was negatively associated with child growth [65]. Collectively, a published paired study can be used to interconvert data from ELISA with mass spectrometry-derived aflatoxin albumin adducts [25].

Other health-related conditions have also been linked to chronic dietary exposure to aflatoxins. It has been suggested that aflatoxins may influence innate and adaptive immunity [54,66], with some human studies providing evidence that aflatoxin can have immunosupressive effects in children and adults [67,68]. Gambian children with higher exposure to aflatoxin had reduced levels of the antibody secretory IgA in their saliva [67]. In adults from Ghana it was found that aflatoxin exposure influences cellular immune status [68]. Further research, particularly in human populations, is required to better understand how aflatoxin exposure affects immunity. Perhaps the results of studies of aflatoxin exposure and oncogenic human papillomaviruses (HPV) are related to effects on the immune system. Studies in both Kenya and Mexico have indicated an association between aflatoxin and oncogenic HPV in women [27,28,69,70]. Aflatoxin exposure may also be related to the development of gallbladder cancer, as reported by studies conducted in Chile and Shanghai [36,37,71,72]. There are also investigations into how aflatoxin-induced oxidative stress and reductions in nuerotransmitter levels may impact neurogenerative disease [54,73].

https://doi.org/10.3390/toxins18010058

6. Toolkit of Interventions to Tackle Aflatoxin Exposure in Latin America

The regulation of aflatoxins in food and the strict enforcement of those regulations are critical components of a primary prevention approach to aflatoxin control. In conjunction with regulatory standards, aflatoxin urinary and blood biomarkers should be used to monitor exposure, providing a metric of the efficacy of the regulatory standards. Urinary biomarkers (AFB_1, AFM_1, and AFB_1-N^7-Gua DNA-adduct) are suitable for measuring short-term exposure [58,74], while serum AFB_1-lys adduct levels are the best estimates of longer-term exposure. In humans, the average lifetime for albumin is approximately thirty days [75]. Therefore, albumin adduct formation provides a more comprehensive picture of aflatoxin exposure that estimates average aflatoxin exposure per day over a 30-day period. Using AFB_1 metabolites to estimate daily aflatoxin exposure in Latin America would be an effective tool to monitor acute exposure or the average daily exposure over a longer time at the individual or population level. Effect monitoring programs could help governments gauge the effectiveness of regulatory measures and aid in making informed decisions about aflatoxin control. To most effectively conduct a monitoring program, there is a demonstrable need for capacity building and infrastructure development to establish aflatoxin monitoring laboratories throughout Latin America.

Due to the importance of preventing crop contamination from aflatoxins, pre-harvest contamination prediction models have been developed [76,77]. The most recent models use a meteorology-driven epidemiological approach, such as the model described by Stutt and colleagues that encompasses the maize supply chain from planting to delivery [76]. Biological control is also a possible approach to pre-harvest aflatoxin management. Some of the pre-harvest techniques include competitive exclusion using non-aflatoxigenic strains and microbial bio-fungicides [2,3,78–80]. During postharvest, proper drying, including such strategies as controlled environment drying, sun drying on platforms, and removing damaged corn, can aid in the reduction of aflatoxin contamination [12]. Field drying of maize under humid conditions in Mexico and northern Central America can result in moisture levels (14–18%), which are higher than the recommended range to reduce aflatoxin contamination (12–14%) [12]. Adequate storage with low humidity and temperature conditions also helps to minimize fungal growth [12].

In addition to pre- and post-harvest strategies for aflatoxin reduction, cooking can also reduce the amount of aflatoxin in foods. Roasting at high temperatures has been shown to decrease aflatoxin levels 50–90% [81]. Boiling can also be an effective strategy, as boiling rice at 100 °C for 12 min has been reported to decrease aflatoxin levels [82]. In Mexico and Central America, nixtamalization of maize is a common practice, and most maize products consumed are nixtamalized [12,39,45,83]. While some studies have found that nixtamalization reduced aflatoxin by 88% (44.99 ppb to 5.26 ppb) [38], the process is not entirely successful as aflatoxin contamination continues to be an issue in Latin America.

While primary prevention is always the optimal strategy, secondary prevention strategies, such as chemoprevention to detoxify consumed aflatoxins, have been proposed. AFB_1 is bioactivated into aflatoxin-8,9-epoxide (AFBO), the metabolite that reacts with DNA to form adducts. To interrupt adduct formation, phase II metabolism then plays an important role in detoxification. Glutathione S-transferases conjugate glutathione to AFBO to facilitate eventual excretion in urine [52,84]. Agents that promote the induction of glutathione S-transferases can therefore assist in the detoxification process. Two agents that have shown a positive effect on glutathione S-transferase induction are the pharmaceutical Oltipraz and a natural compound found in cruciferous vegetables, sulforaphane [85–87]. In a placebo-controlled trial, Oltipraz at a dose of 500 mg taken weekly for one month was demonstrated to decrease median urinary levels of the metabolite AFM_1 by 51% [87,88]. In a study of

https://doi.org/10.3390/toxins18010058

sulforaphane, 2 weeks of broccoli sprout infusion resulted in modest decreases in urinary levels of aflatoxin N^7-guanine [85]. In the study, there was high variability among individuals in sulforaphane levels, which correlated with decreases in aflatoxin N^7-guanine [85]. Other bioactive compounds that have shown promising results are polyphenols from curcumin and green tea [84,89]. To our knowledge, these secondary chemoprevention strategies have not yet been tried in Latin America.

7. Conclusions

Aflatoxins threaten human health in a myriad of ways across the lifespan. The carcinogenic effects of AFB_1 on the liver are of particular concern. In addition, the effects on childhood stunting, oncogenic HPV infection, and gallbladder cancer are of significant concern in areas where contamination is common. Due to fluctuating environmental conditions, this aflatoxin contamination could greatly increase. There is a strong need to implement effective aflatoxin monitoring systems, in areas such as Latin America, where staple dietary foods such as maize are commonly contaminated. Urinary and blood biomarkers produced during aflatoxin metabolism are useful for monitoring exposure in individuals and for measuring the effectiveness of mitigation strategies. The effectiveness of both pre-harvest and post-harvest techniques can be measured by biomonitoring a population's daily aflatoxin exposure. The success of secondary prevention methods can also be determined. Overall, the use of aflatoxin biomarker monitoring in Latin America could guide regulatory efforts and assist in making informed decisions on intervention strategies.

Author Contributions: Conceptualization, K.A.C., J.D.G. and K.A.M.; writing—original draft preparation, K.A.C.; writing—review and editing, C.S.A., M.R.-Z., J.D.G. and K.A.M. All authors have read and agreed to the published version of the manuscript.

Funding: This research received no external funding.

Institutional Review Board Statement: Not applicable.

Informed Consent Statement: Not applicable.

Data Availability Statement: No new data were created or analyzed in this study.

Acknowledgments: The authors wish to thank Alvaro Rivera-Andrade of INCAP, Guatemala City, Guatemala, and the participants of the North American Liver Cancer Study.

Conflicts of Interest: The authors declare no conflicts of interest.

References

1. Kensler, T.W.; Roebuck, B.D.; Wogan, G.N.; Groopman, J.D. Aflatoxin: A 50-year odyssey of mechanistic and translational toxicology. *Toxicol. Sci.* **2011**, *120*, S28–S48. [CrossRef]
2. Pickova, D.; Ostry, V.; Toman, J.; Malir, F. Aflatoxins: History, Significant Milestones, Recent Data on Their Toxicity and Ways to Mitigation. *Toxins* **2021**, *13*, 399. [CrossRef] [PubMed]
3. Jallow, A.; Xie, H.; Tang, X.; Qi, Z.; Li, P. Worldwide aflatoxin contamination of agricultural products and foods: From occurrence to control. *Compr. Rev. Food Sci. Food Saf.* **2021**, *20*, 2332–2381. [CrossRef]
4. Wild, C.P.; Miller, J.D.; Groopman, J.D. (Eds.) *Mycotoxin Control in Low- and Middle-Income Countries;* International Agency for Research on Cancer: Lyon, France, 2015; Volume 9.
5. Liu, Y.; Chang, C.-C.H.; Marsh, G.M.; Wu, F. Population attributable risk of aflatoxin-related liver cancer: Systematic review and meta-analysis. *Eur. J. Cancer* **2012**, *48*, 2125–2136. [CrossRef]
6. EFSA Panel on Contaminants in the Food Chain; Schrenk, D.; Bignami, M.; Bodin, L.; Chipman, J.K.; del Mazo, J.; Grasl-Kraupp, B.; Hogstrand, C.; Hoogenboom, L.; Leblanc, J.-C.; et al. Risk assessment of aflatoxins in food. *EFSA J.* **2020**, *18*, e06040. [CrossRef]
7. Eskola, M.; Kos, G.; Elliott, C.T.; Hajšlová, J.; Mayar, S.; Krska, R. Worldwide contamination of food-crops with mycotoxins: Validity of the widely cited 'FAO estimate' of 25%. *Crit. Rev. Food Sci. Nutr.* **2020**, *60*, 2773–2789. [CrossRef]
8. Nji, Q.N.; Babalola, O.O.; Mwanza, M. Climatic effects on aflatoxin contamination of maize. *Toxicol. Rep.* **2024**, *13*, 101711. [CrossRef]

 https://doi.org/10.3390/toxins18010058

9. European Commission. Commission Regulation (EU) 2023/915 of 25 April 2023 on maximum levels for certain contaminants in food and repealing Regulation (EC) No 1881/2006. *Off. J. Eur. Union* **2023**, *119*, 103–157.
10. Food and Drug Administration. *Compliance Policy Guide Sec. 555.400 Aflatoxins in Human Food: Guidance for FDA Staff*; US Department of Health and Human Services Food and Drug Administration Center for Food Safety and Applied Nutrition and Office of Regulatory Affairs: Silver Spring, MD, USA, 2021.
11. La Moderna, P.A.; De, C.; El Pilar, M.D.T.; De, K.F.D.M.S. ANTEPROYECTO de Norma Oficial Mexicana PROY-NOM-247-SSA1-2005, Productos y Servicios. Cereales y sus Productos. Cereales, Harinas de Cereales, Sémolas o Semolinas. Alimentos a Base de: Cereales, Semillas Comestibles, de Harinas, Sémolas o Semolinas o sus Mezclas. Productos de Panificación. Disposiciones y Especificaciones Sanitarias y Nutrimentales. Métodos de Prueba. PREFACIO. Available online: https://platiica.economia.gob.mx/normalizacion/nom-247-ssa1-2008/ (accessed on 4 January 2025).
12. Odjo, S.; Alakonya, A.E.; Rosales-Nolasco, A.; Molina, A.L.; Muñoz, C.; Palacios-Rojas, N. Occurrence and postharvest strategies to help mitigate aflatoxins and fumonisins in maize and their co-exposure to consumers in Mexico and Central America. *Food Control* **2022**, *138*, 108968. [CrossRef]
13. Comisión Guatemalteca de Normas. Maíz en Grano. Maíz Elaborado. NGO 34 047 1982. Available online: https://cretec.org.gt/wp-content/uploads/2021/03/ngo34047maizelaborado.pdf (accessed on 4 January 2025).
14. Wu, F.; Stacy, S.L.; Kensler, T.W. Global risk assessment of aflatoxins in maize and peanuts: Are regulatory standards adequately protective? *Toxicol. Sci.* **2013**, *135*, 251–259. [CrossRef] [PubMed]
15. Smith, J.W.; Ng, D.K.; Alvarez, C.S.; Egner, P.A.; Burke, S.M.; Chen, J.-G.; Kensler, T.W.; Koshiol, J.; Rivera-Andrade, A.; Kroker-Lobos, M.F.; et al. Assessing the Validity of Normalizing Aflatoxin B1-Lysine Albumin Adduct Biomarker Measurements to Total Serum Albumin Concentration across Multiple Human Population Studies. *Toxins* **2022**, *14*, 162. [CrossRef]
16. Sabbioni, G.; Ambs, S.; Wogan, G.N.; Groopman, J.D. The aflatoxin-lysine adduct quantified by high-performance liquid chromatography from human serum albumin samples. *Carcinogenesis* **1990**, *11*, 2063–2066. [CrossRef] [PubMed]
17. Chen, J.G.; Kensler, T.W.; Zhu, J.; Zhu, Y.R.; Wang, J.B.; Lu, J.H.; Munoz, A.; Groopman, J.D. Profound primary prevention of liver cancer following a natural experiment in China: A 50-year perspective and public health implications. *Int. J. Cancer* **2025**, *156*, 756–763. [CrossRef] [PubMed]
18. Smith, J.W.; Matchado, A.J.; Wu, L.S.; Arnold, C.D.; Burke, S.M.; Maleta, K.M.; Ashorn, P.; Stewart, C.P.; Shaikh, S.; Ali, H.; et al. Longitudinal Assessment of Prenatal, Perinatal, and Early-Life Aflatoxin B1 Exposure in 828 Mother-Child Dyads from Bangladesh and Malawi. *Curr. Dev. Nutr.* **2022**, *6*, nzab153. [CrossRef] [PubMed]
19. Mahfuz, M.; Alam, M.A.; Fahim, S.M.; Gazi, M.A.; Raihan, M.J.; Hossain, M.; Egner, P.A.; Bessong, P.O.; Petri, W.A.; Groopman, J.D.; et al. Aflatoxin exposure in children living in Mirpur, Dhaka: Data from MAL-ED companion study. *J. Expo. Sci. Environ. Epidemiol.* **2019**, *29*, 655–662. [CrossRef]
20. Mahfuz, M.; Hasan, S.M.T.; Alam, M.A.; Das, S.; Fahim, S.M.; Islam, M.M.; Gazi, M.A.; Hossain, M.; Egner, P.A.; Groopman, J.D.; et al. Aflatoxin exposure was not associated with childhood stunting: Results from a birth cohort study in a resource-poor setting of Dhaka, Bangladesh. *Public Health Nutr.* **2021**, *24*, 3361–3370. [CrossRef]
21. Chen, J.G.; Egner, P.A.; Ng, D.; Jacobson, L.P.; Munoz, A.; Zhu, Y.-R.; Qian, G.-S.; Wu, F.; Yuan, J.-M.; Groopman, J.D.; et al. Reduced aflatoxin exposure presages decline in liver cancer mortality in an endemic region of China. *Cancer Prev. Res.* **2013**, *6*, 1038–1045. [CrossRef]
22. Alvarez, C.S.; Hernández, E.; Escobar, K.; Villagrán, C.I.; Kroker-Lobos, M.F.; Rivera-Andrade, A.; Smith, J.W.; Egner, P.A.; Lazo, M.; Freedman, N.D.; et al. Aflatoxin B(1) exposure and liver cirrhosis in Guatemala: A case-control study. *BMJ Open Gastroenterol.* **2020**, *7*, e000380. [CrossRef]
23. Smith, J.W.; Kroker-Lobos, M.F.; Lazo, M.; Rivera-Andrade, A.; Egner, P.A.; Wedemeyer, H.; Torres, O.; Freedman, N.D.; McGlynn, K.A.; Guallar, E.; et al. Aflatoxin and viral hepatitis exposures in Guatemala: Molecular biomarkers reveal a unique profile of risk factors in a region of high liver cancer incidence. *PLoS ONE* **2017**, *12*, e0189255. [CrossRef]
24. Groopman, J.D.; Smith, J.W.; Rivera-Andrade, A.; Alvarez, C.S.; Kroker-Lobos, M.F.; Egner, P.A.; Gharzouzi, E.; Dean, M.; McGlynn, K.A.; Ramírez-Zea, M. Aflatoxin and the aetiology of liver cancer and its implications for Guatemala. *World Mycotoxin J.* **2021**, *14*, 305–318. [CrossRef]
25. McCoy, L.F.; Scholl, P.F.; Sutcliffe, A.E.; Kieszak, S.M.; Powers, C.D.; Rogers, H.S.; Gong, Y.Y.; Groopman, J.D.; Wild, C.P.; Schleicher, R.L. Human Aflatoxin Albumin Adducts Quantitatively Compared by ELISA, HPLC with Fluorescence Detection, and HPLC with Isotope Dilution Mass Spectrometry. *Cancer Epidemiol. Biomark. Prev.* **2008**, *17*, 1653–1657. [CrossRef]
26. Strosnider, H.; Azziz-Baumgartner, E.; Banziger, M.; Bhat, R.V.; Breiman, R.; Brune, M.N.; DeCock, K.; Dilley, A.; Groopman, J.; Hell, K.; et al. Workgroup report: Public health strategies for reducing aflatoxin exposure in developing countries. *Environ. Health Perspect.* **2006**, *114*, 1898–1903. [CrossRef]
27. Tong, Y.; Tonui, P.; Orang'o, O.; Zhang, J.; Maina, T.; Muthoka, K.; Groopman, J.; Smith, J.; Madeen, E.; Ermel, A.; et al. Association of plasma aflatoxin with persistent detection of oncogenic human papillomaviruses in cervical samples from Kenyan women enrolled in a longitudinal study. *BMC Infect. Dis.* **2023**, *23*, 377. [CrossRef]

 https://doi.org/10.3390/toxins18010058

28. Zhang, J.; Orang'o, O.; Tonui, P.; Tong, Y.; Maina, T.; Kiptoo, S.; Muthoka, K.; Groopman, J.; Smith, J.; Madeen, E.; et al. Detection and Concentration of Plasma Aflatoxin is Associated with Detection of Oncogenic Human Papillomavirus in Kenyan Women. In *Open Forum Infectious Diseases*; Oxford University Press: Oxford, UK, 2019; Volume 6. [CrossRef]
29. Solis-Martinez, O.; Monge, A.; Groopman, J.D.; McGlynn, K.A.; Romero-Martinez, M.; Palacios-Rojas, N.; Batis, C.; Lamadrid-Figueroa, H.; Riojas-Rodriguez, H.; Lajous, M. Maize consumption and circulating aflatoxin levels in Mexican middle- and older-aged adults: A cross-sectional analysis. *Am. J. Clin. Nutr.* **2024**, *121*, 454–462. [CrossRef] [PubMed]
30. Monge, A.; Romero, M.; Groopman, J.D.; McGlynn, K.A.; Santiago-Ruiz, L.; Villalpando-Hernández, S.; Mannan, R.; Burke, S.M.; Remes-Troche, J.M.; Lajous, M. Aflatoxin exposure in adults in southern and eastern Mexico in 2018: A descriptive study. *Int. J. Hyg. Environ. Health* **2023**, *253*, 114249. [CrossRef]
31. Chen, C.; Mitchell, N.J.; Gratz, J.; Houpt, E.R.; Gong, Y.; Egner, P.A.; Groopman, J.D.; Riley, R.T.; Showker, J.L.; Svensen, E.; et al. Exposure to aflatoxin and fumonisin in children at risk for growth impairment in rural Tanzania. *Environ. Int.* **2018**, *115*, 29–37. [CrossRef]
32. Chen, C.; Patil, C.L.; Mduma, E.R.; Groopman, J.D.; Riley, R.T.; Wu, F. Mycotoxins were not associated with environmental enteropathy in a cohort of Tanzanian children. *Risk Anal.* **2023**, *43*, 860–866. [CrossRef]
33. Nyikal, J.; Misore, A.; Nzioka, C.; Njuguna, C. *Outbreak of Aflatoxin Poisoning—Eastern and Central Provinces, Kenya, January–July 2004*; 0149–2195; U.S. Center for Disease Control: Atlanta, GA, USA, 2004; p. 790.
34. Azziz-Baumgartner, E.; Lindblade, K.; Gieseker, K.; Helen Schurz, R.; Kieszak, S.; Njapau, H. Case-Control Study of an Acute Aflatoxicosis Outbreak, Kenya, 2004. *Environ. Health Perspect.* **2005**, *113*, 1779–1783. [CrossRef] [PubMed]
35. Probst, C.; Njapau, H.; Cotty, P.J. Outbreak of an acute aflatoxicosis in Kenya in 2004: Identification of the causal agent. *Appl. Environ. Microbiol.* **2007**, *73*, 2762–2764. [CrossRef] [PubMed]
36. Koshiol, J.; Gao, Y.T.; Dean, M.; Egner, P.; Nepal, C.; Jones, K.; Wang, B.; Rashid, A.; Luo, W.; Van Dyke, A.L.; et al. Association of Aflatoxin and Gallbladder Cancer. *Gastroenterology* **2017**, *153*, 488–494 e481. [CrossRef]
37. Nogueira, L.; Foerster, C.; Groopman, J.; Egner, P.; Koshiol, J.; Ferreccio, C. Association of aflatoxin with gallbladder cancer in Chile. *Jama* **2015**, *313*, 2075–2077. [CrossRef]
38. Twagiramungu, J.d.D.; Njoroge, D.; Mburu, M.; Duke, G. Effect of Nixtamalization on Aflatoxins, Functional and Acceptability of Maize from Mulindi, Rwanda. *Eur. J. Agric. Food Sci.* **2024**, *6*, 27–33. [CrossRef]
39. Gilbert Sandoval, I.; Wesseling, S.; Rietjens, I.M.C.M. Aflatoxin B1 in nixtamalized maize in Mexico; occurrence and accompanying risk assessment. *Toxicol. Rep.* **2019**, *6*, 1135–1142. [CrossRef] [PubMed]
40. Guzzon, F.; Arandia Rios, L.W.; Caviedes Cepeda, G.M.; Céspedes Polo, M.; Chavez Cabrera, A.; Muriel Figueroa, J.; Medina Hoyos, A.E.; Jara Calvo, T.W.; Molnar, T.L.; Narro León, L.A.; et al. Conservation and Use of Latin American Maize Diversity: Pillar of Nutrition Security and Cultural Heritage of Humanity. *Agronomy* **2021**, *11*, 172. [CrossRef]
41. Bunny, S.M.; Umar, A.; Bhatti, H.S.; Honey, S.F. Aflatoxin risk in the era of climatic change-a comprehensive review. *CABI Agric. Biosci.* **2024**, *5*, 105. [CrossRef]
42. Wall-Martínez, H.A.; Ramírez-Martínez, A.; Wesolek, N.; Brabet, C.; Rodríguez-Jimenes, G.C.; García-Alvarado, M.A.; Salgado-Cervantes, M.A.; Robles-Olvera, V.J.; Roudot, A.C. Statistical analysis of corn consumption for improved mycotoxin exposure estimates for the population of Veracruz City, Mexico. *Food Addit. Contam. Part A* **2017**, *34*, 864–879. [CrossRef]
43. Zuki-Orozco, B.A.; Batres-Esquivel, L.E.; Ortiz-Pérez, M.D.; Juárez-Flores, B.I.; Díaz-Barriga, F. Aflatoxins Contamination in Maize Products from Rural Communities in San Luis Potosi, Mexico. *Ann. Glob. Health* **2018**, *84*, 300–305. [CrossRef]
44. Alvarez, C.S.; Rivera-Andrade, A.; Kroker-Lobos, M.F.; Florio, A.A.; Smith, J.W.; Egner, P.A.; Freedman, N.D.; Lazo, M.; Guallar, E.; Dean, M.; et al. Associations between aflatoxin B-albumin adduct levels with metabolic conditions in Guatemala: A cross-sectional study. *Health Sci. Rep.* **2022**, *5*, e495. [CrossRef]
45. Kroker-Lobos, M.F.; Alvarez, C.S.; Rivera-Andrade, A.; Smith, J.W.; Egner, P.; Torres, O.; Lazo, M.; Freedman, N.D.; Guallar, E.; Graubard, B.I.; et al. Association between aflatoxin-albumin adduct levels and tortilla consumption in Guatemalan adults. *Toxicol. Rep.* **2019**, *6*, 465–471. [CrossRef]
46. Garsow, A.V.; Torres, O.R.; Matute, J.A.; Voss, D.M.; Miyagusuku-Cruzado, G.; Giusti, M.M.; Kowalcyk, B.B. Dietary, socioeconomic, and maize handling practices associated with aflatoxin and fumonisin exposure among women tortilla makers in 5 departments in Guatemala. *PLoS Glob. Public Health* **2024**, *4*, e0001623. [CrossRef]
47. Cabrera-Meraz, J.; Maldonado, L.; Bianchini, A.; Espinal, R. Incidence of aflatoxins and fumonisins in grain, masa and corn tortillas in four municipalities in the department of Lempira, Honduras. *Heliyon* **2021**, *7*, e08506. [CrossRef]
48. Ranum, P.; Peña-Rosas, J.P.; Garcia-Casal, M.N. Global maize production, utilization, and consumption. *Ann. N. Y. Acad. Sci.* **2014**, *1312*, 105–112. [CrossRef] [PubMed]
49. McGlynn, K.A.; Petrick, J.L.; Groopman, J.D. Liver Cancer: Progress and Priorities. *Cancer Epidemiol. Biomark. Prev.* **2024**, *33*, 1261–1272. [CrossRef]
50. International Agency for Research on Cancer. *Overall Evaluations of Carcinogenicity: An Updating of IARC Monographs (Vols 1–42)*; International Agency for Research on Cancer: Lyon, France, 1987.

 https://doi.org/10.3390/toxins18010058

51. Wang, L.-Y.; Hatch, M.; Chen, C.-J.; Levin, B.; You, S.-L.; Lu, S.-N.; Wu, M.-H.; Wu, W.-P.; Wang, L.-W.; Wang, Q.; et al. Aflatoxin exposure and risk of hepatocellular carcinoma in Taiwan. *Int. J. Cancer* **1996**, *67*, 620–625. [CrossRef]
52. Cao, W.; Pan, Y.; Yang, K.; Cao, D. Aflatoxin B1: Metabolism, toxicology, and its involvement in oxidative stress and cancer development. *Toxicol. Mech. Methods* **2022**, *32*, 395–419. [CrossRef]
53. Rayapati, D.; McGlynn, K.A.; Groopman, J.D.; Kim, A.K. Environmental exposures and the risk of hepatocellular carcinoma. *Hepatol. Commun.* **2025**, *9*, e0627. [CrossRef] [PubMed]
54. Benkerroum, N. Chronic and Acute Toxicities of Aflatoxins: Mechanisms of Action. *Int. J. Environ. Res. Public Health* **2020**, *17*, 423. [CrossRef]
55. Groopman, J.D. Changing Etiology and Epidemiology of Human Liver Cancer. In *Liver Cancer in the Middle East*; Carr, B.I., Ed.; Springer International Publishing: Cham, Switzerland, 2021; pp. 13–29.
56. Chu, Y.J.; Yang, H.I.; Wu, H.C.; Lee, M.H.; Liu, J.; Wang, L.Y.; Lu, S.N.; Jen, C.L.; You, S.L.; Santella, R.M.; et al. Aflatoxin B(1) exposure increases the risk of hepatocellular carcinoma associated with hepatitis C virus infection or alcohol consumption. *Eur. J. Cancer* **2018**, *94*, 37–46. [CrossRef]
57. Díaz, L.A.; Ayares, G.; Arnold, J.; Idalsoaga, F.; Corsi, O.; Arrese, M.; Arab, J.P. Liver Diseases in Latin America: Current Status, Unmet Needs, and Opportunities for Improvement. *Curr. Treat. Options Gastroenterol.* **2022**, *20*, 261–278. [CrossRef]
58. Ross, R.K.; Yu, M.C.; Henderson, B.E.; Yuan, J.M.; Qian, G.S.; Tu, J.T.; Gao, Y.T.; Wogan, G.N.; Groopman, J.D. Urinary aflatoxin biomarkers and risk of hepatocellular carcinoma. *Lancet* **1992**, *339*, 943–946. [CrossRef]
59. Haddad, L.; Gadano, A. HBV elimination in Central and South America: Current status and challenges. *Clin. Liver Dis.* **2024**, *23*, e0226. [CrossRef]
60. Albala, C.; Vio, F. Obesity and Diabetes in Latin America: The Impact of Socioeconomic Status on Programs and Outcomes. In *Global Challenges in Cardiovascular Prevention in Populations with Low Socioeconomic Status*; Romero, T., Nazal, C.N., Lanas, F., Eds.; Springer Nature: Cham, Switzerland, 2025; pp. 51–61.
61. Myers, S.; Neyroud-Caspar, I.; Spahr, L.; Gkouvatsos, K.; Fournier, E.; Giostra, E.; Magini, G.; Frossard, J.L.; Bascaron, M.E.; Vernaz, N.; et al. NAFLD and MAFLD as emerging causes of HCC: A populational study. *JHEP Rep.* **2021**, *3*, 100231. [CrossRef] [PubMed]
62. Ssentongo, P.; Ssentongo, A.E.; Ba, D.M.; Ericson, J.E.; Na, M.; Gao, X.; Fronterre, C.; Chinchilli, V.M.; Schiff, S.J. Global, regional and national epidemiology and prevalence of child stunting, wasting and underweight in low- and middle-income countries, 2006–2018. *Sci. Rep.* **2021**, *11*, 5204. [CrossRef] [PubMed]
63. Voth-Gaeddert, L.E.; Torres, O.; Maldonado, J.; Krajmalnik-Brown, R.; Rittmann, B.E.; Oerther, D.B. Aflatoxin exposure, child stunting, and dysbiosis in the intestinal microbiome among children in Guatemala. *Environ. Eng. Sci.* **2019**, *36*, 958–968. [CrossRef]
64. Rasheed, H.; Xu, Y.; Kimanya, M.E.; Pan, X.; Li, Z.; Zou, X.; Shirima, C.P.; Holmes, M.; Routledge, M.N.; Gong, Y.Y. Estimating the health burden of aflatoxin attributable stunting among children in low income countries of Africa. *Sci. Rep.* **2021**, *11*, 1619. [CrossRef]
65. Matchado, A.; Smith, J.W.; Schulze, K.J.; Groopman, J.D.; Kortekangas, E.; Chaima, D.; Arnold, C.D.; Maleta, K.; Ashorn, U.; Ashorn, P.; et al. Child Aflatoxin Exposure is Associated with Poor Child Growth Outcomes: A Prospective Cohort Study in Rural Malawi. *Curr. Dev. Nutr.* **2023**, *7*, 101962. [CrossRef] [PubMed]
66. Gong, Y.Y.; Watson, S.; Routledge, M.N. Aflatoxin Exposure and Associated Human Health Effects, a Review of Epidemiological Studies. *Food Saf.* **2016**, *4*, 14–27. [CrossRef]
67. Turner, P.C.; Moore, S.E.; Hall, A.J.; Prentice, A.M.; Wild, C.P. Modification of immune function through exposure to dietary aflatoxin in Gambian children. *Environ. Health Perspect.* **2003**, *111*, 217–220. [CrossRef]
68. Jiang, Y.; Jolly, P.E.; Ellis, W.O.; Wang, J.S.; Phillips, T.D.; Williams, J.H. Aflatoxin B1 albumin adduct levels and cellular immune status in Ghanaians. *Int. Immunol.* **2005**, *17*, 807–814. [CrossRef]
69. Carvajal, M.; Berumen, J.; Guardado-Estrada, M. The presence of aflatoxin B1-FAPY adduct and human papilloma virus in cervical smears from cancer patients in Mexico. *Food Addit. Contam. Part. A* **2012**, *29*, 258–268. [CrossRef]
70. de León-Martínez, L.D.; López-Mendoza, C.; Terán-Figueroa, Y.; Flores-Ramírez, R.; Díaz-Barriga, F.; Alcántara-Quintana, L. Detection of aflatoxin B1 adducts in Mexican women with cervical lesions. *World Mycotoxin J.* **2021**, *14*, 327–338. [CrossRef]
71. Koshiol, J.; Hildesheim, A.; Zhu, B.; Wang, R.; Gao, Y.; Egner, P.; Yuan, J.; Groopman, J. Longitudinal analysis of aflatoxin and gallbladder cancer. *HPB* **2019**, *21*, S20–S21. [CrossRef]
72. Koshiol, J.; Zhu, B.; Wang, R.; Hildesheim, A.; Gao, Y.T.; Egner, P.A.; Yuan, J.M.; Groopman, J.D. Association of aflatoxin with gallbladder cancer in a case-control study nested within a Chinese cohort. *Int. J. Cancer* **2024**, *154*, 801–806. [CrossRef]
73. Dai, C.; Tian, E.; Li, H.; Das Gupta, S.; Hao, Z.; Wang, Z.; Velkov, T.; Shen, J. Molecular mechanisms of aflatoxin neurotoxicity and potential neuroprotective agents. *Food Sci. Hum. Wellness* **2024**, *13*, 2445–2455. [CrossRef]
74. Mitchell, N.J.; Kumi, J.; Johnson, N.M.; Dotse, E.; Marroquin-Cardona, A.; Wang, J.S.; Jolly, P.E.; Ankrah, N.-A.; Phillips, T.D. Reduction in the urinary aflatoxin M1 biomarker as an early indicator of the efficacy of dietary interventions to reduce exposure to aflatoxins. *Biomarkers* **2013**, *18*, 391–398. [CrossRef]

75. Skipper, P.L.; Tannenbaum, S.R. Protein adducts in the molecular dosimetry of chemical carcinogens. *Carcinogenesis* **1990**, *11*, 507–518. [CrossRef]
76. Stutt, R.O.J.H.; Castle, M.D.; Markwell, P.; Baker, R.; Gilligan, C.A. An integrated model for pre- and post-harvest aflatoxin contamination in maize. *Npj Sci. Food* **2023**, *7*, 60. [CrossRef]
77. Dövényi-Nagy, T.; Rácz, C.; Molnár, K.; Bakó, K.; Szláma, Z.; Jóźwiak, Á.; Farkas, Z.; Pócsi, I.; Dobos, A.C. Pre-Harvest Modelling and Mitigation of Aflatoxins in Maize in a Changing Climatic Environment—A Review. *Toxins* **2020**, *12*, 768. [CrossRef] [PubMed]
78. Peles, F.; Sipos, P.; Kovács, S.; Győri, Z.; Pócsi, I.; Pusztahelyi, T. Biological Control and Mitigation of Aflatoxin Contamination in Commodities. *Toxins* **2021**, *13*, 104. [CrossRef]
79. Ortega-Beltran, A.; Bandyopadhyay, R. Aflatoxin biocontrol in practice requires a multidisciplinary, long-term approach. *Front. Sustain. Food Syst.* **2023**, *7*, 1110964. [CrossRef]
80. Alaniz Zanon, M.S.; Bossa, M.; Chiotta, M.L.; Oddino, C.; Giovanini, D.; Cardoso, M.L.; Bartosik, R.E.; Chulze, S.N. Pre-harvest strategy for reducing aflatoxin accumulation during storage of maize in Argentina. *Int. J. Food Microbiol.* **2022**, *380*, 109887. [CrossRef]
81. Kortei, N.K.; Osei, S.; Addae, A.A.; Akonor, P.T.; Manaphraim, N.Y.B.; Annan, T. Impact of some Ghanaian local roasting methods on aflatoxin reduction in groundnuts (*Arachis hypogaea* L). *Sci. Afr.* **2024**, *23*, e02022. [CrossRef]
82. Romero-Sánchez, I.; Gracia-Lor, E.; Madrid-Albarrán, Y. Aflatoxin detoxification by thermal cooking treatment and evaluation of in vitro bioaccessibility from white and brown rice. *Food Chem.* **2024**, *436*, 137738. [CrossRef]
83. Montenegro-Benthancourt, G.; Glesener, H.; Torres, O.; Seegmiller, E.; Rohloff, P.; Voth-Gaeddert, L.E. Practices of maize handling and nixtamalization to reduce fungal toxin exposure in rural Guatemala. *J. Agric. Food Res.* **2024**, *18*, 101512. [CrossRef]
84. Deng, J.; Zhao, L.; Zhang, N.-Y.; Karrow, N.A.; Krumm, C.S.; Qi, D.-S.; Sun, L.-H. Aflatoxin B1 metabolism: Regulation by phase I and II metabolizing enzymes and chemoprotective agents. *Mutat. Res./Rev. Mutat. Res.* **2018**, *778*, 79–89. [CrossRef] [PubMed]
85. Kensler, T.W.; Chen, J.G.; Egner, P.A.; Fahey, J.W.; Jacobson, L.P.; Stephenson, K.K.; Ye, L.; Coady, J.L.; Wang, J.B.; Wu, Y.; et al. Effects of glucosinolate-rich broccoli sprouts on urinary levels of aflatoxin-DNA adducts and phenanthrene tetraols in a randomized clinical trial in He Zuo township, Qidong, People's Republic of China. *Cancer Epidemiol. Biomark. Prev.* **2005**, *14*, 2605–2613. [CrossRef]
86. Chen, J.-G.; Zhu, Y.-R.; Qian, G.-S.; Wang, J.-B.; Lu, J.-H.; Kensler, T.W.; Jacobson, L.P.; Muñoz, A.; Groopman, J.D. Fifty Years of Aflatoxin Research in Qidong, China: A Celebration of Team Science to Improve Public Health. *Toxins* **2025**, *17*, 79. [CrossRef]
87. Wang, J.S.; Shen, X.; He, X.; Zhu, Y.R.; Zhang, B.C.; Wang, J.B.; Qian, G.S.; Kuang, S.Y.; Zarba, A.; Egner, P.A.; et al. Protective alterations in phase 1 and 2 metabolism of aflatoxin B1 by oltipraz in residents of Qidong, People's Republic of China. *J. Natl. Cancer Inst.* **1999**, *91*, 347–354. [CrossRef] [PubMed]
88. Jacobson, L.P.; Zhang, B.C.; Zhu, Y.R.; Wang, J.B.; Wu, Y.; Zhang, Q.N.; Yu, L.Y.; Qian, G.S.; Kuang, S.Y.; Li, Y.F.; et al. Oltipraz chemoprevention trial in Qidong, People's Republic of China: Study design and clinical outcomes. *Cancer Epidemiol. Biomark. Prev.* **1997**, *6*, 257–265.
89. Wang, X.; Wang, T.; Nepovimova, E.; Long, M.; Wu, W.; Kuca, K. Progress on the detoxification of aflatoxin B1 using natural anti-oxidants. *Food Chem. Toxicol.* **2022**, *169*, 113417. [CrossRef]

 https://doi.org/10.3390/toxins18010058

MDPI AG
Grosspeteranlage 5
4052 Basel
Switzerland
Tel.: +41 61 683 77 34

Toxins Editorial Office
E-mail: toxins@mdpi.com
www.mdpi.com/journal/toxins